D1710314

SKIN
Resurfacing

SKIN
Resurfacing

William P. Coleman III M.D.
Clinical Professor of Dermatology
Tulane University School of Medicine
New Orleans, Louisiana

Naomi Lawrence, M.D.
Assistant Professor of Clinical Medicine
Director of Dermatologic Surgery
University of Medicine and Dentistry of New Jersey
Cooper Hospital
Marlton, New Jersey

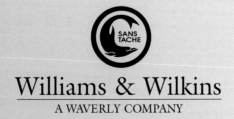

Williams & Wilkins
A WAVERLY COMPANY

BALTIMORE • PHILADELPHIA • LONDON • PARIS • BANGKOK
BUENOS AIRES • HONG KONG • MUNICH • SYDNEY • TOKYO • WROCLAW

Editor: Jonathan W. Pine, Jr.
Managing Editor: Leah Ann Kiehne Hayes
Marketing Manager: Lorraine A. Smith
Production Coordinator: Danielle Hagan
Project Editor: Jeffrey S. Myers
Designer: Graphic World, Inc.
Illustration Planner: Lorraine Wrzosek
Cover Designer: Joan Cox
Typesetter: Graphic World, Inc.
Printer/Binder: RR Donnelley & Sons Company

Copyright © 1998 Williams & Wilkins

351 West Camden Street
Baltimore, Maryland 21201-2436 USA

Rose Tree Corporate Center
1400 North Providence Road
Building II, Suite 5025
Media, Pennsylvania 19063-2043 USA

Accurate indications, adverse reactions and dosage schedules for drugs are provided in this book, but it is possible that they may change. The reader is urged to review the package information data of the manufacturers of the medications mentioned.

Printed in the United States of America

First Edition,

Library of Congress Cataloging-in-Publication Data

Skin resurfacing / [edited by] William P. Coleman III, Naomi Lawrence.
— 1st ed.
     p.   cm.
   Includes bibliographical references and index.
   ISBN 0–683–30165–9
   1. Skin—Surgery.   2. Dermabrasion.   3. Chemical peel.   4. Face—
Laser surgery.   I. Coleman, William P.   II. Lawrence, Naomi.
   [DNLM: 1. Skin—surgery.   2. Skin Diseases—surgery.
3. Chemexfoliation.   4. Dermabrasion.   5. Laser Surgery.   WR 650
S6275 1998]
RD520.S556   1998
617.4′7—dc21
DNLM/DLC
for Library of Congress   97–48638
                                                                 CIP

The publishers have made every effort to trace the copyright holders for borrowed material. If they have inadvertently overlooked any, they will be pleased to make the necessary arrangements at the first opportunity.

To purchase additional copies of this book, call our customer service department at **(800) 638-0672** or fax orders to **(800) 447-8438.** For other book services, including chapter reprints and large quantity sales, ask for the Special Sales department.

Canadian customers should call **(800) 665-1148,** or fax **(800) 665-0103.** For all other calls originating outside of the United States, please call **(410) 528-4223** or fax us at **(410) 528-8550.**

Visit Williams & Wilkins on the Internet: **http://www.wwilkins.com** or contact our customer service department at **custserv@wwilkins.com** Williams & Wilkins customer service representatives are available from 8:30 am to 6:00 pm, EST, Monday through Friday, for telephone access.

98 99 00 01 02
1 2 3 4 5 6 7 8 9 10

This book is dedicated to our families
—
William P. Coleman III
Naomi Lawrence

FOREWORD

Laser resurfacing is the "new kid on the block" compared to older techniques like dermabrasion and chemical peel. There is nothing quite like the excitement of watching extensive facial peel rhytides tighten and disappear during carbon dioxide (CO_2) laser resurfacing. Laser resurfacing works well for photoaging and rhytides, but not for acne scars; it does not provide the consistent results that are possible using dermabrasion and other techniques. Laser resurfacing is effective for superficial acne scars and also for tightening the skin in patients with soft undulating acne scars. Dermabrasion has also been used with great success for photoaging and rhytides, especially on the upper lip. Medium-depth and deep chemical peels are also proven and effective for treating photoaging and wrinkles.

The mechanism of injury is clearly different for laser resurfacing, dermabrasion, and chemical peel, although the final results at times can be identical. Dermabrasion involves the physical removal of the papillary dermis and sometimes a portion of the reticular dermis. Chemical peel involves the application of various acids that penetrate to a depth which produces the desired amount of epidermal and/or dermal necrosis. CO_2 laser resurfacing involves ablation of tissue and a varying amount of adjacent thermal damage. The upper dermis is replaced with a new layer of collagen following dermabrasion, chemical peel, or laser resurfacing.

Regrettably, some physicians who are relatively new to skin resurfacing do not have experience with dermabrasion and chemical peel. We have heard the old adage, "if all you have is a hammer, everything looks like a nail." In my opinion, if all a physician has is a CO_2 laser, he or she is at a distinct disadvantage and cannot offer the full spectrum of quality skin resurfacing to his or her patients. In addition, the lessons of dermabrasion and chemical peel must be learned anew by these physicians for laser resurfacing.

Dermatology is a relatively small speciality. However, the contributions of dermatologists to skin resurfacing have been huge, and cannot be overstated. Kurtin revolutionized dermabrasion techniques in the early 1950s. MacKee published his 50-year experience with phenol peels in 1952. The initial descriptions of the three medium-depth chemical peels that are currently used were published in *Dermatologic Surgery* by Brody, Monheit, Coleman, and co-workers from 1986-1994. In 1961, Goldman was the first physician to treat patients with laser. David was the first to perform laser resurfacing with the continuous wave CO_2 laser in the mid-1980s. David and Fitzpatrick pioneered laser resurfacing techniques with the high energy, short-pulsed CO_2 laser in the early 1990s. Let us not forget that all of these physicians are dermatologists.

Similarly, the contributions of the editors and contributors to this book cannot be overstated. They all have been leaders and innovators in skin resurfacing. The goal of this book is understanding, not the teaching of cookbook technique. We are all grateful to Dr. Coleman and Dr. Lawrence and their contributors for taking the trouble to educate us all in this important subject area.

C. William Hanke, MD, FACP
Professor of Dermatology and Vice Chairman
Professor of Pathology and Laboratory Medicine
Professor of Otolaryngology, Head & Neck Surgery
Indiana University School of Medicine
Indianapolis, Indiana

PREFACE

Controlled wounding to improve the appearance of the skin has been used at least since the time of the Egyptian Pharaohs. Just like our ancient forbearers, we as cosmetic surgeons, try to control a delicate balance to the patients' best advantage: to destroy enough but not too much; to stimulate a healthy reparative process. Our goal is to get the best possible result with the least risk of complication. The tools we use to accomplish this are chemicals, cold steel (or other) abrasive instruments, and the laser. Although the laser is the newest and most precise of these instruments, its precision makes our ignorance more stark. How much destruction is best? Does the method of destruction itself portend different results or is depth the only critical factor? Is there a way to eliminate complications, individual variations, and morbidity?

We practice in a society where the media sensationalizes every new cosmetic technique well before the technique has a clinical track record or has been tested by prospective controlled studies. As physicians and scientists, we need to approach new tools and procedures with both enthusiasm and skepticism. Efficacy must be proved dispassionately by evaluation of objective parameters. Safety should be the top priority (Primum non nocere). Consideration should be given to appropriate training standards for new procedures. To date, we have not developed an adequate system for dissemination of new technology that is all inclusive, non-restrictive and meets the highest standard of care. Dermatologic surgeons, with their knowledge of skin histology and wound healing, combined with a broad resurfacing experience, are the natural leaders in resurfacing techniques. But these are procedures that have been adopted by several other surgical specialities. Interspecialty dissemination of information is not only appropriate, but essential to future advances.

This text begins with a comprehensive history of skin resurfacing. As medicine is a scientific field, physicians are most often interested in the newest developments and less concerned with the historical evolution of a technique. However, one must understand history as not merely a regurgitation of the past, but a vital tool to understanding the origin of our procedures to both enhance further development and avoid past mistakes.

We have selected a brilliant and highly respected group of contributors for many of the chapters in this book. Seth Materasso, the well-known lecturer and writer, lends his experience and wisdom to the introductory chapter "Indications for Skin Resurfacing," which puts the rest of the text in perspective. "Home Treatment Alternatives to Skin Resurfacing" are detailed in a chapter co-authored by the editors and Patrick Coleman, Dr. Coleman's son and a biology major at SMU. David Harris, a highly experienced cosmetic dermatologist, contributes a thought-provoking chapter on the nuances of "The Selection and Education of the Resurfacing Patient." Critical to a successful and enjoyable resurfacing practice is the selection of a patient who has attainable, realistic expectations and fully understands the risks and benefits.

Each of the next three major sections (Chemical Peeling, Dermabrasion, and Laser Resurfacing) begins with a chapter on clinicopathologic correlation. These chapters highlight the literature on the histologic response of the skin to each of the different types of skin resurfacing. Harold Brody, well known for his expertise in chemical peeling and for joining the science of peeling to the art, contributes "Skin Response to Chemical Peeling." Chris Harmon, a promising young dermatologic surgeon and researcher reviews "Skin Response to Abrasive Resurfacing." Sue Ellen Cox, a young dermatologic surgeon with considerable cosmetic experience, collaborates with Clay J. Cockerell, an energetic and astute dermatopathologist for "Skin Response to Laser Resurfacing." In the appendix, David Margolis, an expert in wound healing provides an insightful commentary on the dermapathologic similarities and differences of these three resurfacing modalities.

Section II, Chemical Peeling, and Section III, Dermabrasion, present fresh approaches to these established techniques that confirm to the reader that chemical and abrasive resurfacing are vibrant, evolving techniques that are not made obsolete by the advent of laser resurfacing. Lawrence and Coleman explain the niche occupied by "Superficial Chemical Peeling." Gary Monheit, a wise dermatologic surgeon and well known peeling expert, provides an excellent update on "Medium Depth Chemical Peeling." William Beeson, an esteemed facial plastic surgeon and president of the American Academy of Cosmetic Surgery contributes a nicely detailed review of "Facial Rejuvenation: Phenol-Based Chemexfoliation."

John Yarborough, the acknowledged world expert on wire brush dermabrasion and past president of the American Society for Dermatologic Surgery, is the lead author on "Wire Brush Dermabrasion." Coleman and Lawrence follow this with "Diamond Fraise Dermabrasion." In "Manual Dermasanding," David Harris shows how we can use tools of the past to develop new techniques.

In Section IV, Elizabeth McBurney, a laser pioneer and also a past president of the American Society for Dermatologic Surgery, provides an elegantly readable chapter on the "Physics of Resurfacing Lasers."

Tina Alster, a dynamic laser expert who has made many significant contributions to the literature provides useful pearls in "Preoperative Preparations for CO_2 Laser Resurfacing." Fitzpatrick, Smith, and Goldman, international leaders in laser research, contribute "Treatment Techniques Common to All Laser Systems" with practical guidelines for resurfacing. Kauver and Geronemus, the highly respected laser researchers and teachers, look at tissue effects to compare CO_2 lasers currently in use. They also provide an overview of the new Erbium:YAG resurfacing lasers available. Lawrence and Coleman review the approaches, available dressings, and topicals used for "Postoperative Care After Laser Resurfacing." In "The Future of Laser Resurfacing," Ron Wheeland, one of the most experienced laser experts in the world, concludes the laser section with an exciting preview of new lasers on the horizon.

Section V highlights combined approaches to the aging face. Lawrence and Coleman illustrate how resurfacing techniques can be used both in discriminating and complimentary fashion. In "Combining Skin Resurfacing with Soft tissue Augmentation," the editors join Greg Goodman, an innovative Australian dermatologic surgeon, in addressing the sequencing and combination of these techniques. Alistair and Jean Carruthers, the inventors of BOTOX for wrinkles, combine their dermatologic and ophthalmologic expertise to provide an excellent chapter on "Combining Botulinum Toxin and Laser Resurfacing for Facial Rhytides." Greg Goodman contributes a beautifully illustrated review on "Combining Laser Resurfacing and Blepharoplasty." Cynthia Weinstein, also from Australia and one of the pioneers of laser resurfacing, provides the latest information on "Laser Assisted Endoscopic Forehead Lifting Combined with CO_2 Laser Resurfacing." Section V ends with a thoughtful presentation of "Resurfacing Complications and their Management" by Goldman, Fitzpatrick and Smith and a practical approach to "The Use of Postoperative Cosmetics" by Zoe Draelos, a highly acclaimed expert in the science of cosmetics.

In the appendix, the editors present the interesting results of a survey on resurfacing sent to all book contributors. As in any multi-authored book, each chapter is presented from the viewpoint and expertise of that author. The survey was done to give balance to other viewpoints, styles of practice, and to illustrate general trends in care. We hope you enjoy reading this book as much as we have enjoyed preparing it.

William P. Coleman III
Naomi Lawrence

ACKNOWLEDGMENT

No endeavor as time consuming as editing a book occurs without a tremendous amount of support from those around us. We would like to thank our spouses, Kerry and Jerry and sons Patrick, Kyle, Stuart, Casey, Michael, Mark, and Lucas for their love and tolerance. Thanks to our parents, Barbara, Bill, Mary K, and Fran for setting the example of excellence, and to our siblings Grant, Lissy, Chris and Jenny, for an environment of friendly competition. We have been lucky enough to learn from the best, including Vincent Derbes, Larry Millikan, John Yarborough, Elizabeth McBurney, Hal Brody, Bill Hanke, and Will Cottel. Our Administrative Assistants, Barbara Tregre and Mary Cook, did a beautiful job of transcribing and pulling everything together. Through the diligent efforts of Jonathan Pine, Editor; Leah Hayes, Managing Editor; Jeff Myers, Project Editor; and Danielle Hagan, Production Coordinator, this book was brought to fruition.

CONTRIBUTORS

Tina S. Alster, MD
Clinical Assistant Professor of Dermatology
Georgetown University School of Medicine
Director, Washington Institute of Dermatologic Laser Surgery
Washington, D.C.

William H. Beeson, MD
Clinical Assistant Professor of Dermatology and
    Otolaryngology
Head and Neck Surgery
Indiana University
Indianapolis, Indiana

Harold J. Brody, MD
Clinical Associate Professor of Dermatology
Emory University School of Medicine
Atlanta, Georgia

Alastair Carruthers, MD, FRCPC
Clinical Professor of Dermatology
University of British Columbia Faculty of Medicine
Vancouver, British Columbia, Canada

Jean Carruthers, MD, FRCS(C)
Clinical Professor of Ophthalmology
University of British Columbia Faculty of Medicine
Vancouver, British Columbia, Canada

Clay J. Cockerell, MD
Clinical Professor of Dermatology and Pathology
Director, Division of Dermatopathology
University of Texas Southwestern Medical Center
Dallas, Texas

William P. Coleman III, MD
Clinical Professor of Dermatology
Tulane University School of Medicine
New Orleans, Louisiana

William P. Coleman IV
Department of Biology
Southern Methodist University
Dallas, Texas

Sue Ellen Cox, MD
Clinical Assistant Professor of Dermatology
University of North Carolina at Chapel Hill School of
    Medicine
Chapel Hill, North Carolina

Zoe Diana Draelos, MD
Clinical Associate Professor of Dermatology
Wake Forest University
Bowman Gray School of Medicine
Winston-Salem, North Carolina

Richard E. Fitzpatrick, MD
Associate Clinical Professor of Medicine
Division of Dermatology
University of California, San Diego, School of Medicine
San Diego, California

Roy G. Geronemus, MD
Clinical Associate Professor of Dermatology
New York University Medical Center
Director, Laser and Skin Surgery Center of New York
New York, New York

Mitchel P. Goldman, MD
Associate Clinical Professor of Medicine
Division of Dermatology
University of California, San Diego, School of Medicine
San Diego, California

Gregory Goodman, MBBS, FACD
Senior Lecturer in Community Medicine
Monash University
Cayon, Victoria, Australia
Director, Micrographic Surgery Unit
Skin and Cancer Foundation
Melbourne, Victoria, Australia

Christopher B. Harmon, MD
Clinical Instructor in Dermatology
University of Alabama School of Medicine
Birmingham, Alabama

David R. Harris, MD
Clinical Professor of Dermatology
Stanford University School of Medicine
Palo Alto, California

Arielle N.B. Kauvar, MD
Clinical Assistant Professor of Dermatology
New York University School of Medicine
Associate Director, Laser and Skin Surgery Center of
    New York
New York, New York

Naomi Lawrence, MD
Assistant Professor of Clinical Medicine
Director of Dermatologic Surgery
University of Medicine and Dentistry of New Jersey
Cooper Hospital
Marlton, New Jersey

David J. Margolis, MD, FACP
Assistant Professor of Dermatology
Senior Scholar in the Center for Clinical Epidemiology and
    Biostatistics
University of Pennsylvania School of Medicine
Philadelphia, Pennsylvania

Seth L. Matarasso, MD
Associate Clinical Professor of Dermatology
University of California, San Francisco, School of
    Medicine
San Francisco, California

Elizabeth I. McBurney, MD, FACP
Clinical Professor of Dermatology
Tulane University School of Medicine
Louisiana State University School of Medicine
New Orleans, Louisiana

Gary D. Monheit, MD
Assistant Clinical Professor of Dermatology
University of Alabama at Birmingham School of Medicine
Birmingham, Alabama

Stacy R. Smith, MD
Clinical Instructor in Dermatology
University of California, San Diego, School of Medicine
Clinical Consultant in Dermatology
Naval Medical Center
San Diego, California

Cynthia Weinstein, MBBS, FACD, FRACP
Director, Cosmetic Laser Centre
Freemasons Hospital
Freemason's Medical Centre
East Melbourne, Victoria, Australia

Ronald G. Wheeland, MD, FACP
Professor of Dermatology
University of New Mexico School of Medicine
Albuquerque, New Mexico

John B. Yarborough, MD
Clinical Professor of Dermatology
Tulane University School of Medicine
New Orleans, Louisiana

CONTENTS

SECTION I

Introduction

CHAPTER 1

The History of Skin Resurfacing

■ William P. Coleman III
Naomi Lawrence

Since ancient times, man has practiced the art of removing layers of skin to obtain a specific cosmetic result. Scarification has been practiced by primitive people for thousands of years and has survived among some cultures into this century. Abrasive or sharp implements were used to scrape the skin to intentionally produce scars or keloids in a decorative pattern (1).

CHEMICAL RESURFACING

Recorded history tells us that the Egyptians were quite interested in peeling agents to rejuvenate skin. The Edwin Smith and Ebers Papyruses contain descriptions of several substances for resurfacing skin to obtain cosmetic improvement (2). They became quite sophisticated in using a variety of acids, balms, and oils for chemical peeling. Greek and later Roman physicians used sour milk, grape juice, and lemon extracts for skin rejuvenation. The active ingredients in these substances were the alpha hydroxy acids: lactic acid, tartaric acid, and citric acid. A number of Greek physicians restricted their practice to care of the skin. These forbearers of modern dermatologists were primarily women. They wrote extensively on the use of acids to beautify the skin (3).

Meanwhile, in Babylonia and India physicians used pumice to exfoliate the stratum corneum. In the middle ages, poultices of mustard, lime stone, and sulphur were applied to rejuvenate the skin. The Turks singed the skin with fire followed by light exfoliation. Itinerant gypsies moved from village to village offering peels with a variety of chemicals. They passed their formulas from generation to generation. At some point, the gypsies began using phenol (4).

The latter half of the 19th century witnessed an increased interest in chemical peeling by physicians. The German dermatologist, Unna, reviewed techniques for chemical peeling in 1882 (5). He reported treatment with salicylic and trichloroacetic acid (TCA) as well as resorcinol and phenol. In England, Mackee began using phenol as a peeling agent to treat facial scarring as early as 1903. He summarized a half century of experience with these techniques in 1952 (6). In France, LaGasse also worked with phenol to treat facial burns during World War I (7). His daughter Antoinette, moved to Los Angeles and practiced lay chemical peeling in the 1930s and 40s using a phenol formula with adhesive taping. Sloughs and scars were commonly seen during this period.

In the 1940s, physicians again became interested in using phenol for chemical peeling. Eller and Wolff reviewed the use of phenol as well as resorcinol and sulphur pastes, salicylic acid, and carbon dioxide ice peels (8). Urkov described occluded phenol peels in 1946 (9). Winter studied the use of phenol in ether for removing lentigines in 1950 (10). Monash described his experience using TCA for scarring in 1949 (11). Ayres studied the histology of TCA versus phenol peels (12).

Until 1960, most of the work in chemical peeling had been done by dermatologists. However, in 1960, the British plastic surgeon Brown published his clinical experience using phenol formulas (13). In the United States, Baker and Gordon developed a modified phenol peel adding water, septisol, and croton oil (14). Litton in 1962 described his formula which substituted glycerin for septisol allowing the emulsion to be stored; however, Baker and Gordon's formula, which was easier to prepare, became the standard procedure for deep chemical peeling and is still in use today (15).

The 1970s witnessed a rebirth in interest in TCA peeling primarily by dermatologists. Resnik, Lewis, and Cohen reviewed their work with TCA peels in 1976 (16). Stegman published a comparative histologic study of the effects of various peeling agents and dermabrasion demonstrating the histologic depth of injury (17). This became the basis for a more scientific approach to chemical peeling. Meanwhile, VanScott began his work on alpha hydroxy acids publishing extensively on this in the 1970s and 80s (18). His initial work gradually led to widespread use of alpha hydroxy acids in the 1990s. Collins advanced the science of non-facial chemical peeling using TCA, publishing his techniques in 1984.

The use of two milder agents to produce a medium depth chemical peel was introduced by Brody and Hailey in 1985 when they published their experience on combining carbon dioxide ice with TCA (19). Other combination chemical peels followed. Monheit described the concept advanced by Bloom of using Jessner's solution before TCA to produce a medium depth chemical peel in 1989 (20). Coleman and Futrell developed and published the concept of the glycolic acid and TCA combination peel for medium depth injury in 1994 (21). Interest in chemical peeling remains high and undoubtedly other approaches or variations of existing ones will appear in the future.

ABRASIVE RESURFACING

Ancient people used rocks or shells to abrade the skin and alter its appearance. The first written descriptions of dermabrasion are found in Egyptian papyruses from 1500 BC (2). The modern age of dermabrasion began with Kromayer, a German dermatologist who reported on using power driven instruments in 1905 (22). He published extensively on the use of abrasion to treat scarring from acne. He used rapidly rotating burs after solidifying and anesthetizing the skin with carbon dioxide snow. He studied the effects of dermabrasion to various depths and established that scarring would not result if the dermabrasion did not penetrate the reticular dermis (23).

After World War II, Iverson, an American plastic surgeon, reported on the use of sand paper for removal of traumatic tattoos and acne scars (24). However, this technique was soon overshadowed by work of the dermatologist Kurtin who modified power dental equipment for use in dermabrasion (25). He first employed this technique for removal of tattoos from concentration camp survivors but later expanded his experience to the treatment of acne scars.

Kurtin's work created an explosion of interest among American dermatologists who enthusiastically embraced dermabrasion. Orentreich, Burks, Luikart, Ayres, Wilson, Pierce, and Rattner widely expanded the use of dermabrasion after Kurtin's premature death in 1955

(26). Lowenthal developed the technique of punch grafting for removal of scars prior to dermabrasion (1953) (27). Wilson, Ayres, and Luikart conducted extensive experiments with various skin refrigerants before finally settling on dichlorotetrafluoroethane (28). They also introduced diamond fraises in 1957 with Noel Robbins who had collaborated with numerous dermatologists in developing new tools. The enormous interest in dermabrasion began to fade in the 1960s, but was soon resurrected by a second generation of dermatologic surgeons who were trained by the original pioneers. Yarborough determined the optimal interval after a skin injury for obtaining maximal scar recontouring with dermabrasion (29). He proposed the use of this technique after traumatic accidents as well as surgical repairs. Stegman and Tromovitch studied the histologic depth of injury of motorized dermabrasion (17). Alt refined the use of the diamond fraise (30).

In the 1980s, Johnson repopularized Lowenthal's approach to punch grafting and modernized the technique (31). Hanke and others studied the increased scarring from newly introduced colder refrigerant sprays prior to dermabrasion (32). Pinski reported the use of biologic dressings for more rapid healing after skin abrasion (33). Mandy proposed preoperative tretinoin to enhance re-epithelialization after dermabrasion (34). In 1991, Coleman and Klein introduced the concept of tumescent anesthesia for dermabrasion after adopting this approach from dermatologic work with liposuction (35). Goodman further refined this approach adding the use of topical anesthetics (36). Harris repopularized manual dermabrasion using silicone carbide sandpaper after chemical peel or laser resurfacing (37).

LASER RESURFACING

Leon Goldman, a former chairman of dermatology at the University of Cincinnati, was the first physician to employ lasers for treating skin disorders (1961) (38). He helped to develop a number of laser systems including the Neodymium: Yttrium-Aluminum-Garnet (Nd:YAG), copper vapor, and ruby lasers. The development of the carbon dioxide laser in the 1970s provided a new technique for removal of skin lesions. McBurney pioneered the use of the carbon dioxide laser for a variety of dermatologic lesions and Bailin and Ratz described the use of this laser for Mohs' Surgery (39, 40). Wheeland and Bailin researched the use of carbon dioxide lasers as a tool for scalp reduction and as an alternative to dermabrasion for removal of multiple trichoepitheliomas (41). David described ablation of the vermillion in actinic cheilitis using the carbon dioxide laser (42).

In the 1990s, the development of pulsed carbon dioxide lasers led to much less charring than previously feasible and allowed lasers to become an effective method for skin resurfacing, similar to chemical peels and derm-abrasion but with more precision. A number of dermatologists helped pioneer techniques with these new systems. Alster, David, Dover, Fitzpatrick, Geronemus, Goldman, Hruza, Lask, Lowe, Kauvar, Waldroff, Weinstein and others wrote and lectured extensively on these new instruments (43-48). As of this writing, an increasing number of pulsed laser systems are being introduced for skin resurfacing.

AN INTEGRATED APPROACH TO SKIN RESURFACING

Although the initial enthusiasm over laser resurfacing encouraged some laser experts to predict that dermabrasion and chemical peeling were now dead, their demise has been greatly exaggerated. Many of the early researchers on laser resurfacing were primarily experienced in the use of vascular lasers (49). As this technique was embraced by others with long experience in chemical and abrasive resurfacing, a new perspective was developed. Chemical peeling and dermabrasion remain excellent modalities for skin resurfacing. These techniques may be used sequentially or concomitantly in a segmental fashion (50). Some cosmetic units of the face respond better to one of these techniques than another. Likewise, patients of different genetic backgrounds and with varying degrees of aging or actinic damage may respond better to one of these techniques. The informed physician who practices skin resurfacing should have training in chemical peeling, dermabrasion, and laser resurfacing in order to offer patients the broadest possible array of resurfacing techniques. Undoubtedly, other approaches to skin resurfacing will be introduced in the future to take their place along the currently practiced ones.

REFERENCES

1. Durant W. Our Oriental heritage. New York: Simon and Schuster, 1934.
2. Saags H. Civilization before Greece and Rome. New Haven, CT: Yale University Press, 1989.
3. Durant W. The life of Greece, New York: Simon & Schuster, 1939.
4. Lawrence N, Brody H, Alt T. Chemical Peeling. In: Coleman WP III, et al, eds. Cosmetic Surgery of the Skin. St. Louis: Mosby, 1997:85.
5. Hanke CW, Coleman WP III, Francis LA. History of dermatologic cosmetic surgery. Am J Cosmet Surg 1992;9:231-234.
6. Mackee GM, Karp FL. The treatment of post acne scars with phenol. Br J Dermatol 1952;64:456-459.
7. Gross BG, Maschek F. Phenol chemosurgery for removal of deep facial wrinkles. Int J Dermatol 1980;19:159.
8. Eller JJ, Wolff S. Skin peeling and scarification. JAMA 1941;116:934.
9. Urkov J. Surface defects of skin: treatment by controlled exfoliation. Ill Med J 1946;89:75-81.
10. Winter L. Method of permanent removal of freckles. Br J Dermatol Syph 1950;62:83.
11. Monash S. The uses of diluted trichloracetic acid in dermatology. Urol Cutan Rev 1949;49:119-120.
12. Ayres S. Superficial chemosurgery in treating skin. Arch Dermatol 1962;85:125-133.
13. Brown AM, Kaplan LM, Brown ME. Phenol induced histological skin changes: hazards, techniques, and uses. Br J Plast Surg 1960;13:158.
14. Baker TJ. Chemical face peeling and rhytidectomy. Plast Reconstr Surg 1962;29:199.
15. Litton C. Chemical face lifting. Plast Reconstr Surg 1962;29:371.
16. Resnik SS, Lewis LA, Cohen BH. Trichloroacetic acid peeling. Cutis 1976;17:127-129.
17. Stegman S. A comparative histologic study of the effects of three peeling agents and dermabrasion on normal and sun damaged skin. Aesthetic Plast Surg 1982;6:123-135.
18. Van Scott EJ, Yu RJ. Hyperkeratinization, corneocyte cohesion, and alpha hydroxy acids. J Am Acad Dermatol 1984;11:867-879.
19. Brody H, Halley C. Medium-depth chemical peeling of the skin: a variation of superficial chemosurgery. J Dermatol Surg Oncol 1989;15:953-963.
20. Monheit GD. The Jessner's + TCA peel: a medium depth chemical peel. J Dermatol Surg Oncol 1989;15:945-950.
21. Coleman WP III, Futrell JM. The glycolic trichloroacetic acid peel. J Dermatol Surg Oncol 1994;20:76-80.
22. Kromayer E. Rotationsinstrumente: ein neues techisches Verfahren in der dermatologischen Kleinchirurgic. Dermatol Z 1905;12:26.
23. Kromayer E. Cosmetic treatment of skin complaints. New York: Oxford University Press, 1930 (English translation of the second German edition, 1929).
24. Iverson PC. Surgical removal of traumatic tattoos of the face. Plast Reconstr Surg 1947;2:427.
25. Kurtin A. Corrective surgical planning of the skin. Arch Dermatol Syph 1953;68:389.
26. Coleman WP, Hanke CW. The history of dermatologic cosmetic surgery. In: Coleman WP III, et al, eds. Cosmetic Surgery of the Skin. St. Louis: Mosby, 1997.
27. Lowenthal L. Punch biopsy with autograft. Arch Dermatol Syph 1953;67:629-631.
28. Wilson J, Ayres S, Luikart R. Mixtures of fluorinated hydrocarbons as refrigerated anesthetic. Arch Dermatol 1956;74:310-311.
29. Yarborough JM. Scar revision by dermabrasion. In: Dermatologic surgery. Roenigk RK, Roenigk HH, eds. New York: Marcel Dekker, 1989.
30. Alt T. Facial dermabrasion: advantages of the diamond fraise technique. J Dermatol Surg Oncol 1987;13:618-624.
31. Johnson W. Treatment of pitted scars. Punch transplant techniques. J Dermatol Surg Oncol 1986;12:260.
32. Hanke CW, O'Brian JJ, Salow EB. Laboratory evaluation of skin refrigerants in dermabrasion. J Dermatol Surg Oncol 1985;11:45-49.
33. Pinski J. Dressings for dermabrasion: new aspects. J Dermatol Surg Oncol 1987;13:673-677.

34. Mandy SH. Tretinoin in the preoperative and postoperative management of dermabrasion. J Am Acad Derm 1986; 35:878-879.

35. Coleman WP, Klein JA. Use of tumescent technique for scalp surgery, dermabrasion, and soft tissue augmentation. J Dermatol Surg Oncol 1992;18:130-135.

36. Goodman G. Dermabrasion using tumescent anesthesia. J Dermatol Surg Oncol 1994;20:802-807.

37. Harris DR, Noodleman FR. Combining manual dermasanding with low strength trichloroacetic acid to improve actinically injured skin. J Dermatol Surg Oncol 1994;20: 436-442.

38. Goldman L, Wilson R, Hornby P. Radiation from a Q-switched ruby laser. Effect of repeated impacts of power output of 10 megawatts on a tattoo of man. J Invest Dermatol 1965;44:69-71.

39. McBurney EI. Carbon dioxide laser surgery of dermatologic lesions, South Med J 1978;71:795-797.

40. Bailin PL, Ratz JL, Lutz-Nagey L. CO_2 laser modification of Mohs' surgery. J Dermatol Surg Oncol 1981;7:621-623.

41. Wheeland RG, Bailin PL, Kronberg E. Carbon dioxide (CO_2) laser vaporization for the treatment of multiple trichoepithelioma. J Dermatol Surg Oncol 1984;10:470-475.

42. David LM. Laser vermillion ablation for actinic chelitis. J Dermatol Surg Oncol 1985;11:605.

43. David LM, Sarne AJ, Unger WP. Rapid laser scanning for facial resurfacing. Dermatol Surg 1995;21:1031-1033.

44. Fitzpatrick RE, Tope WD, Goldman MP, et al. Pulsed carbon dioxide laser, trichloroacetic acid, Baker Gordon phenol, and dermabrasion: a comparative clinical and histologic study of cutaneous resurfacing in a porcine model. Arch Dermatol 1996;132:469-471.

45. Waldrof HA, Kauvar ANB, Geronemus ARG. Skin resurfacing of fine to deep rhytides using a char-free carbon dioxide laser in 47 patients. Dermatol Surg 1995;21: 940-946.

46. Hruza GJ. Skin resurfacing with lasers. Fitzpatrick's J Clin Dermatol 1995;3(4):38-41.

47. Weinstein C. Ultrapulse carbon dioxide laser removal of periocular wrinkles in association with laser blepharoplasty. J Clin Laser Med Surg 1994;12:205-209.

48. Lowe N, Lask G, Griffin ME, et al. Skin resurfacing with the Ultrapulse carbon dioxide laser: observations on 100 patients. Dermatol Surg 1995;21:1025-1029.

49. Wheeland RG. History of lasers in dermatology. Clin Dermatol 1995;13:3-10.

50. Coleman WP III, Narins RS. Combining surgical methods for skin resurfacing. Sem Cut Med Surg 1996;15(3): 194-199.

CHAPTER 2

Indications for Skin Resurfacing

■ Seth L. Matarasso

The definition of cutaneous resurfacing is to make the skin smooth again, and to attain this goal there is a vast array of treatment options. Topical preparations primarily address the epidermis and remove superficial pathology. Acids, abrasive modalities, and the new generation of lasers not only remove the epidermis, but can also penetrate to the mid-reticular dermis, affecting deeper pathology and collagen remodeling. These many resurfacing options must be matched to an array of indications for resurfacing. The indications range from reconstruction and therapeutic to aesthetic concerns including scar revision surgery, removal of both benign and preneoplastic lesions, and the effacement of rhytides in the treatment of the aging face.

Many of the indications and pathology addressed with resurfacing can be treated with any number of tools, either alone or simultaneously. It is the physician's responsibility to correctly identify the defect and its histologic location and, with the patient, select the appropriate resurfacing tool that will produce the optimal result with the corresponding lowest morbidity.

CONTRAINDICATIONS

As important as it is to recognize the indications for resurfacing, it is equally important to be familiar with absolute and relative contraindications. Perhaps one of the more subtle and correspondingly harder contraindications to identify is psychological instability. While an in-depth psychological profile and patient analysis is generally beyond the realm of most physicians, establishing a strong doctor/patient rapport will often eliminate patients who are unacceptable resurfacing candidates (Table 2.1). The patient should specifically identify their concerns, and the physician has the responsibility of explaining the limits of resurfacing, tempering patient expectations so that they are appropriate. Generally, a properly educated patient with realistic expectations reduces the potential for dissatisfaction.

Similarly, any patient interested in resurfacing needs to accept the responsibility of sun protection and sun avoidance. Discussing the patient's recreational or occupational outdoor activities and ultraviolet light exposure is important. Casual sun exposure increases the risk of pigmentary changes, and is also counterproductive to any progress made with resurfacing. Daily and generous use of broad-spectrum, high sun-protective factor sunscreens and a fundamental knowledge of peak sun hours is a basic foundation for all resurfacing.

Active cutaneous infection is recognizable, and appropriate treatment should be instituted and resurfacing delayed until the infection is resolved. Herpes labialis is quite prevalent in the adult population, and patients with active lesions should refrain from initiating therapy. There are many effective oral antivirals, and a history of herpes simplex virus should not preclude resurfacing. Should resurfacing be anticipated, however, prophylaxis before treatment and until re-epithelialization is completed is appropriate to suppress reactivation. While chemical resurfacing is helpful in treating facial human papilloma virus, any other type of resurfacing is contraindicated due to the potential for dissemination of the virus. Similarly, active bacterial or fungal infections warrant culture and preclude resurfacing until there is complete resolution.

TABLE 2.1

POTENTIAL PROBLEM PATIENTS

The patient with unrealistic expectations
The obsessive-compulsive patient
The sudden whim patient
The indecisive patient
The rude patient
The over-flattering patient
The overly familiar patient
The unkempt patient
The patient with minimal or imagined deformity
The careless or poor historian
The "VIP" patient
The uncooperative patient
The overly talkative patient
The surgeon shopper
The depressed patient
The "plastic surgicoholic"
The price haggler
The patient involved in litigation
The patient you or your staff dislike

Reprinted with permission from Tardy ME, Klimsensmith M. Face-lift surgery: Principles and variations. In: Roenigk RK, Roenigk HH (eds). Dermatologic Surgery. New York: Dekker, 1988; p 1249.

Medications and past medical and surgical history should be carefully reviewed. Any medications with photosensitizing capabilities should be substituted. The use of isotretinoin has become common, and its mechanism of action is atrophy of the pilosebaceous unit. Re-epithelialization following resurfacing originates from adnexal structures, and alteration of these structures can retard wound healing, with subsequent adverse sequelae including scarring. Prior to any dermal injury, it is recommended that isotretinoin be discontinued at last six months preoperatively. Similarly, patients with diminished adnexae on facial skin and patients who have altered adnexae from previous facial radiation therapy are at higher risk for scarring following resurfacing. Any questions regarding the patient's general health and medical suitability for a procedure should be evaluated and approved by the appropriate medical specialist. In addition, allergies to medication should be noted and potential drug interactions should be anticipated and avoided.

Previous surgery and the appearance of the prior incisions may be predictive of a patient's response to resurfacing. A poor quality scar, dyspigmentation, or any evidence of poor wound healing would be a contraindication to resurfacing. However, because resurfacing is not a full thickness injury, previous scarring is not always completely predictive, a test spot with the proposed resurfacing modality may be helpful in assessing response to wounding. Finally, as resurfacing can cause vascular compromise and tissue contraction, any facial surgery that would further compromise blood supply or affect skin laxity should be scheduled with an adequate time interval for healing and recovery.

TOPICAL RESURFACING AGENTS

Topical resurfacing preparations are products that are applied at home, and although some are over-the-counter, the stronger agents are given by prescription (Table 2.2). These products, which have different mechanisms of action, can be used alone or together and usually cause some level of epidermal desquamation. Long used as the mainstay in the treatment of acne, topical resurfacing preparations are now also indicated for the treatment of the early signs of photodamage such as dyschromia and pathology restricted to the epidermis (Fig. 2.1). However, there is mounting evidence that with long-term treatment there is an effect on the upper papillary dermis resulting in softening of fine, nondynamic rhytides.

These agents are also useful prior to and following other resurfacing procedures. Preoperatively, the use of these agents in a skin care regimen promotes uniform desquamation, and subsequent uniform resurfacing and accelerated wound healing postoperatively (Table 2.3). Upon complete re-epithelialization, resuming this topical regimen reduces potential complications and further sustains the result of the resurfacing.

Within this category, the topical retinoids and alpha hydroxy acids have been studied extensively. Tretinoin (Retin-A, Ortho Pharmaceuticals Corp., Raritan, NJ) is a Vitamin A-based product that is available as a cream (0.025%, 0.05%, 0.1%), a gel (0.01%, 0.025%, and 0.1%), a solution (0.1%), and an emollient-based cream (Renova

TABLE 2.2

TOPICAL RESURFACING PREPARATIONS

Alpha-hydroxy acids	Salicylic acid
Azelaic acid	Tretinoin cream
5-Fluorouracil	

TABLE 2.3

PRE- AND POSTOPERATIVE RESURFACING SKIN CARE REGIMEN

A.M.
Bland cleanser
8-12% Glycolic acid or kojic acid or ascorbic acid
Sunscreen (broad-spectrum, SPF >15)

P.M.
Bland cleanser
0.025-1% Tretinoin compounded with 4% hydroquinone

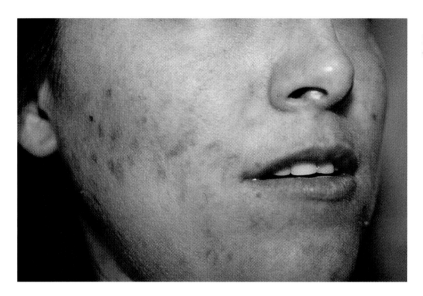

FIGURE 2.1
Postinflammatory pigment that can be treated with topical resurfacing products.

TABLE 2.4	
ALPHA-HYDROXY ACIDS	
Glycolic acid	Citric acid
Lactic acid	Tartaric acid
Malic acid	

TABLE 2.5	
JESSNER'S (COMBES) SOLUTION	
Resorcinol 14 g	Lactic acid (85%) 14 g
Salicylic acid 14 g	Ethanol 95% q.s.a.d., 100 ml

0.05%). To maximize compliance and avoid skin irritancy and sun sensitivity, patients are started on small amounts of low-concentration creams in conjunction with daily sunscreen. Frequency, amount, and concentration are adjusted according to individual patient tolerance.

Tretinoin has been shown to thin the stratum corneum, stimulate keratinocytes, normalize epidermal atypia, and redistribute epidermal pigment. Tretinoin stimulates proliferation of fibroblasts in the dermis and production of elastin and Type I collagen and new blood vessels. Clinically, the application of tretinoin results in superficial resurfacing, with an improvement in skin color and fine rhytides. Most of the clinical effects are dose-related and require at least 6 months to realize improvement.

Perhaps fueled in part by the lay press and the perception that they are a "natural" alternative to rejuvenation, alpha hydroxy acids have witnessed an impressive revival in their popularity (Table 2.4). The two most commonly used alpha hydroxy acids are glycolic and lactic acids. At a concentration of 5% to 20%, lactic acid acts primarily as a humectant, with secondary properties causing desquamation of the stratum corneum. Lactic acid can also be compounded with resorcinol and salicylic acid into Jessner's solution to produce a superficial chemical peel (Table 2.5). Recently, salicylic acid, a beta hydroxy acid, has generated interest as a topical resurfacing agent.

Glycolic acid has clearly received the most interest of the alpha hydroxy acids and has been enthusiastically accepted by the general public. Nevertheless, there is no consensus as to what is the most effective formulation, concentration, and acid bioavailability. Almost all of the commercially available products range from 2% to 20% glycolic acid and are buffered to a pH of 3.5 to 4.5. Unbuffered solutions have a pH close to 1.9 and are more irritating. At low concentrations in topical preparations, glycolic acid causes keratinocyte detachment and reduction in stratum corneum thickness, and increases the ability to disperse melanin granules. Although through a different mechanism of action, glycolic acid has a similar superficial resurfacing effect as retinoic acid, but can be less irritating and photosensitizing.

Whether these topical preparations can reverse early photodamage to the degree that is clinically desirable by patients who seek a more youthful appearance is somewhat controversial, and most physicians consider them as a useful adjunct to other resurfacing procedures.

CHEMICAL PEELS

Chemical peels are defined as the application of an acid to the skin to produce a controlled injury to the epidermis and/or dermis. Subsequent re-epithelialization by second intention wound healing produces a rejuvenated appearance. Broadly classified into superficial, medium, and deep peels depending upon their depth of cutaneous injury, there is actually a continuum between categories and there is a large overlap in the indications for chemical peeling.

There are a number of superficial chemical peeling agents, all with similar indications (Table 2.6). With a single peel, the superficial agents cause desquamation and are primarily indicated for pathology that is epidermal or restricted to the superficial dermis, such as active acne and its sequelae. Regular serial superficial chemical peels can affect the upper papillary dermis with subsequent improvement in the early signs of photoaging and fine rhytides. Superficial chemical peels are also used as an initial keratolytic prior to the application

of a second acid in an effort to produce an upper papillary medium depth chemical peel. They are also used as the primary resurfacing modality for nonfacial skin (Fig. 2.2).

Three of the commonly used superficial chemical peels are low concentrations of trichloroacetic acid (TCA) (10% to 30%), Jessner's solution, and high concentrations of glycolic acid (35% to 70%). TCA is prepared as a weight-to-volume solution, and upon application turns the skin white, indicating coagulative necrosis and protein denaturation. TCA is neutralized by the serum upon absorption, and its effects cannot be diluted or attenuated after application. Jessner's solution has a variety of names and consists of three superficial chemical peeling agents compounded in ethanol. Superficial chemical peeling with Jessner's solution is accomplished through microvesiculation of the stratum corneum. Depending upon concentration and exposure time, glycolic acid can cause corneocyte detachment to frank epidermolysis. As TCA, Jessner's solution and glycolic acid can increase epidermal and dermal glycosaminoglycans and skin thickness, they have the same indications for treating early photodamage and epidermal pathology. While subtle differences exist in recuperation within this class, agent selection is largely based on operator preference.

MEDIUM DEPTH CHEMICAL PEELS

Medium depth chemical peels were developed as a means to get deeper cutaneous penetration without the associated systemic risks of deep chemical peels. The agents in this class have the capability to penetrate to the papillary dermis and the upper reticular dermis; and they include 35% to 50% TCA (alone or in conjunction with an initial superficial keratolytic), and 88% phenol. Used by itself, 35% TCA produces a medium depth

TABLE 2.6

CLASSIFICATION OF CHEMICAL PEELS

Type of Peel	Approximate Depth of Wound
Superficial Chemical Peel Alpha-hydroxy acids CO_2 (+/− alcohol, +/− sulfur) Jessner's (Combes) solution Resorcinol Salicylic acid TCA (10-30%) Unna's paste TCA 10-30%	0.06 mm (stratum granulosum to superficial papillary dermis)
Medium-Depth Chemical Peel 88% Phenol 35-50% TCA +/− a second keratolytic	0.45 mm (papillary to upper reticular dermis)
Deep Chemical Peel Baker-Gordon formula (open or closed)	0.6 mm (midreticular dermis)

FIGURE 2.2

Extensive nonfacial keratosis that could be addressed with several superficial chemical peels.

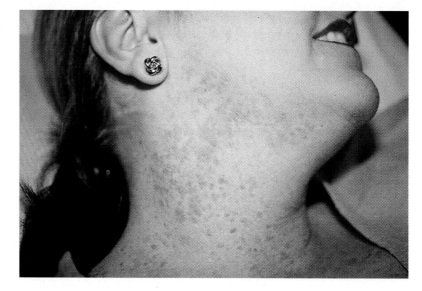

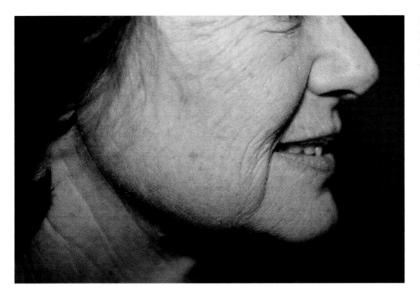

FIGURE 2.3
Moderate rhytidosis and dyschromia secondary to chronic ultraviolet light exposure can be improved with a medium-depth chemical peel, dermabrasion, or carbon dioxide laser resurfacing.

peel; however, its penetration can be further enhanced with prior application of a superficial chemical peeling agent such as carbon dioxide, Jessner's solution, or glycolic acid. Concentrations of TCA that exceed 40% are somewhat unpredictable and have a higher risk profile. A phenol peel using concentrations of 45% to 50% penetrates to the mid-reticular dermis and is considered a deep chemical peel, but at 88%, phenol only penetrates to the papillary dermis and upper reticular dermis and is still considered a medium depth peel. However, due to its absorption and inherent associated cardiac, hepatic, and renal risks, 88% phenol carries the same systemic precautions as deep chemical peels.

The primary indications for medium depth chemical peels are the cutaneous changes associated with chronic photodamage. Static rhytides, diffuse actinic keratoses, and solar lentigines respond well to medium depth peels (Fig. 2.3). Dynamic wrinkles, deep furrows, and frank neoplasia are generally less responsive to a medium-depth peel and require supplemental treatment. Postinflammatory pigmentation and other superficial pigmentary anomalies are an appropriate indication for medium depth peels. Melasma, however, can have a variable location, and if it is superficial, can resolve with a medium depth chemical peel. Pigment that is deeper is often recalcitrant to treatment and is associated with a higher incidence of postoperative pigmentary abnormalities. Medium depth peels are also used to soften the appearance of vitiligo and leukoderma by reducing the color contrast of surrounding skin. Similarly, they can be used with deep resurfacing as blending agents to avoid sharp color demarcation between treated and untreated skin. Molluscum contagiosum, acne rosacea, and neurotic excoriations have been successfully treated with medium depth peels. Improvement may be temporary, and maintenance with topical preparations and repeat peels may be necessary to sustain the results.

TABLE 2.7

THE BAKER-GORDON SOLUTION

Phenol 88% U.S.P., 3 ml	Septisol liquid soap, 8 drops
Distilled water, 2 ml	Croton oil, 3 drops

DEEP CHEMICAL PEELS

The most commonly used deep chemical peel is the Baker-Gordon solution, a mixture of phenol, Septisol (Vestal Laboratories, Inc., St Louis, MO), and croton oil (Table 2.7). The formula results in a phenol concentration of 45% to 55% and penetrates to the mid reticular dermis. Postoperative occlusion prevents phenol evaporation, promotes maceration, and therefore further enhances penetration of the solution deeper into the dermis. Deep chemical peels are used to improve both intrinsic and extrinsic changes associated with the aging face. Intrinsic or chronological characteristics such as rhytidosis can be improved or eliminated. Extrinsic photoaging changes inclusive of dyschromia, keratotic lesions, and solar elastosis can also be improved. While rhytides from gravitational changes and dynamic motion can be improved from tissue contraction, it is a mistake to undertake any type of deep resurfacing as a substitute for face lifting surgery. Nevertheless, deep chemical peels are an appropriate ancillary procedure to rejuvenating facial surgery and complement procedures such as blepharoplasty, rhytidectomy, brow lifts, and soft tissue augmentation. However, when anticipating both a full-face deep chemical peel and facial surgery, an adequate time interval should be scheduled. Both deep chemical peels and facial undermining can cause vasoconstriction, and when performed simultaneously can impede the blood supply leading to a skin slough.

Recently, preliminary reports of simultaneous deep chemical peeling and transconjunctival blepharoplasty or deep plane face lifts were found not to be associated with an increase of skin necrosis.

DERMABRASION

Dermabrasion uses a rapidly rotating hand-held apparatus attached to either a coarse wire brush or diamond fraise to produce a controlled mechanical injury. With second intention healing, there is an improvement in superficial pathology and reorganization of dermal collagen and elastin fibers.

Removal of unwanted tattoos remains one of the primary indications for dermabrasion. Amateur home-made tattoos are often made up of carbon-based India ink that is typically less dense and unevenly dispersed throughout the skin. This latter characteristic makes removal somewhat unpredictable. Conversely, professional tattoos made with a tattoo gun contain more ink, but the ink placement is in a more uniform distribution and is often responsive to removal with dermabrasion. Tattoos should be partially removed in stages at 2 to 3 month intervals. An attempt to remove all of the ink initially risks injury to the reticular dermis and resultant scar formation. Application of gentian violet or salt (salabrasion) postoperatively prolongs wound healing and creates continued inflammation. This can stimulate phagocytosis of additional pigment and further reduce the appearance of the tattoo.

Facial tumors, either solitary or multiple, respond well to dermabrasion, however, it is often prudent to document either by clinical inspection, historical in-formation, or histopathologic examination, the non-metastasizing nature of the lesion prior to ablation (Table 2.8). In addition, patients must be informed that treatment is often aimed at temporary cosmetic improvement as repeat treatment may be needed when new lesions appear or previous lesions recur.

Dermabrasion is indicated for restoring facial architecture. Dramatic improvement can be obtained by reshaping the external appearance of a rhinophymatous nose. In addition, scars from previous surgery, trauma, or varicella can not only be cosmetically disfiguring, but can also carry a negative emotional connotation. Scars respond best to dermabrasion 6 to 8 weeks after the injury, when the collagen is still in the remodeling phase. Perhaps more than any other resurfacing modality, facial acne scars are well-suited to dermabrasion (Fig. 2.4). Shallow, atrophic, distensible scars can be erased or substantially improved. However, deep ice-pick or bound-down acne scars are ideally treated initially with surgical scar revision by punch excision or grafting, and then dermabrasion 6 weeks postoperatively.

Possibly under-used, dermabrasion remains an effective tool for improving photodamage associated with the aging face. Dermabrasion effectively removes ac-

TABLE 2.8

TUMORS RESPONSIVE TO RESURFACING

Adenoma sebaceum	Syringoma
Dermatosis papulosis nigra	Trichoepithelioma
Sebaceous hyperplasia	Xanthoma

FIGURE 2.4
Facial acne scarring that would be responsive to dermabrasion. Dermabrasion test spot is evident in the preauricular sulcus.

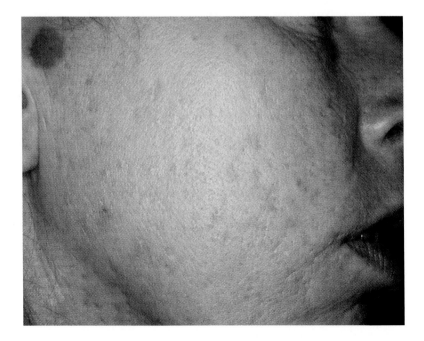

tinic keratoses, prevents the formation of new lesions, and can adequately eradicate superficial basal cell carcinomas in cosmetically difficult areas. Nondynamic facial rhytides can be effaced and deep perioral rhagades can also be improved with dermabrasion. Extra care should be exercised when operating around the periocular and perioral areas, and precautions with blood-borne aerosolized particles should be enforced.

LASERS

Although lasers have been used for nearly four decades, it is only in the past few years that they have gained widespread acceptance in medicine. The recent development of carbon dioxide (CO_2) lasers that use high-peak powers and pulse durations shorter than the thermal relaxation time of water-containing tissue allow for diminished thermal conduction to normal cutaneous structures. Although water is the common absorbing chromophore for the CO_2 lasers, the delivery method, power, pulse duration, and energy can vary greatly. Nevertheless, the indications for all of the resurfacing lasers are similar, and with continued experience and long-term follow up, the list will continue to evolve.

Isolated cutaneous lesions such as lentigines and actinic keratoses can be eliminated by skin resurfacing. Pulsed laser systems minimize damage to normal perilesional skin structures by vaporizing the lesion faster than heat can be conducted to the surrounding area. In a bloodless field, the laser precisely vaporizes tissue with each pass and avoids sharp demarcation between treated and untreated skin. However, the laser is best used for treating diffuse lesions and obtaining a uniform field effect.

Atrophic scars secondary to acne, trauma, or surgery are readily amenable to high-energy laser resurfacing. The procedure can be made very precise by sculpting the scar edges, vaporizing more tissue only in the area of the scar, and doing superficial resurfacing on the remaining area. The thermal effects of the laser appear to cause collagen shrinking and appreciable improvement can be seen perioperatively. The appearance of the scars, however, continues to improve up to 1 year postoperatively due to collagen remodeling. Deep, pitted acne scars may also show some degree of improvement with laser resurfacing, but often require preoperative scar revision. Hypertrophic or keloidal scars do not respond well to laser resurfacing due to the high risk of recurrence, and are best treated with the 585 nm pulsed dye laser.

Perhaps one of the more common indications for laser resurfacing is for photodamage and the cutaneous changes associated with aging. Epidermal and preneoplastic lesions respond to many destructive modalities, including CO_2 lasers. Actinic cheilitis is particularly well-suited to laser ablation. With one pass on low power settings, the CO_2 laser can effectively vaporize the lip epidermis and eliminate or improve actinic cheilitis. However, as with most resurfacing, the role of CO_2 laser resurfacing in the removal of frank neoplasia remains limited.

Finally, laser resurfacing is an optimal treatment for facial rhytidosis. Successive laser passes precisely remove tissue layer by layer, flattening elevations by vaporization and tightening the skin by collagen remodeling. With the first pass, the epidermis is removed, and the tissue changes in color with each additional pass as resurfacing proceeds into the dermis. Entry into the papillary dermis is evident as a pink color, the deeper papillary dermis as a gray color, and the upper reticular dermis as a yellow color. The periocular and perioral areas generally require multiple passes due to the extent of photodamage and profound rhytidosis. When resurfacing an isolated aesthetic unit, it is important to follow the wrinkle out to its end and feather it (lightly vaporize the edges) to blend into the untreated area as resurfacing one anatomic area can be obvious. Full-face blending can reduce color contrast and promote a more uniform tissue contraction, hence effacing more rhytides. Similarly, preoperative use of chemical denervation with botulinum toxin (BOTOX, Allergan Inc., Irvine, CA) in the upper one-third of the face prevents animation and may further promote collagen reorganization and enhance the clinical results (Fig. 2.5).

CONCLUSION

There is a large and diverse gamut of indications for cutaneous resurfacing, ranging from elective cosmetic improvement to restoration of diseased tissue. Regardless, the ultimate goal is the same: an improvement in the appearance of the skin. Paralleling the numerous indications is the current availability of a wide spectrum of resurfacing tools. All of the resurfacing tools have a similar endpoint: destruction and replacement of the epidermis, and injury to the dermis with subsequent new collagen deposition.

The art of cutaneous resurfacing is to match the indication with the appropriate tool. Ironically, more often than not, multiple resurfacing techniques are appropriate for any one indication. Rather than being mutually exclusive, these approaches can be complementary, and the use of different modalities together can enhance the final result. The ultimate selection of the resurfacing tool or tools is contingent upon the physical parameters and psychological profile of the patient as well as the expertise of the physician. Clearly, a risk/benefit ratio should be strictly adhered to, and maximal cosmesis should not be sacrificed for unacceptable risks.

FIGURE 2.5
A, Early periocular rhytides (crow's feet) that can be treated with topical preparations. B, Deep wrinkles that would require deeper resurfacing with a chemical peel or carbon dioxide laser. Preoperative treatment with BOTOX could enhance clinical improvement.

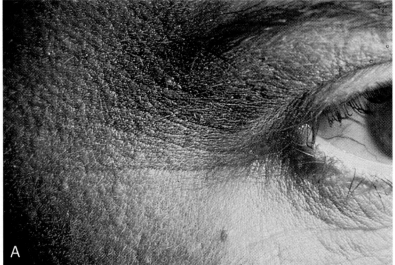

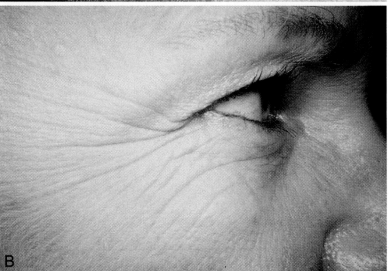

REFERENCES

Alster TS, West TB. Resurfacing of atrophic acne scars with a high-energy, pulsed CO2 laser. Dermatol Surg 1996;22: 151-155.

Alster TS. Comparison of two high-energy, pulsed carbon dioxide lasers in the treatment of periorbital rhytides. J Dermatol Surg 1996;22:541-545.

Alster TS. Improvement of erythematous and hypertrophic scars by the 585-nm flashlamp-pumped pulsed dye laser. Ann Plast Surg 1993;31:1-5.

Alt TH. Occluded Baker/Gordon chemical peel: review and update. J Dermatol Surg Oncol 1989;15:980-993.

Asken S. Unoccluded Baker/Gordon phenol peels: review and update. J Dermatol Surg Oncol 1989;15:998-1008.

Baker TJ, Gordon HL. The ablation of rhytides by chemical means: a preliminary report. J Fla Med Assoc 1961;48:541.

Baker TJ. Chemical face peeling and rhytidectomy. Plast Reconstr Surg 1962;29:199.

Baker TJ. Discussion on simultaneously deep-plane face lift and trichloroacetic acid peel. Plast Reconstr Surg 1994;93: 94-95.

Becker FF, Langford FPJ, Rubin MG, et al. a histological comparison of 50% and 70% glycolic acid peels using solutions with various pHs. Dermatol Surg 1996;22:463-468.

Brody HJ, Hailey CW. Medium depth chemical peeling of the skin: A variation of superficial chemosurgery. J Dermatol Surg Oncol 1986;12:1268.

Brody HJ. Trichloroacetic acid application in chemical peeling. Operative Techniques Plast Reconstr Surg 1995;2:127-128.

Brody HJ. Variations and comparisons in medium depth chemical peeling. J Dermatol Surg Oncol 1989;15:953-963.

Coleman WP, Futrell JM. The glycolic acid 1 trichloroacetic acid peel. J Dermatol Surg Oncol 1994;20:76-80.

Coleman WP, Yarborough JM, Mandy SH. Dermabrasion for prophylaxis and treatment of actinic keratoses. J Dermatol Surg Oncol 1996;22:17-21.

Collins PS. Trichloroacetic acid peels revisited. J Dermatol Surg Oncol 1989;15:933-940.

Colven RM, Pinnell SK. Topical Vitamin C in aging. In: Ledo A (ed). Clinics in Dermatology, Skin Aging and Photo-aging 1996;14:227-234.

Combes FC, Sperber PA, Reisch M. Dermal defects: treatment by a chemical agent. NY Physician Am Med 1960;56:36.

DiNardo JD, Grove GL, Moy LS. Clinical and histological effects of glycolic acid at different concentrations and pH levels. Dermatol Surg 1996;22:421-428.

Ditre CM, Griffin TD, Murphy GF, et al. The effects of alpha hydroxy acids on photoaged skin: a pilot clinical, histological and ultrastructural study. J Am Acad Dermatol 1996;34:187-195.

Fitzpatrick RE, Goldman MP, Ruiz-Esparza J. Clinical advantage of the CO2 laser superpulsed mode. Treatment of verruca vulgaris, seborrheic keratoses, lentigines, and actinic cheilitis. J Dermatol Surg Oncol 1994;20:449-56.

Fitzpatrick RE, Goldman MP, Sauter NM, et al. Pulsed carbon dioxide laser resurfacing of photoaged facial skin. Arch Dermatol 1996;132:395-402.

Fitzpatrick RE, Ruiz FJ, Goldman MP. The depth of thermal necrosis using the CO2 laser: a comparison of the superpulsed mode and conventional mode. J Dermatol Surg Oncol 1991;17:340-344.

Fitzpatrick RE, Tope WD, Goldman MP, et al. Pulsed carbon dioxide laser, trichloroacetic acid, Baker-Gordon phenol, and dermabrasion: a comparative clinical and histologic study of cutaneous resurfacing in a porcine model. Arch Dermatol 1996;132:469-471.

Garcia A, Fulton JE. The combination of glycolic acid and hydroquinone or kojic acid for the treatment of melasma and related conditions. Dermatol Surg 1996;22:443-444.

Garrett SJ, Robinson JK, Roenigk HH Jr. Trichloroacetic acid peel of molluscum contagiosum in immunocompromised patients. J Dermatol Surg Oncol 1992;18:855-858.

Glogau RG, Matarasso SL. Chemical peels. Dermatol Clin 1995;13:263-276.

Goldman MP, Fitzpatrick RE. Laser treatment of scars. Dermatol Surg 1995;21:685-687.

Greenbaum SS, Krull EA, Watnich K. Comparison of CO_2 laser and electrosurgery in the treatment of rhinophyma. J Am Acad Dermatol 1988;18:363-368.

Griffiths CEM, Kang S, Ellis CN, et al. Two concentrations of topical tretinoin (retinoic acid) cause similar improvement of photoaging but different degrees of irritation. Arch Dermatol 1995;131:1037-1044.

Hayes DK, Berkland ME, Stambaugh KI. Dermal healing after local skin flaps and chemical peel. Arch Otolaryngol Head Neck Surg 1990;116:794-797.

Hevia O, Nemeth AJ, Taylor JR. Tretinoin accelerates healing after trichloroacetic acid chemical peel. Arch Dermatol 1991;127:678-682.

Hruza GJ, Dover JS. Laser skin resurfacing. Arch Dermatol 1996;132:451-455.

Humphreys TR, Werth V, Dzubow L, et al. Treatment of photodamaged skin with trichloroacetic acid and topical tretinoin. J Am Acad Dermatol 1996;34:638-44.

Karam PG. 50% resorcinol peel. Int J Dermatol 1993;32:569-574.

Kligman AM, Grove GL, Hirose R, et al. Topical tretinoin for photoaged skin. J Am Acad Dermatol 1986;15:836-859.

Lawrence NL, Cox SE, Brody HJ. A comparison of Jessner's solution and glycolic acid in the treatment of melasma in dark skinned patients: a double blind study. J Am Acad Dermatol 1997 (in press).

Leyden JJ, Lavker RM, Grove G, et al. AHAs are more than moisturizers. J Geriatr Dermatol 1995;3(Suppl A):33A-37A.

Mandy SH. Tretinoin in the preoperative and postoperative management of dermabrasion. J Am Acad Dermatol 1986;15:878-879.

Matarasso SL, Glogau RG, Markey AC. Wood's lamp for superficial chemical peels. J Am Acad Dermatol 1994;30:988-992.

Matarasso SL, Glogau RG. Chemical face peels. Dermatol Clin 1991;9:131-150.

Matarasso SL, Glogau RG. The role of chemical peeling in the treatment of photodamaged skin. J Dermatol Surg Oncol 1991;17:622-623.

Matarasso SL. Cutaneous resurfacing. Seminars in Cutaneous Med Surg 1996;15:131-214.

Monheit G. The Jessner's 1 TCA peel: A medium depth chemical peel. J Dermatol Surg Oncol 1989;15:945.

Moy LS, Murad II, Roy RL. Glycolic acid peels for the treatment of wrinkles and photoaging. J Dermatol Surg Oncol 1993;19:243-246.

Nazzaro-Porro M. The depigmenting effect of azelaic acid. Arch Dermatol 1990;126:1649-1653.

Nelson BR, Fader DJ, Gillard M, et al. Pilot histologic and ultrastructural study of the effects of medium-depth chemical facial peels on dermal collagen in patients with actinically damaged skin. J Am Acad Dermatol 1995;32:475-476.

Newman J, Brandow K, Petmecky F. Transconjunctival blepharoplasty with simultaneous lower lid skin peel. Int J Aesth Restor Surg 1995;3:43-52.

Olsen EA, Katz HI, Levine N, et al. Tretinoin emollient cream: a new therapy for photodamaged skin. J Am Acad Dermatol 1992;26:215-224.

Phillips CL, Combs SB, Pinnel SS. Effects of ascorbic acid on proliferation and collagen synthesis in relation to the donor age of human dermal fibroblasts. J Invest Dermatol 1994;103:228-232.

Ridge JM, Siegle RJ, Zuckerman J. Use of alpha-hydroxy acids in the therapy for "photoaged" skin. J Am Acad Dermatol 1990;23:932.

Robinson JK. Actinic cheilitis. Arch Otolaryngol Head Neck Surg 1989;115:848-852.

Rubenstein R, Roenigk HH, Stegman SJ, et al. Atypical keloids after dermabrasion of patients taking isotretinoin. J Am Acad Dermatol 1986;15:280-285.

Rubin MG. Chemical peeling as an adjuvant therapy for facial neurotic excoriations. J Am Acad Dermatol 1995;32:296-297.

Spira M, Gerow FJ, Hardy SB. Complications of chemical face peeling. Plast Reconstr Surg 1974;54:397-403.

Stagnone JJ. Superficial peeling. J Dermatol Surg Oncol 1989;15:924-930.

Stegman SJ. A comparative histologic study of the effects of three peeling agents and dermabrasion on normal and sundamaged skin. Aesth Plast Surg 1982;6:123.

Stegman SJ. A study of dermabrasion and chemical peels in an animal model. J Dermatol Surg Oncol 1980;6:490.

Van Scott EJ, Yu RJ. Hyperkeratinization, corneocyte cohesion and alpha hydroxy acids. J Am Acad Dermatol 1984;11:867-879.

Waldorf HA, Kauvar AN, Geronemus RG. Skin resurfacing of fine to deep rhytides using a char-free carbon dioxide laser in 47 patients. Dermatol Surg 1995;21:940-946.

Weinstein C. Ultrapulse carbon dioxide laser removal of peri-ocular wrinkles in association with laser blepharoplasty. J Clin Laser Med Surg 1994;12:205-209.

Weiss JS, Ellis CN, Headington JT, et al. Topical tretinoin improves photoaged skin: a double-blind, vehicle-controlled study. JAMA 1988;259:527-532.

Wentzell J, Michael J. Physical properties of aerosols produced by dermabrasion. Arch Derm 1989;125:1637-1643.

Yu RJ, Van Scott EJ. Alpha-hydroxy acids: science and therapeutic use. Cosmet Dermatol 1994;7(Suppl):12-20.

CHAPTER 3

Home Treatment Alternatives to Skin Resurfacing

■ William P. Coleman III
William P. Coleman IV
Naomi Lawrence

Often, people first try topical therapeutic regimens at home before turning to skin resurfacing. In many cases, these therapeutic regimens are pseudoscientific formulations promoted by cosmetic companies. The marketing strategy of these companies seems to include convincing customers to employ multiple, local potency, high cost formulations "in a daily system" as recommended by a sales representative. Other patients devise a home therapy program of their own, relying on consumer magazines, television infomercials and local "skin care specialists" such as cosmetologists, health food stores, and friends. Often these product lines are more expensive and less effective than scientifically proven formulations.

Other people consult their physicians before embarking on a home therapeutic skin regimen. Many of these individuals are simply not interested in skin resurfacing because of costs, fears of side effects, or inconvenience. These individuals are comfortable applying therapeutic agents that have proven scientific efficacy in order to obtain minor improvement in their skin appearance with minimal costs and inconvenience. Other patients request therapeutic skin care regimens as a pretreatment option prior to anticipated skin resurfacing. These individuals are usually busy and do not have the time to recover from a resurfacing procedure at the current time but hope to do so later. In the interim, they are motivated to improve their skin by using approaches that do not require time off work. Currently, there are a number of topical agents for physicians to recommend

which have a scientific basis for their use. They have been proven in controlled studies to improve the texture, thickness, and pigmentation of the skin. These few compounds stand in stark contrast to the thousands of other products promoted for skin improvement that have absolutely no scientific substantiation.

TRETINOIN

Topical tretinoin is currently the gold standard for skin rejuvenation products. Tretinoin (all-trans-retinoic acid) is a naturally occurring metabolite of Vitamin-A. Originally patented as Retin-A (Ortho Pharmaceutical Corp., Raritan, NJ) it has been used for the treatment of acne for over two decades. More recent clinical studies have demonstrated that this substance is effective for long term use as a treatment of photodamaged skin [1-4]. These findings have been verified by histologic studies including light and electron microscopy [5, 6]. Studies of tretinoin have demonstrated normalization of damaged skin with thickening of previously atrophic epidermis, reduction of dysplasia, more uniform dispersion of melanin and the production of new dermal collagen and blood vessels [7]. The changes translate into a reduction of fine wrinkles and skin roughness, as well as improvement in melasma and postinflammatory hyperpigmentation through reduction in skin melanin content [8, 9]. Long term studies have confirmed a sustained increase in dermal mucin and a decrease in elastosis [10]. The main side effect encountered was a mild

17

dermatitis (2, 4). Tretinoin naturally occurs in small amounts in human plasma and there were concerns about toxicity. However, studies have confirmed that long term use of topical tretinoin had no detectable effect on endogenous plasma levels (11).

Tretinoin is available in a 0.05% liquid, a 0.025%, 0.05% and 0.1% cream as well as a 0.01%, 0.025%, and 0.1% gel. It also recently became available in a 0.05% emollient cream (Renova, Ortho Pharmaceutical Corp., Raritan, NJ). In general, the liquid form is the most irritating. The gel is also more irritating to most patients than the cream formulations. Recently, a microsphere 0.1% gel has been marketed as a less irritating gel formulation. Tretinoin has come off patent and new forms are likely to be developed.

Retin-A is best introduced into a home care regimen after a careful discussion with the patient about the use of ancillary cosmetic products. Mild soaps are recommended with instructions to avoid scrubbing. For this reason, abrasive pads and wash cloths should be discouraged. Astringents are commonly used by female patients as part of cosmetic programs. These should also be eliminated prior to using tretinoin. Patients must also be counseled about avoidance of sun exposure since increased photosensitivity is commonly seen with this agent.

Tretinoin is usually best applied as a solo agent at night. During the initial phases of use, patients should wait at least 30 minutes after washing the skin before applying the preparation. Milder formulations such as 0.025% cream are better tolerated in sensitive patients. Patients with oily skin may be started on a higher concentration. The concentration of tretinoin can then be increased as tolerated.

Patients are urged to carefully inspect their skin prior to applying tretinoin each evening. Areas of dryness or dermatitis should be avoided. However, there is no reason to omit applying the tretinoin to most of the face just because a small portion is inflamed. In some patients, the chin area is particularly sensitive and can only tolerate applications of tretinoin every second or third night. However, even in these individuals, the rest of the face can usually be treated nightly. Xerosis is common in dry climates especially in the winter time and may reduce the frequency of application. Patients with seborrheic dermatitis may experience irritation especially around the nose or glabellar area and should avoid these areas until the dermatitis has resolved. Patients who are excessively sensitive or dry should apply a moisturizer instead of tretinoin until the dryness has faded. The long term goal is to use the highest strength tolerated on a nightly basis.

ADAPALENE

Adapalene is a naphthoic acid derivative that has potent retinoid and anti-inflammatory properties. Its affinity for cellular retinoic acid receptors is similar to tretinoin. Studies in acne patients indicate that adapalene gel 0.1% is more effective and better tolerated than tretinoin gel 0.025%. The skin irritation seen with tretinoin was markedly reduced with adapalene (12). Adapalene rapidly penetrates the follicular structures, which is an advantage in treating acne (13).

Adapalene gel is a relatively new product and physicians are still fine-tuning its role for the treatment of acne. It has also become attractive as an alternative to tretinoin for the treatment of photodamage. Some patients are intolerant of tretinoin regardless of the formulation or concentration. Many patients who are intolerant to tretinoin do tolerate adapalene, and some physicians are substituting this product for tretinoin in these individuals. It remains to be seen whether the same degree of retinoid benefit will occur in these individuals. Until these studies are completed, it is unknown to what extent adapalene may play a future role in retinoid therapy for photoaging.

ALPHA HYDROXY ACIDS

The concept of using alpha hydroxy acids (AHAs) for the topical treatment of skin disorders was reintroduced by Van Scott and Yu in 1974 (14). However, these agents have been used throughout history even in ancient times for improving aging skin. Tartaric acid from the bottom of wine barrels and lactic acid from sour milk were used as skin rejuvenating agents by the Egyptians, including Cleopatra.

AHAs include glycolic acid, lactic acid, citric acid, malic acid, mandelic acid, and tartaric acid. These products all occur naturally, however, they are now produced synthetically for cosmetic use (Table 3.1). Many over the counter products now contain AHAs. Some of these products have such a low concentration of AHAs that they have minimal effects on the skin. Since AHAs are acidic, many formulations employ organic or inorganic alkali to partially neutralize them by raising the pH to match the skin surface pH of 4.2 to 5.6 (15). The bioavailability of an AHA is dependent on the fraction that is in a free acid form. Partially neu-

TABLE 3.1

ALPHA HYDROXY ACIDS

Alpha Hydroxy Acids	Source
Glycolic acid	Sugar cane
Lactic acid	Fermented milk
Citric acid	Citrus fruits
Malic acid	Unripened apples
Mandelic acid	Bitter almonds
Tartaric acid	Fermented grapes

tralizing these substances to higher pH levels reduces the bioavailability, but decreases their skin irritation potential. Seventy percent formulations of glycolic acid have a pH of 0.6. Likewise, 90% formulations of lactic acid have a pH of 0.5. The bioavailability of these low pH–high concentration formulations is very high and makes them quite suitable for superficial chemical peeling. However, they are far too potent to be tolerable in a home therapeutic regimen and if left in contact with the skin for several minutes can have the potential to cause prolonged erythema or even scarring. Therefore, home products must be adjusted to a higher pH and a lower concentration, thus delivering a lower bioavailability of the AHA.

The vehicle that the AHA is formulated in also plays an important role. Many AHAs are water soluble and work best in oil-in-water emulsions. In an oil-in-water emulsion of glycolic acid, most of the acid will be present in the water phase. This would put the acid in direct contact with the stratum corneum when it is applied to the skin. Some vehicle components can interfere with the topical effects of an AHA (15). Glycerin has a strong affinity for water soluble AHAs such as glycolic acid; thus, it would compromise the effects of these AHAs. Propylene glycol, on the other hand, can enhance penetration of AHAs by alternating the permeability of the stratum corneum. Other chemical compounds may have undefined effects on the bioavailability of AHAs; therefore, simpler vehicles are preferable.

AHAs produce enhanced desquamation of the stratum corneum and are thus touted as exfoliants. Glycolic acid for instance, causes decreased keratinocytic cohesion (14). This desquamation gradually decreases in time as the skin acclimates to the stimulatory effects of AHAs (16). This ability to exfoliate is promoted by cosmetic companies and valued by patients. However, exfoliation is not the primary desired effect of these compounds. AHAs increase mucopolysaccharide and collagen synthesis, which translates into smoother skin with improvement of minor wrinkles (17, 18). Continued improvement has been noted in long term studies well after the exfoliating effect had faded (16).

The chief complication of AHAs is skin irritation. As with tretinoin, this is variable and depends on the patient's skin sensitivity. Using higher pH–lower concentration formulations decreases the benefits of AHAs but allows sensitive patients to use them regularly. The physicians who use these products in a home therapy program must balance this equation of irritability and effect.

Glycolic Acid

Glycolic acid is the most popular AHA in home therapeutic programs. Double blind vehicle controlled studies have demonstrated that use of an 8% oil-in-water emulsion compound of glycolic acid achieves mild improvement in photodamage (19). Clinical improvement is usually manifested by reduced hyperpigmentation, skin sallowness and minor wrinkles. Patients using these compounds should be counseled to use proper sun precautions. Photodamage due to the sun is a primary cause of aging and thus sun exposure should be reduced and sunscreens employed if any progress is to be made in rehabilitated aging skin (20). Also, AHAs may increase phototoxicity so that patients will sunburn more easily when using these compounds.

Glycolic home formulations are typically prescribed in an 8% to 10% gel. Some formulations also contain topical bleaching agents. Stronger concentrations of up to 20% may also be employed on less sensitive areas of the body such as the extremities. The skin sensitivity of each patient must be determined to avoid irritation. There is evidence that a therapeutic regimen that combines the use of topical glycolic acid and topical tretinoin enhances the effect of both agents (21). Therefore, it is common to prescribe tretinoin for nightly use and an AHA formulation, such as 10% glycolic acid gel, each morning. The combined effects of these two agents typically produce visible improvement within 3 months. Patients who continue to employ these agents can expect further improvement in skin thickness, minor wrinkles, and dyspigmentation.

Lactic Acid

Lactic acid salts have been hypothesized to be part of the skin's natural moisturizing system (22). Lactic acid compounds have been popularized as moisturizers and exfoliants for many years (23). A buffered 12% ammonium lactate lotion (Lac-Hydrin, Westwood Squibb Pharmaceuticals, Buffalo, NY) has been successfully used for years as a potent skin moisturizer. However, it has been recently discovered that this formulation also causes an increase in dermal ground substance and increased glycosaminoglycan synthesis (24). Lower concentrations of topical lactic acid (5%) increase epidermal thickness but have little effect on the dermis (25). In another study, 8% L-lactic acid cream was similar to 8% glycolic acid cream in improving cutaneous photodamage (19).

Although lactic acid is less popular than glycolic acid in home therapeutic programs, it can be quite useful. 12% ammonium lactate lotion is well tolerated by patients with severe dry skin. It is one of the most powerful moisturizers available. Many patients cannot tolerate glycolic acid formulations and may also not tolerate tretinoin, even in low concentration creams. Alternatively, sensitive individuals can use lactic acid lotions on days when they develop irritancy from glycolic acid or tretinoin. This is particularly useful for patients who live in dry climates.

OTHER HYDROXY ACIDS

Salicylic acid (ortho hydroxy benzoic acid) has been used by dermatologists for many decades. In higher concentrations (50%), it can be used for chemical peeling. At 3% to 5%, salicylic acid is keratolytic and may be useful in enhancing topical penetration of other agents. Salicylic acid also has some efficacy as a fungicide (Whitfield's ointment) and 2% to 5% creams are available as antiacne products.

Recent studies have indicated that salicylic acid products in a concentration of 1% to 2% increase epidermal cell turnover (26). Irritation associated with salicylic acid appears to be less than that of many AHA products. As with AHAs, lower pH formulations of salicylic acid produce greater bioavailability. The chief problem with salicylic acid is the potential for salicylate intoxication (27). Salicylism is indicated by disturbed consciousness, hyperpyrexia, and eventual coma. Salicylates can induce liver damage. Therefore, salicylic-based substances are better used in low concentrations over small body areas or in high concentrations for brief periods of time as in chemical peeling.

TOPICAL VITAMINS

Vitamins C, E, and beta carotene act as natural antioxidants. When these vitamins are consumed in foods or capsules, they apparently act to reduce the formation of hydrogen peroxide, superoxide anions, and hydroxy radicals that damage living cells (28). However, it is still unsubstantiated whether or not topical vitamins function in a similar way to prevent damage within the dermis.

Vitamin C (ascorbic acid), is a hydrophilic compound that is light sensitive, is unstable in aqueous solutions, and has short-lived effects on the skin (29, 30). Attempts to increase the penetration and stability of Vitamin C have resulted in formulations such as Cellex-C (Cellex-C Corp., Dallas, TX). Initial studies indicate that hydrophilic compounds may protect skin from ultraviolet radiation (31). However, there are no substantiated claims that topical Vitamin C reduces wrinkles. Some of the hydrophilic compounds are quite expensive, but trendy, and whether or not they will become a mainstay of cutaneous home therapy remains to be determined. Magnesium L-Ascorbyl-2-Phosphate (VC-PMG), a more stable ascorbic acid compound, has been used in Japan as a depigmenting agent (32).

Vitamin E (tocopherol) has been shown to decrease erythema after sunburn (33). This may be due to scavenging of ultraviolet radiation induced oxygen free radicals. However, Vitamin E is a fat soluble vitamin with minimal penetration into the stratum corneum. Enhancing the penetration of topical vitamins by occlusion or barrier modification may increase the potential for these agents (34). At this time there is not enough scientific evidence to recommend the regular use of topical vitamins.

BLEACHING AGENTS

For centuries man has sought an ideal agent for reducing hyperpigmentation or to lighten skin color. This trend has been particularly prominent among darker skinned individuals who often have problems with uneven skin pigmentation. Those with lighter complexions may develop uneven pigmentation and frank cutaneous pigmentary lesions such as lentigenes due to photodamage. Integrating bleaching agents into a home skin care regimen can be quite useful for patients of all colors. Although tretinoin and AHAs help to lighten skin discoloration, the addition of a bleaching cream can accelerate this process.

The bleach currently used by most physicians is hydroquinone. This agent acts by inhibiting tyrosinase and decreases the formation of melanosomes. When used in concentrations between 3% and 5%, hydroquinone can improve both dermal and epidermal pigmentation (35). When hydroquinone is used in combination with tretinoin, this effect is enhanced (36). Hydroquinone can be combined with AHAs, such as glycolic acid, to heighten the effects of these agents.

The chief problems associated with the use of hydroquinone are contact dermatitis and the potential for ochronosis. Ochronosis is produced by using high concentrations of hydroquinones for extended periods of time and is characterized by blue-black pigmentation often in a splattered form that can occur far from the site of the hydroquinone application. This disorder appears to be much more common in South Africans than in American blacks (37).

Kojic acid, which is related to hydroquinone chemically, is a byproduct of an aspergillus species fungus that grows on corn in Japan (38). Kojic acid is typically used as a 1% to 2% cream and may be combined with glycolic acid. Whether or not it is as effective as hydroquinone is controversial (39). Kojic acid appears to be better tolerated than hydroquinones in Asian patients.

Azelaic acid was developed as an acne therapeutic agent. A 20% cream is available as Azelex (Allergan Hebert, Inc., Irvine, CA). This formulation is also moderately helpful in reducing hyperpigmentation. This straight chained dicarboxylic acid inhibits DNA synthesis in the melanocyte (40). 20% azelaic acid is well tolerated by most patients, but may cause minor skin irritation. It is probably not as effective as hydroquinone but further studies are needed to compare the two agents (41). Azelaic acid is primarily useful as a bleaching agent in individuals who are intolerant of hydroquinone.

Patients with severe postinflammatory hyperpigmentation may respond to a combination of bleaches.

Hydroquinone and kojic acid can be formulated in a glycolic acid 10% gel. Azelaic acid can also be used provided skin irritation does not develop.

FORMULATING A HOME THERAPEUTIC REGIMEN

Every patient is different and has different needs. The physician must carefully determine what skin pathology exists and what the best options are for treating it. The mainstay of any home skin care regimen is tretinoin. Other rejuvenating agents may be added as needed. Patients should be observed on a regular basis to determine the benefits of treatment and the need for changing the regimen. Ultimately, many patients who begin their journey with the physician on a home skin care regimen end up as resurfacing patients.

REFERENCES

1. Klingman AM, Grove GL, Hirose R, et al. Topical tretinoin for photoaged skin. J Am Acad Dermatol 1986;15:836-859.
2. Weiss JS, Ellis CN, Headington JT, et al. Topical tretinoin improves photodamaged skin: a double-blind vehicle-controlled study. JAMA 1988;259:527-532.
3. Leyden JJ, Grove GL, Grove MJ, et al. Treatment of photo-damaged facial skin with topical tretinoin. J Am Acad Dermatol 1989;21:538-544.
4. Lever L, Kumar P, Marks R. Topical retinoic acid for treatment of solar damage. Br J Dermatol 1990;122:91-98.
5. Bhawan J, Olsen E, Lufrano L, et al. Histologic evaluation of the long term effects of tretinoin on photodamaged skin. J Dermatol Sci 1996;11:177-182.
6. Yamamoto O, Bhawan J, Solares G, et al. Ultrastructual effects of topical tretinoin on dermo-epidermal junction and papillary dermis in photodamaged skin: a controlled study. Exp Dermatol 1995;4:146-154.
7. Gilchrest B. Treatment of photo damage with topical tretinoin: An overview. J Am Acad Dermatol 1997;36:S25-S36.
8. Bulengo-Ransby SM, Griffiths CEM, Kimbrough-Green CK, et al. Topical tretinoin (retinoic acid) therapy for hyperpigmented lesions caused by inflammation of the skin in black patients. N Engl J Med 1993;328:1438-1443.
9. Kimbrough-Green CK, Griffiths CEM, Finkel LJ, et al. Topical retinoic acid (tretinoin) for melasma in black patients. Arch Dermatol 1994;130:727-733.
10. Bhawan J, Gonzalez-Serva A, Nehal K, et al. Effects of tretinoin on photodamaged skin: a histologic study. Arch Dermatol 1991;127:666-672.
11. Latriano L, Tzimas G, Wong F, et al. The percutaneous absorption of topically applied tretinoin and its effect on endogenous plasma tretinoin concentration following single doses or long term use. J Am Acad Dermatol 1997;36:S37-S46.
12. Shalita A, Weiss JS, Chalker DK, et al. A comparison of the efficacy and safety of adapalene gel 0.1% and tretinoin gel 0.025% in the treatment of acne vulgaris, a multicenter trial. J Am Acad Dermatol 1996;34:482-485.
13. Allec J, Chatelus A, Wagner N. Skin distribution and pharmaceutical aspects of adapalene gel. J Am Acad Dermatol 1997;36:S119-S125.
14. Van Scott EJ, Yu RJ. Control of keratinization with alphahydroxy acids and related compounds: I. Topical treatment of ichthyotic disorders. Arch Dermatol 1974;110:586-590.
15. Yu RJ, Van Scott EJ. Bioavailability of alphahydroxy acids and topical formulations. Cosmet Dermatol 1996;9,No.6:54-62.
16. Smith WP. Hydroxy acids and skin aging. Cosmet Toilet, September 1994;109:41-48.
17. Ditre CM, Griffin TD, Murphy GF, et al. Effects on alpha hydroxy acids on photoaged skin: a pilot clinical, histologic, and ultrastructual study. J Am Acad Dermatol 1996;34;187-195.
18. Van Scott EJ, Yu RJ. Alpha-hydoxy acids: Procedures for use in clinical practice. Cutis 1989;43:222-228.
19. Stiller MJ, Bartolone J, Stern R, et al. Topical 8% glycolic and 8% L-lactic acid creams for the treatment of photo-damaged skin. Arch Dermatol 1996;132:631-636.
20. Gilchrest B, Blog F, Szabo G. Effects of aging and chronic sun exposure on melanocytes in human skin. J Invest Dermatol 1979;73:141-143.
21. Klingman AM. Compatibility of a glycolic acid cream with topical tretinoin for the treatment of the photodamaged face of older women. J Geriatr Dermatol 1993;1:179-181.
22. Middleton JD. Sodium lactate as a moisturizer. Cosmet Toiletries 1978;93:85-86.
23. Stern EC. Topical application of lactic acid in the treatment and prevention of certain disorders of the skin. Urol Cutan Rev 1946;50:106-107.
24. Lavker RM, Kaidbey K, Leyden JJ. Effects of topical ammonium lactate on cutaneous atrophy from a potent topical corticosteroid. J Am Acad Dermatol 1992;26:535-544.
25. Smith WP. Epidermal and dermal effects of topical lactic acid. J Am Acad Dermatol 1996;35:388-391.
26. Berger R. Initial studies show salicylic acid promising as antiaging preparation. Cosmet Dermatol 1997;10:31-32.
27. Peck J, Stmenova M, Palencarova E, et al. Salicylate intoxication after use of topical use of salicytic acid ointment by a patient with psoriasis. Cutis 1992;50:307-309.
28. Draelos ZD. The value of vitamins on the skin. Cosmet Dermatol 1995;8:17-20.
29. Bast A, Haenen GRMM, Doelman DJA. Oxidants and antioxidants: State of the art. Am J Med 1991;91:2S-13S.
30. Nomura H, Ishiguro T, Morimoto S. Studies on L-ascorbic acid derivatives. II. L-Ascorbic acid 3-phosphate and 3-pyrophosphate. Chem Pharm Bull (Tokyo) 1989;17:381-386.
31. Darr D, Combs S, Dunston S, et al. Topical vitamin C protects porcine skin from ultraviolet radiation-induced damage. Br J Dermatol 1992;127:247-253.
32. Kameyama K, Sakai C, Kondoh S, et al. Inhibitory effect of magnesium L-ascorbyl 2-phophate (VC-PMG) on melogenesis in vitro and in vivo. J Am Acad Dermatol 1996;34:29-33.
33. Mayer P, Pittermann W, Wallat S. The effects of vitamin E on the skin. Cosmet Toilet 1993;108:99-109.
34. Zatz JL. Enhancing skin penetration of actives with the vehicle. Cosmet Toilet 1994;109:27-36.

35. Spencer MC. Topical use of hydroquinone for depigmentation. JAMA 1965;194:962-964.
36. Kligman AM, Willis I. A new formula for depigmenting human skin. Arch Dermatol 1975;111:40-48.
37. Weiss RM, del Fabbro E, Kolisang P. Cosmetic ochronisis caused by bleaching creams containing 2% hydroquinone. S Afr Med J 1990;77:373.
38. Kim S, Suh K, Chae Y, et al. The effect of arbutin, glycolic acid, kojoic acid and pentadecenoic acid on the in vitro and in vivo pigmentary system after ultraviolet irradiation. Korean J Dermatol 1994;32(6):977-989.
39. Garcia A, Fulton JE. The combination of glycolic acid and hydroquinone or kojic acid for the treatment of melasma and related conditions. Dermatol Surg 1996;22:443-448.
40. Nazzaro-Porro M. Beneficial effect of 15% azelaic acid cream on acne vulgaris. Br J Dermatol 1983;109:45.
41. Grimes PE. Melasma: etiologic and therapeutic considerations. Arch Dermatol 1995;131:1453-1457.

CHAPTER 4

The Selection and Education of the Resurfacing Patient

■ David R. Harris

After years spent in the clinical practice of peeling and resurfacing scars and rhytides, it is clear that the most important skill that must be learned is not procedural. The art of communication is both more critical and difficult to master than any particular surgical technique. Moreover, the careful selection of an appropriate candidate and the subsequent education of this individual for realistic expectations and possible untoward consequences is the vital element in a successful outcome (1).

What is the definition of success when undertaking a cosmetic procedure? Success is an elusive sense of satisfaction defined by the patient, not the physician. Therefore, a thorough appreciation of a potential candidate's motivation and that person's desires is of paramount importance. In addition, the patient must have a complete understanding of not only the rewards of the procedure and the risks inherent, but also the limitations of the desired treatment (2). In this regard, the physician must be brutally honest about what he or she can realistically improve and what cannot be accomplished (3). When the physician offers the service of peeling or resurfacing, the candidate is being introduced to a process, which over time, may provide a satisfactory result. Only the patient will know when the process is complete. This chapter explores the elements of patient selection and education that are valuable and add to the likelihood of a successful outcome.

THE PROPER SETTING

Interaction with a potential resurfacing patient begins before the patient is ever seen by the physician. Someone will answer the phone and make the appointment for this important person. That someone, part of the front office personnel, is the physician's surrogate. How the potential cosmetic patient is greeted, and what is said by the employee will set the stage for further interaction. In addition, when the patient arrives, the facility's appearance creates a first and lasting impression. Finally, the setting for the interview itself is important, as is the time and effort invested in this first interaction. Each of these issues will be reviewed.

Staff

Before the potential cosmetic patient is educated, the office staff must be appropriately trained. A cosmetic procedure is much different from traditional medical tasks that are frequently accomplished in the same setting. The cosmetic patient who seeks a satisfying result from a peel or resurfacing does not have a need, but wants to have this anticipated improvement. The decision to seek a physician's services constitutes an elective desire to bestow what is in fact, a kind of "gift" to oneself. The staff member who interacts with the potential patient must have a thorough understanding of these psychological and social "wants." It is imperative for the staff to completely understand that the wants of a potential cosmetic patient are on a decidedly different level than the needs of the traditional patient. Staff must also know not only what the physician does and how it is done, but why the physician does peeling and resurfacing procedures. All front and back office personnel would benefit by receiving the same discussion of the procedure and anticipated outcome as do potential cosmetic patients. Moreover, all involved staff members would do well to view the procedures, to see what happens to the patients and interact with the physician and the patients during follow-up visits. Most important, the staff must be imbued with an enthusiastic attitude and be excited about what is accomplished by the physician. Nothing motivates a staff member more than undergoing a successful cosmetic procedure by the physician. A successfully treated staff member becomes the physician's greatest ally, each day verifying the results of a beneficial outcome.

The staff member responsible for answering the phones needs additional skills in dealing with a potential cosmetic patient. First, the cosmetic patient must be identified. This necessitates careful training because a large percentage of callers may not identify themselves as such. Thus, the front office personnel must be oriented to recognizing a potential cosmetic patient during the first contact. Staff should be trained to ask an appropriate question when a patient calls, such as, "Are you seeing the doctor about a cosmetic procedure to improve your skin?" or, "Are you calling about skin or body enhancement?" If so, the candidate can then be scheduled for an interview. Potential cosmetic patients who have made the decision to call and who have already had a long dialogue with themselves about wanting a procedure, are not often willing to wait several weeks for an appointment like a psoriasis or acne patient. Therefore, it is necessary to block appropriate time in the schedule and leave that time open only for these types of patients. They should receive an appointment within a week.

THE APPROPRIATE TIME

Depending on the physician's office, the time allotted for traditional patient interaction will vary with the problem or task at hand. Whatever time is given to a potential peel or resurfacing candidate must be "enough." This means that the physician and/or the staff must be available for any period required to interview a potential candidate, discuss the desired procedure in depth in its entirety, noting its limitations and side effects, and what is required by the candidate in terms of preparation, healing and cost (4). Educational materials, such as written explanations and before and after photographs, should be used during the interview. All of this takes a good deal of time and generally varies from one-half hour to an hour. Moreover, in many settings, this consultation may be provided free of charge, especially if the patient decides to go ahead with the procedure. In the traditional practice paradigm, a free consultation is often unacceptable; however, since the patient has sought the physician's services for something he or she wants and has a perceived outcome, often the consultation fee is waived.

It is difficult to mix cosmetic and traditional patients during the same practice day because their needs are

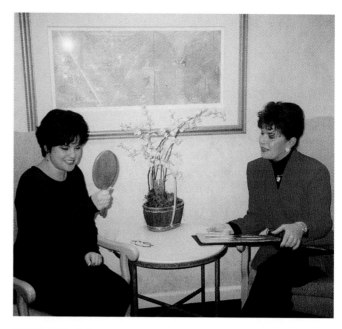

FIGURE 4.1

A comfortable, home-like consultation room offers a more inviting, relaxed environment than does an examination room.

different. Thus, a system where cosmetic consultation and procedure times are blocked only for these tasks can be helpful. In addition, trained staff members can aid in the initial interview. Sometimes, appointments are made initially with the physician, but can be carried out by a staff member who is thoroughly trained in the interview process. The potential candidate sees one of these "care coordinators" or the physician and is introduced to the peeling or resurfacing process in a nonthreatening, comfortable environment. Small consultation rooms with decor like a home library or living room can aid in easing patient comfort levels during the consultation (Fig. 4.1). If the patient meets with the physician, and the physician does not have the full time necessary, the patient can be given over to one of the staff members to complete the educational process.

THE FACILITY

An attractive office, clean and comfortable, designed in a tasteful and upscale manner is an important consideration in the decision to provide cosmetic services. Along with staff members who first greet the patient, the facility will also make an impression. A pleasing facility, appropriately trained and attired staff, and a focus on providing the time needed to allow a potential peeling or resurfacing candidate to make an informed decision, constitutes the proper setting for the most important part of the peeling or resurfacing procedure, patient selection and education.

MINI SYMPOSIUMS

In addition to the traditional consultation, cosmetic mini symposiums are a new consultation format. The symposiums can be conducted several times a month, last no more than one to one and a half hours, and cover both limited topics (laser resurfacing or liposuction) as well as general themes (e.g., "beautiful eyes") covering all skin rejuvenation procedures. Presentations begin with the physician giving an overview of indications, procedures, and before and after slides showing expected improvement. A video can also be helpful. Candidates are not screened at the symposium, but staff should be available to make appointments for personal consultation. It has been noted that screening patients on the evening of a symposium is less satisfactory than a longer, more focused time period scheduled within the next few days.

The symposium format provides a different environment to explain cosmetic procedures that is both time efficient and appeals to the apprehensive or less committed patient. A group comradery can develop among the participants which can support the individual decision to seek cosmetic improvement.

THE CANDIDATE

To whom do you speak? Before the educational process can begin, it is imperative to become acquainted with the individual seeking peeling or resurfacing. The entire thrust of the initial interaction should attempt to answer whether the person is an appropriate candidate. Many will present with the declarative, "I need a peel or lasering or etc." As a matter of fact, the potential candidate does not know what procedure will help most, he or she only knows what they desire or want! At this early juncture, it is helpful to give the candidate a hand mirror and ask them to identify the problem they want to correct (Fig. 4.2). The surgically-appropriate peel candidate will point out areas that would obviously be improved by chemosurgical peeling of one kind or another. These areas might include signs of dyschromia and actinic injury, areas that would respond with improved uniformity of tone and luster, and a softening of finer rhytides and darker spots including melasma and lentigines. An appropriate candidate for resurfacing would point out areas of scarring or actinic injury including keratoses and rhytides, which would respond well to this procedure (5).

However, patient identification of skin areas that they would like to see changed is only the first step. The fact that the potential candidate has problems that can be improved by cosmetic service does not necessarily make the person an ideal or even a desirable patient. The patient's motivation for peeling or resurfacing must be identified. Questioning why the individual wants a procedure done, has this person had multiple cosmetic procedures in the past, is the person satisfied with previous procedures, and how the individual feels about other physicians who have been interviewed or provided services can provide valuable information on the candidate. Other questions to ask include what are the individual's expectations coming in, is there a perception that the person wishes to simply improve a cosmetically offensive issue or does this person want the physician to change their life. If the latter is sensed, all efforts will be unsuccessful. During this get acquainted period, certain responses could cause a measure of concern and are important to clarify. Patients with a history of multiple (and perhaps unnecessary) cosmetic procedures may be less satisfactory candidates. For instance, a face or brow lift done on a young person in their early 30s, or resurfacing on an individual with obviously flawless skin is not appropriate. Some individuals are cosmetic surgery "junkies" who constantly strive for perfection, which in their eyes, will never exist. Watch out for those who complain about the failure of previous cosmetic surgeons or those who angrily point out trivial or invisible defects in the work of others. Some will try to ingratiate themselves by saying, "Doctor so-and-so didn't solve my problem, but I know you are the best and that everything you do will come out perfect."

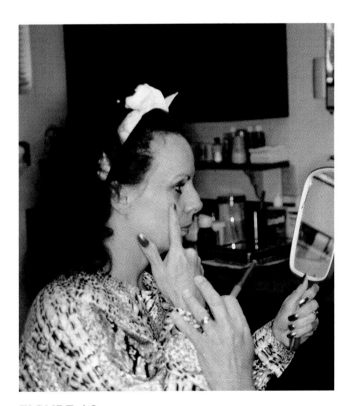

FIGURE 4.2
Early in the consultation, give the cosmetic procedure candidate a hand mirror and ask him or her to identify each problem for which they have presented.

This is a candidate who is not apt to find a satisfactory experience!

If a patient seems to be fixated on one area of skin, such as a virtually imperceptible pitted scar on the nose, and indicates that this "hideous defect" is the source of all personal problems, this is probably another unsatisfactory candidate. Many times, this type of patient is a sad, obviously depressed person. A monotone, flattened affect in such an individual quickly alerts the physician that this person is unhappy with him or herself, life in general, and their social situation in particular. This person wants the physician's cosmetic procedure to make all this right.

Conversely, the appropriate candidate is not just a patient who presents with a problem that can be corrected by peeling or resurfacing, but one who has other characteristics which are likely to provide a satisfactory outcome for patient and physician. These would include evidence of a mature and realistic attitude and a general demeanor which suggests a satisfactory, content life. This patient makes eye contact, and smiles when the physician is introduced. They readily talk about their life, job and relationships and have come to the office at this point, not because their life is bad, but because things are good. They wish to correct or improve an old problem or a new one about which they have some discomfort. While this candidate is proactive, they are not particularly focused on a perfect outcome. When procedure limitations are discussed, instead of the perception that what is said has gone unheard, the appropriate candidate acknowledges that perfection is not expected and that some measure of improvement is satisfactory. This candidate may have had other cosmetic procedures that were appropriate for this particular person. The desired patient would, in general, have praise for the cosmetic surgeon who may have served them previously. They may point out something about which they find a measure of disappointment but might add they are reasonably pleased in general. This is a good candidate!

The desired candidate is intent on listening to what is said and acknowledges, by facial expression or verbal response, the points made and how they feel about them. The appropriate candidate is one with realistic expectations and a mature sense of self.

In summary, many who seek peeling or resurfacing are good candidates on a technical level because they have a facial defect or anomaly they want changed. But some patients are poor candidates and will cause long-lasting difficulty, because they will never be satisfied with the result, no matter how superior.

THE EDUCATION

Materials

Patients must see what the physician has to say, and not just hear the discussion. Not only does this have impor-

tance medicolegally, but most patients remember only a portion of anything that is discussed in a medical setting. Few have complete recall concerning matters that they do not wish to hear. Whatever is written out should be as succinct as possible, like paragraphs in a newspaper, or like the abbreviated subject treatment one sees in headline news shows. All of the text should be in easily understood nonmedical terms, divided into sections, with titles in bold type (Fig. 4.3).

Appropriate written discussions include an explanation of the procedure and why it is done. This succinct paragraph should include a mission statement concerning the problems that are usually addressed with a peel or resurfacing. In any cosmetic procedure, the most important legal document is the Informed Consent form. This form should be tailored to the needs of each practice and developed in the physician's own words. Some states require specific language and this must of course be followed, but a statement with less legal language may be used additionally. Any consent form should be concise and important areas again in bold type (Fig. 4.3).

A third written statement that can help minimize disappointment with post treatment sequelae, is a document called "What to Expect After . . ." (Fig. 4.4). This document again discusses the procedure goals in one short paragraph and goes on to a series of bullet statements describing what the patient should expect following the procedure. All of these documents are given to the patient during the first interview, whether or not the patient is seriously interested in a procedure or the decision has been made concerning the candidacy.

Another set of important materials that must be included are reasonable before and after photographs of prior patients, including a realistic cross section of what a patient should expect from a peeling or resurfacing procedure. For instance, when showing before and after photographs of a dyschromia patient, do not use ones that show a patient with perfect results; instead, select a more realistic group of photos showing some area of residual pigmentation which may need further peeling. This is a more likely event following one peel than complete or perfect elimination of all hyperpigmentation (Fig. 4.5A and B). In like manner, a photo series of resurfacing patients before and after scar revision or rejuvenation for actinic injury should include patients that have residual scarring and scattered remaining rhytides. These patients may have enjoyed remarkable improvement, but it is far more important to illustrate possible areas of remaining problems for which further treatment may be indicated. It is also helpful to show photos of what patients look like during the healing period, and especially in the case of resurfacing, noting how the erythema fades over time (Fig. 4.6A and B).

In summary, the prepared physician at the interview time has a set of materials that document, in a realistic fashion, what the potential patient will experience, what can and cannot be accomplished, and what the

OUR SKIN BUFFING AND PEELING PROCEDURE
WHAT OUR PATIENTS SHOULD KNOW FIRST

Why do we do this procedure?   We introduced our skin buffing and peeling procedure to counteract the major effects of sunlight and aging on facial skin. Some of these problems include a loss of luster, with a flat, opaque-appearing skin, irregular pigmentation (brown spots), and the onset of superficial as well as deep wrinkle lines. This procedure can also be used in an attempt to lessen scars from acne, chickenpox, or other causes. In addition to looking better, the skin actually becomes healthier with less precancerous, sun damaged cells.

What is this procedure?   Sterile buffing material and/or a power driven abrasive wheel is utilized to remove a superficial layer of facial skin in those areas which require attention. A peeling solution is then applied to the entire surface. The procedure is usually accomplished in a quiet office setting under light sedation and local anesthetic. Most patients perceive some discomfort during the buffing procedure and some degree of a transient burning sensation during the application of the peeling solution; iced compresses are then applied to soothe the skin. Alternatively, the procedure may be done in a surgery center with sedation/anesthesia administered by an anesthesiologist at additional cost. If this is done, any additional risks will be discussed with you by the anesthesiologist prior to the procedure. The whole procedure usually takes about one-half to one hour, after which the patient rests a while before returning home. The patient must obtain a ride to and from the office for the procedure. Because of the medications used prior to and during the procedure, the patient cannot drive him/herself.

What happens after this procedure?   Most patients experience a period of warmth for the first hour or two. Over the first 3–5 days there is a degree of swelling over the entire face and especially the eyelids. A thin, flexible brown crust forms which feels somewhat tight. Some patients experience some itching, but few complain of burning and severe discomfort. During the following 5–7 days the swelling quickly disappears and the thin crust peels off, much like the peeling after a severe sunburn. Complete separation occurs in about 7–14 days, allowing the patient to return to normal activity.

Infection during healing is possible but unlikely if postoperative care instructions are followed and follow up visits are kept. If healing is delayed, pus drains from the skin or you have a history of cold cores, you must notify your doctor since these signs may indicate a potential infection problem. Although unlikely, an allergic reaction is always possible to the topical and oral medications used in connection with this procedure.

Patient's initials_____

What can patients expect over a longer period?   After the swelling disappears and the crust separates, most patients note areas of pinkness or redness, much like one would expect after any scab falls off. For the most part this color difference is appreciated in the areas that have received the buffing. While the pink discoloration is easily covered with most foundation and makeup programs, some patients note persistence of color change for several months. On occasion, some people gain a degree of brown or excessive pigmentation of the skin. This varies from individual to individual and is most commonly seen in darker skin types. We have found that brown excessive pigmentation can be treated with lightening preparations and generally improves in a matter of months. A few people are prone to loss of pigmentation, which can be permanent in a few cases. Because of this, we first buff and peel a hidden test site to check for these pigmentary problems. However, these tests may not be totally predictive of what will occur when the entire face is treated. Although unlikely, scarring may occur especially if there is a problem with healing (such as an infection).

Can we guarantee satisfaction?   No cosmetic surgeon can guarantee to make a patient happy but can only promise to do the best work possible. We offer this procedure because the majority of our patients are pleased with the outcome. Satisfaction is based on a realistic expectation. No one should expect our efforts will remove every abnormal pigment spot, every wrinkle or smooth skin perfectly. Moreover, deeper folds are not affected by this procedure. If there are problems with healing, preexisting scars may be made worse or new ones created.

Patients should understand that friends and family generally appreciate beneficial changes less than they do. This is because we are much more critical of our own appearance than we are of other people. Moreover, some people seek this kind of procedure expecting it to make them happier; not only happier about personal appearance but about life in general. If one feels that a satisfactory result will change his or her life, meet someone new or get a better job, disappointment is bound to occur. A realistic attitude is absolutely necessary for satisfaction.

What can we do to make our patients satisfied?   We do everything within our power to maximize patient satisfaction. We consider this procedure part of an overall continuing skin rejuvenation program which may include topical care, collagen augmentation, further procedures or "touch ups".

I have read the above and discussed this information with my doctor. I feel I have a clear understanding of the procedure and the possible side effects. I have been informed that this procedure will not be covered by insurance and that payment is my responsibility before the procedure is done.

_____   _____
            Patient   Witness

_____
            Date

FIGURE 4.3
Written materials should be succinct and divided into short, well-identified sections. A customized informed consent form should be concise and written in easily understood short sections.

WHAT TO EXPECT AFTER YOUR SKIN RESURFACING

When sun damaged or acne scarred skin is treated with our special resurfacing procedures, our patients are given complete instructions concerning postoperative care. Here is a reminder of the important changes that may occur during the healing phase.

1. OOZING.   When the old skin is removed, and before the new fresh, smooth surface is restored, there is a measure of oozing and draining for the first two to four days. Most of the fluid is either clear or slightly yellow-tinged over a surface which is moist and light pink. Because we apply ointments to keep the skin moist, this drainage is entirely appropriate.

2. SWELLING.   Swelling occurs and is most intense between day two and five. For some, the swelling occurs most intensely around the eyes and upper cheeks. At times, for a day or so, the eyes may be swollen almost shut. This is an entirely natural phenomenon and is in no way detrimental to healing or harmful to you, the patient.

3. A ROSY HUE.   When the skin has finished growing, usually by day six to ten, the skin takes on a rosy or pink color. This pinkness is the new fresh skin before it assumes its natural color tones. The pinkness fades a lot over the first several weeks, but some people will note a measure of pinkness for some months. The rosy or pink tones can be easily camouflaged with appropriate foundation or make-up and will not be a problem with daily activities.

4. ITCHINESS AND DISCOMFORT.   Some patients note a degree of itchiness during the healing phase, totally normal, for skin which is regrowing or healing. However, increased *PAIN* after the first 48 hours is a important sign that there may be a problem. While rare, increasing pain after 48 hours should be reported immediately to the physician or nurse in charge of your case.

5. RESIDUAL LINES OR SCARS.   Your physician has discussed the fact that not every scar or wrinkle line will be removed by our resurfacing procedure. This is because each scar and wrinkle is a separate problem and some are far more resistant to our treatment than others. While we enjoy a high degree of patient satisfaction, some measure of disappointment may occur when the patient recognizes that not every line or scar has been removed. As we discussed, we then can further improve those residual wrinkle lines and scars by a "touch-up" procedure at a later time.

6. CHANGE IN PIGMENTATION.   In spite of appropriate preparation, some darker skinned patients will recognize a measure of deeper pigmentation after the resurfacing procedure. This darkening, which may occur at any of the resurfaced areas, will be treated and will fade over time.

   An occasional patient, in spite of our efforts to test beforehand, may note over some months the occurrence of a lighter than normal spot in the resurfaced skin. This occurs in a few because of unusual response to the healing process. While this is rare, it can occur and remain permanently. These areas can be covered with make-up and at times can be blended satisfactorily to the surrounding skin.

FIGURE 4.4
A hand-out explaining "What to Expect" after a cosmetic procedure in a "laundry list" form saves a lot of questions later.

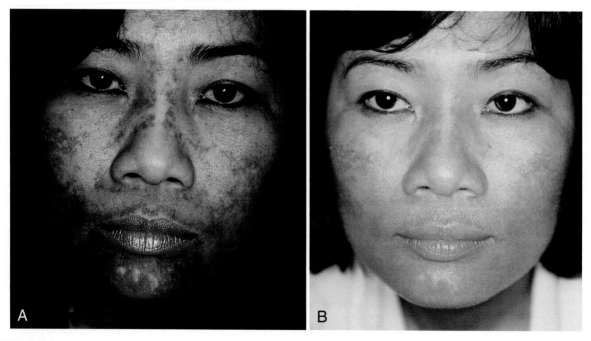

FIGURE 4.5
A, Dyschromia pre-peel. B, Residual dyschromia following treatment. This is a more realistic illustration than a photo of complete eradication of pigment.

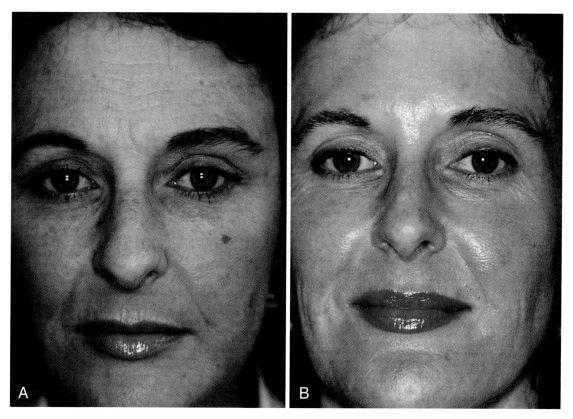

FIGURE 4.6
Showing photos of residual erythema give resurfacing candidates realistic expectations of the procedure. A, Before resurfacing. B, Ten days following procedure.

potential hazards, side effects and sequelae are (both short and long term) for each procedure.

The Interview

The first interview can be conducted in several ways. Some who enjoy a cosmetically oriented practice use patient educators who, while not being trained physicians or nurses, have been thoroughly acquainted with patient needs, the treatment process, discussion of options, the fee schedule and the need for realistic expectations. Since the first interview is time consuming, involving both written and oral explanations, many have found this strategy successful. Other physicians prefer to conduct the interview entirely themselves. If the physician prefers to be an important part of the interview process, it is useful to block a portion of a day, such as an hour or two or a whole morning or afternoon, to focus just on patient interviews. This promotes a relaxed, comfortable state, so that the physician is not rushing between appointments, running behind schedule or otherwise being preoccupied in the middle of a cosmetic procedure. It is of benefit to quickly decide whether a patient is technically a candidate for a procedure and then focus on whether the patient is emotionally well suited before proceeding with an in-depth dis-

cussion of the peeling or resurfacing procedure. This process may take 10 or 15 minutes, and after which, a trained staff member can take over, presenting the written materials and describing before and after photographs. Whoever is responsible for the educational process should thoroughly cover several critical aspects of the procedure, the understanding of which is paramount for patient satisfaction.

What The Patient Needs to Know

The candidate must come away with an understanding that he or she is engaging in a process of care to improve a skin problem. Realistically, the improvement of tone or texture or the elimination of rhytides or scars, demands a number of activities to result in consistent patient satisfaction. These might include a program of topical care before and after a peel or resurfacing; this is especially true if the patient is prone to hyperpigmentation or has an ongoing problem with regard to acne. In addition, few practitioners can carry out a peel or resurfacing procedure with complete satisfaction after one session. Residual pigmentation and scars or rhytides must be anticipated and explained (6). It is important to stress to the patient at the beginning of the interview that he or she is engaging in a process of

---

OUR IMAGE ENHANCING "TOUCH-UP" PROGRAM

A Special Service for Dermasanding and Peel Patients

Improving wrinkled skin lines, abnormal pigmentation, or scarring, involves a skilled type of texturing of the skin. We are proud of the results of our dermasanding and peeling procedures, the success of which is a product of over 20 years of experience.

However, no single texturing procedure can guarantee 100 percent satisfaction. We tell our patients they will generally appreciate anywhere from 30 up to 80% improvement in scars, pigmentation or wrinkle lines. This is to say that in some spots there may be a complete eradication, but in other areas there may be less satisfactory improvement.

This means that for some people there may be a measure of *dissatisfaction* with any one procedure.

Because of this fact and our desire to continue working with each patient to find the greatest level of satisfaction possible, we offer our "Touch-up" program. Simply stated, we will continue to work for one year on those areas where scars and wrinkles remain, for $_____ per "touch-up" session. We encourage our patients to participate in a quest for continued improvement by keeping "touch-ups" affordable. This entire program is an investment in one's own sense of self image. To have an unwanted spot here and there is a continuing disappointment. With our "Touch-up" program, the physician and patient work with one another to enhance satisfaction with a modest investment of time and money.

I have read the above, discussed and understand the "Touch-up" program.

_____   _____
Date   Patient

                                                              _____
                                                              Witness

---

FIGURE 4.7
A specific "touch-up" discussion underlines the fact that any one procedure may be part of an ongoing process.

care and explain this thoroughly. One important aid when discussing a continued program for improvement over time is the concept of "touch-up" or repeat procedures. During this part of the interview, the probability of the patient's desire to repeat peeling or resurfacing in areas where the outcome was less than satisfactory is emphasized both by photos and another written statement that can explain a "touch-up" program (Fig. 4.7). Thus, the candidate understands how the procedure is done and what can be reasonably expected, and can anticipate further procedures as part of an ongoing process.

THE ISSUE OF FEAR

During the interview it is helpful not only to describe what happens before, during and after a procedure and what the patient can expect, but also to explore why some people choose to reject cosmetic surgery after the initial interview. Many patients have a basic fear of proceeding following a discussion of chemosurgical peeling or resurfacing, whether it is laser or abrasion. Few patients vocalize this during an interview, especially if they have had no previous cosmetic procedures. Fears can include what others might think, the degree of pain during and after the procedure, the patients' appearance through the healing process, or how long the erythema will last following resurfacing. Some are frightened to hear the words "acid" or "abrasion," or by the concept of skin removal with a "laser beam." These all have connotations of serious injury such as caused by thermal burning and some worry that they may heal in a manner that will be disfiguring. It is interesting that the pragmatic issues of cost and time off work figure less in this process of generic fear than unrealistic perceptions of pain, ridicule and untoward results. This is the time for the practitioner or staff to allay these unstated fears and to reaffirm that the physician intends to "do no harm," and that the process of care, over time, is safe and effective. During this part of the discussion each of these unstated, possible areas of concern can be discussed frankly and openly after a preface such as, "I know many patients have some unstated concerns or worries about this type of procedure." Many candidates visibly relax, smile and acknowledge that some of these issues are indeed on their minds.

TIME TO REASSESS

It is appropriate to proceed immediately with candidates chosen for a light peel with little or no down side sequelae, with the exception that the procedure may need to be repeated or topical care may be indicated. However, for deeper peels and for resurfacing, a prudent strategy after the initial interview is to schedule time for reflection. A substantial subset of potential candidates need further topical care and doctor/patient interaction to assess whether they will find satisfaction with the procedure. Patients must come to term with the nature of the process and gain an understanding that any one procedure may not be totally satisfactory and that their wants may not be totally realized. There are several strategies for appropriate delay that can be utilized.

A Topical Program

Virtually every patient benefits from pre- and postoperative topical care. The actinically injured patient can be supplied with an armamentarium to protect and enhance the effects of the peeling or resurfacing procedure using modern dermatological skin care including physiologically active substances such as retinoids, alpha hydroxy acids, anti-oxidants, lightening agents such as hydroquinone and 5 fluorouracil (5). Topical care can be explained to a patient by likening it to buying a new car and then giving that new car a protective wax coating. Obviously, a patient with a degree of active acne will need a measure of control and those who are prone to dyschromia, including all patients of Asian, African, Mediterranean or Latino descent, and many Nordic blood groups, will need a lightening program (6). These customized programs should begin at least 1 to 2 months prior to the procedure and be resumed shortly after healing. Most every patient regardless of how impatient, will agree with this approach.

The "Test Site"

All patients being considered for rejuvenation or scar revision with deeper peeling or resurfacing have the potential to permanently lose pigment. For some, especially those prone to vitiligo, this untoward sequela is common. The patient must be forewarned and a helpful delay tactic and important medicolegal exercise is to perform a test peel or resurfacing in the post auricular area. Patients are assessed 8 weeks later. Again, the strategy is two-fold; first to allow time for reflection and reassessment, and second to test the patient for a potential problem. The practitioner should understand that much post-inflammatory hypopigmentation results from delayed healing due to a variety of variables and may not be evident for several months after the procedure is completed. However, patients who are prone to this problem because of a disposition to vitiligo may be identified in as little as 8 weeks. It should be acknowledged that, because the response to treatment is not clearly predictable, many cosmetic surgeons do not favor test sites.

Nonetheless, during this reassessment time the patient is provided with a reason for waiting, and applying topical care and preparing the skin for the procedure. All this becomes part of the process.

AVOIDING DISAPPOINTMENT

The preceding discussion focused on selecting the appropriate patient and providing complete and realistic information so that both physician and patient can make an informed choice. All of this is done to maximize the opportunity for patient satisfaction. Part of this educational process is designed implicitly to avoid disappointment. During an interview the single most important plan for avoiding disappointment is acknowledging that it does occur. Patients should be told to reasonably expect both a good deal of satisfaction and a measure of disappointment. Give examples of what patients might say postoperatively. These include pointing to the skin while the patient looks in a hand mirror and stating, "I'm really pleased with my forehead doctor, but I still see a few lines around my eyes," or "You got all of these scars and I only see a little of those, but this one hardly went away at all." This type of example graphically illustrates what, in fact, commonly occurs. Patients will often see what is left and not what is gone after a procedure.

The concept of a "touch-up" procedure and the entire issue of a process for improvement should be reviewed and the "touch-up" handouts and "What to Expect After..." written materials reintroduced. Photos showing less than complete improvement should be shown again to the prospective candidate. It is not a surprise to the experienced cosmetic surgeon that in spite of all of these efforts there is a subset of patients who come back with bitter disappointment. Often, these type of patients admit that they were told, shown, and that all of the possible ramifications of the procedure were discussed with them, including the possibility of bitter disappointment.

Dealing With Disappointment

Part of the strategy to avoid disappointment is a skillful approach to dealing with disappointment when it occurs. The patient must be reassured in a gentle and persuasive manner that the physician stands ready to continue the process and to make every effort to reach the most satisfactory result possible over time. Following a first peel or resurfacing, the "touch-up" or repeat procedure should be reviewed with the patient.

When discussing the next step, the entire issue of what to expect in terms of further improvement must again be thoroughly reviewed. It is beneficial to have several before and after photos showing people who have had their initial procedure and following that, the further improvement they enjoyed with "touch-ups." It has been noted that further scar or rhytid improvement with subsequent resurfacing tends to be minimal after three resurfacing procedures. Part of this may be due to muscle movement under the resistant rhytid or the fact that valley and pitted scars are tough to completely eliminate. It is not possible to predict how many peels may be necessary to eradicate dyschromia. Complete removal of hyperpigmentation may occur with one light peel, but, it is possible that 4 to 6 peels might still result in a persisting problem. The candidate needs to know all these things, because realistic expectations and ultimate satisfaction depends more on this interview than it does on the execution of a chemosurgical peel or resurfacing procedure.

THE PREOPERATIVE VISIT

For those who undergo a more aggressive peel or resurfacing procedure, a preoperative consultation and review is very useful. The best time for this interaction, which takes place entirely with a nurse or trained staff member, is about 48 hours before the procedure. If possible, the person who cares for the patient postoperatively should be present. At this time, the entire procedure should be explained again with emphasis on what the patient will do in the next 48 hours to prepare for the procedure, what will occur during the procedure, and what is expected afterwards. All of the written materials should be reviewed and signed including all informed consent forms. This is an appropriate time for photographs to be taken.

During the preoperative visit, it may be helpful to provide patients with a tote bag containing all the necessary prescriptions and topical preparations. Depending on the wishes of the physician, these might include a dose of steroid, antibiotics, antiviral agents and pain medication (Fig. 4.8). Other written materials necessary for postoperative instructions such as another copy of

the "What to Expect After . . ." handout, a postoperative instruction sheet including detailed descriptions of how the patient is to care for his or her skin (Fig. 4.9), and copies of the signed informed consent forms can be included in the bag.

THE POSTOPERATIVE PHONE CALL

Anyone who has practiced medicine has been impressed by the positive impact made when a patient receives an unsolicited call from the physician. After cosmetic surgery, this postoperative phone call, which may be made several hours after the patient leaves the facility, should be considered mandatory. Although preferable, the call need not be made by a physician but can be done by skilled personnel. Primarily this call is to reassure and show concern. Almost always there will be some kind of question which either the care giver or the patient needs to have clarified. It is wise to call once or twice during the first 2 or 3 postoperative days. Many physicians like to see the patient at 24 or 48 hours, again for reassurance and to emphasize the depth of concern as well as for medical reasons. Early intervention can also begin if complications have occurred. Since the cosmetic surgeon should expect some measure of disappointment, an effort to cement a strong bond in a caring manner at this point in the process is prudent.

SUMMARY

The selection of the appropriate peeling or resurfacing candidate demands time and effort on the part of the physician and staff. This patient is not just one with a

FIGURE 4.8
During a preoperative visit, it is helpful to review all necessary pre- and postsurgical instructions, and to provide both these and topical preparations and prescriptions in a handy "tote bag."

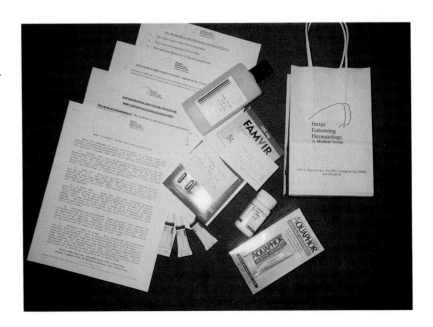

TIPS FOR BUFF-PEEL PATIENTS DURING THE HEALING STAGE

1. Immediately after your buff-peel you will be partially sedated when you return home. During this first day you will need to take several different kinds of pills.

   It is important that your eat and drink a normal amount of food and water during the course of the first day. We recommend an eight ounce glass of fluid each hour, even if a family member must wake you.

2. Sometimes patients are concerned about swelling around the face and eyes. This is a part of the healing process and perfectly normal. At times the eyes may swell completely shut for a few hours or even a day. We have given you special medication to decrease the swelling and ice compresses also help. This usually decreases significantly by day 4 or 5. Scabs usually separate by day 7 to 10.

3. Occasionally some patients find a mild degree of nausea over the first two or three days. We have given you a prescription for Tigan suppositories for the nausea if necessary. Note the list of drug stores in the Santa Clara Valley that are open overnight to fill any prescription.

FACIAL CARE INSTRUCTIONS

1. Cleanse face three to four times daily with our soap-free cleansing lotion, using a soft wash cloth moistened with water. Rinse your face several times with tepid water after cleansing and gently pat dry. You may shower and shampoo as usual. Many patients find the shower a convenient way to cleanse the skin.

2. After patting dry, apply a thin film of Silvadene cream and Elta melting moisturizer mixed together in equal amounts. Continue to apply mixture three to four times daily, until all scabbed areas have fallen off. If you experience burning or stinging for more than a minute or two—call. You may be sensitive to the Silvadene.

3. A few patients become sensitive to the cream which you have been given. If you become sensitive you will note an increase in stinging and irritation rather than a cool relief when the medicine is applied. If this occurs, please call and we will make an adequate adjustment.

ALL NIGHT PHARMACIES

(Physicians can provide a list for patients)

FIGURE 4.9
Detailed postoperative instructions should be provided in writing.

surgical problem that can be corrected, but is also an individual with maturity, a positive attitude and a good self-image that will allow for realistic expectations and ultimately a substantial measure of satisfaction. The education of such a patient involves a series of steps that include verbal and written discussion, review of realistic photographic results and a period of reflection before the procedure is undertaken. Both before and following the procedure, this educational process must once again be visited and an inevitable measure of disappointment must be met with a concerned and caring attitude. When the cosmetic surgeon works at mastering these necessary tasks, then the process leading to a satisfying result for both physician and patient will commence.

REFERENCES

1. Harris DR, Noodleman FR. Combining manual dermasanding with low strength trichloroacetic acid to improve actinically injured skin. J Dermatol Surg Oncol 1994;20:436-442.
2. Roenigk HH. Treatment of the aging face. Derm Clinics 1995;13:245-261.
3. Fournier PF. Body sculpturing through syringe liposuction and autologous fat reinjection. Samuel Rolf Intern 1987;7-9.
4. Stegman SJ, Tromovitch TA, Glogau RG. Cosmetic dermatologic surgery. 2nd Ed, Littleton: Year Book Medical Publishers, 1990:1-4.
5. Harris DR. Treatment of the aging skin with glycolic acid. In: Elson ML, ed. Evaluation and treatment of the aging skin. New York: Springer-Verlag, Inc., 1995:22-33.
6. Ho C, Quan N, Low NJ, et al. Laser resurfacing in pigmented skin. Dermatol Surg 1995;21:1035-1037.

SECTION II

Chemical Peeling

CHAPTER 5

Skin Response to Chemical Peeling

◼ Harold J. Brody

Controlled wounding with chemical agents produces a partial-thickness wound that heals by secondary intention. Recognizing the conditions that lead to proper re-epithelialization and wound reorganization helps to minimize the risk factors that may impede proper healing. Wound healing combines a series of complex events that lead to the resurfacing, reconstitution and restoration of tensile strength of wounded skin (1). Partial-thickness wounds penetrate partially, but not completely, into the dermis and these defects heal by re-epithelialization from residual adnexal epithelium or epithelium derived from adjacent uninjured skin. Healing is rapid, and scarring is clinically imperceptible since contraction does not generally occur.

CHEMICAL PEELING WOUND HEALING STAGES (TABLE 5.1)

Coagulation and Inflammation

Coagulation and inflammation, the initial phases of wound healing in excisional surgery, are intimately related and practically instantaneous in the first stages of chemical peeling. Soluble factors are elaborated in clotting that activate the kinin and complement inflammatory pathways. Inflammatory mediators derived from these pathways function as chemoattractants for neutrophils, macrophages, and lymphocytes. Neutrophils enter the wound at the time of injury and are present for 3 to 5 days or longer. Macrophages are present from 3 to 10 days after injury and direct the subsequent development of granulation tissue. The lymphocyte is present later at days 6 to 7 after injury and may augment fibroblast accumulation and proliferation (1).

Re-epithelialization

An important factor in dermal wounding after the initial epidermal necrosis from chemical peel is the initial migration of undamaged keratinocytes from the wound margins and from residual adnexal epithelia at the base of the wound (2-5). This process of re-epithelialization begins within 24 hours of wounding and is a directed event that does not require an initial increase in cellular proliferation (Fig. 5.1). Certain mediators released during inflammation such as fibronectin, laminin and platelet-derived growth factor may stimulate keratinocyte cell movement. Migrating keratinocytes rely on a matrix of fibronectin (which is cross-linked to fibrin, collagen, and elastin) at the wound bed to spread. Fibronectin is a dimer that allows simultaneous adhesion to fibrin, collagen and a variety of cells. After migration begins, cell proliferation at the wound margins increases to provide additional cells for wound coverage.

The water content of the wound bed is a major factor in the epithelial cell migration rate. Occluded wounds re-epithelialize faster than open, dry wounds (6-7). This occurs partially because the epidermis does not need to grow as deeply into the dermis. After inducing partial-thickness epidermal wounds with Jessner's resorcinol-based solution, many physicians allow the epidermis to dry out for 24 hours, allegedly to promote separation. However, dermal wound healing mechanisms are not activated with these very superficial peeling agents. The classic medium-depth and deep wounding agents heal most rapidly when maximum hydration is applied to the skin. In the original descriptions of deep peeling from the 1960s, the application of thymol iodide powder 48 hours after peeling formed a crust. The migrating epidermal cells then move beneath this crust to seek a plane of hydration. This delays wound resurfacing. The wound surface migration plane produces more rapid epithelialization when wounds are treated with topical ointments.

Biosynthetic occlusive dressings are used to decrease pain and speed healing with dermabrasion and laser resurfacing. The dressings are not necessary after chemical peeling because the epidermis, while nonviable, is still intact immediately following the peel. However, these dressings can be valuable after deep peeling when the entire necrotic epidermis is stripped off with the optional removal of occlusive tape.

Whether dermal quality is enhanced or lessened with more rapid epithelialization is unknown. Both oxygen-permeable and impermeable dressings stimulate increased collagen synthesis in the dermis. Tensile strength, however, is related to collagen maturity and intermolecular cross-linking, not to the amount of collagen synthesized. Any beneficial effects from increased collagen synthesis are unknown. The exact relationship between the rate of epidermal resurfacing and collagen synthesis remains to be determined (8).

Granulation Tissue Formation

Granulation tissue is a loose collection of cellular components including fibroblasts, fibronectin, inflammatory cells, glycosaminoglycans (GAGs) and collagen. Granulation tissue formation begins on the second or third day after peeling and is maintained until re-epithelialization is complete (9-12). The chief cell in the formation of granulation tissue is the fibroblast, which produces fibrillar collagen and elastin, fibronectin, GAGs and proteases such as collagenase. Collagenase is important in dermal remodeling while GAGs help to maintain wound hydration and may assist in cellular migration and proliferation within the wound.

Angiogenesis

After chemical peeling, the resumption of blood flow is essential for supplying oxygen and nutrients to the healing wound (13, 14). Endothelial cells migrate directly into the wound and travel along the fibronectin matrix. Interference with this matrix formation may delay wound healing. Angiogenic growth factors may be important in this directed migration. They are released from fibroblasts, macrophages and endothelial cells.

Collagen Remodeling

Collagen and matrix remodeling begin when granulation tissue formation begins and continues for months after re-epithelialization (1, 15). As collagen is laid down, fibronectin gradually disappears. Collagen fibers, particularly fibers of collagen types I and III, lie closer together as water is resorbed and reorient in a parallel fashion to the skin surface. Collagen is progressively digested by collagenase and other locally produced proteases. The neovasculature gradually regresses, leaving a less vascular dermis. This remodeling is responsible for the texture of the skin after peeling and is not complete in medium-depth or deep peeling until well after 60 days, usually 90 days, after peeling.

TABLE 5.1
CHEMICAL PEELING WOUND HEALING STAGES
1. Coagulation and Inflammation
2. Re-epithelialization
3. Granulation tissue formation
4. Angiogenesis
5. Collagen remodeling

FIGURE 5.1
Histology of re-epithelialization showing migration of new cells from the hair follicle with overlying necrotic epidermis present.

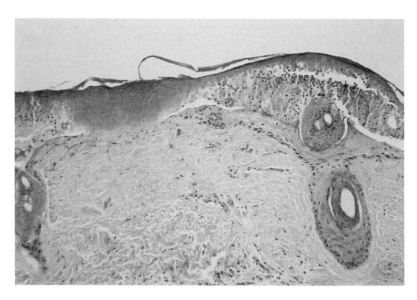

TABLE 5.2

**TOPICAL MEDICATIONS THAT
AFFECT RE-EPITHELIALIZATION**

**Postoperative Medications that Accelerate
Re-epithelialization**

Bacitracin ointment	Eucerin cream
Polysporin ointment	Petrolatum USP (variable)
Silvadene cream	Aloe Vera (variable)

**Postoperative Medications that Retard
Re-epithelialization**

Povidone-Iodine full strength solution
Tretinoin
Fluorinated corticosteroid ointments and creams

MEDICATIONS THAT AFFECT RE-EPITHELIALIZATION

Local wound care in the form of topical creams or ointments or a different vehicle may affect both epithelial cell migration and wound healing time (1, 16-19) (Table 5.2). The zinc moiety in bacitracin may stimulate re-epithelialization directly. Even certain antiseptics such as 1% povidone-iodine, 0.5% chlorhexidine, or 3% hydrogen peroxide have been shown to delay the development of granulation tissue formation in pig skin (18, 19). However, the use of a more dilute surgical scrub rather than the direct application of antiseptic solution may divert infection and not delay the healing process after peeling. A solution of 0.1% iodine is bactericidal (20). Lathering 1 tbsp. of 7.5% povidone-iodine scrub solution USP (United States Pharmacopeia) in a basin of water is sufficient. Polysporin ointments contain both polymyxin sulfate and zinc bacitracin, but lack the sensitizer neomycin and seem to promote wound healing with minimal complications. The incidence of contact dermatitis in chemical peeling is less than that found in abrasive or laser resurfacing, probably due to the protection provided by the nonviable epidermis retained during the initial healing period. Therefore, mild sensitizers can be, and have been used without excessive risk in chemical peeling. Sulfadiazine silver (Silvadene [Merion Merrell Dow, Kansas City, MO]) cream is rarely used due to its excessive sensitization and expense.

Petrolatum

Petrolatum, a mixture of long-chain aliphatic hydrocarbons, is effective in treating dry skin with damaged stratum corneum by permeating throughout the horny layer interstices, accelerating normal barrier recovery despite its occlusive properties (21). In an open, randomized study, petroleum jelly did not seem to retard healing after trichloroacetic acid (TCA) chemical peeling and may hasten healing time (22). The petrolatum

vehicle of Neosporin (Burroughs Wellcome, Research Triangle Park, NC) ointment has a lower melting point than petroleum jelly and therefore an improved healing rate (17). If petrolatum application is desired, the use of petrolatum-based moisturizers without the low molecular weight hydrocarbons that are associated with grease and oil may be well tolerated by most patients after healing. Recent studies suggest that there is no difference with the healing time or infection rate between petrolatum (Vaseline [Beiersdorf, Inc., S. Norwalk CT], Aquaphor [Chesebrough-Pond's, Inc., Greenwich CT]) and the antibacterial ointments in wound healing (23).

Aloe Vera

Aloe vera gel in a patented formula with a polyethylene oxide-water gel dressing (Second Skin) has been reported to reduce wound healing time after dermabrasion in a human model (24). Previously, the scientific results documenting the benefits of Second Skin aloe gel have been unsatisfactory, perhaps due to a destabilized product or poor penetration of the aloe. Its usage and mechanism in chemical peeling is undetermined.

Tretinoin

Tretinoin is used topically prior to chemical peeling as part of a routine photoaging prophylaxis program. When used in adequate concentrations and consistency for greater than 4 months, an orthokeratotic compaction of actinically damaged stratum corneum with improvement of actinic dysplastic keratinocytes is observed in concert with granular cell layer hyperplasia (25). Widened vascular lumina, increased collagen formation and fibroblasts seen ultrastructurally are found in the dermis. Continued treatment beyond one year widens the papillary dermal Grenz zone to create a sharp interface between old and new tissue. After 24 weeks of tretinoin treatment, the epidermal hyperplasia, the increase in granular layer thickness, and the appearance of compact orthokeratosis return to baseline and then reverse after 48 weeks of treatment, suggesting that continued clinical improvement is not histologically correlated. The initial epidermal alterations may reflect a retinoid effect for which accommodation occurs (26).

In a double-blind, placebo study, the daily application of tretinoin cream for 2 weeks prior to a 35% TCA peel enhanced healing of the face, forearms and hand (27-29). In guinea pig skin pretreated with tretinoin prior to 50% phenol application and dermabrasion, the tretinoin group showed 1.5 times more epidermal regeneration histologically than the control group 1 week after wounding and twice the amount of epidermal hyperplasia at 2 weeks. At 6 weeks, the thickness of the epidermis was 4 to 5 cell layers in controls and 7 to 8 layers in the tretinoin group. Collagen regeneration appeared to be faster in the tretinoin group than in the control group. The acceleration of epidermal regeneration may be the mechanism of tretinoin to speed healing when used prior to peeling (30). If used inappropriately in the immediate postoperative period as part of an aftercare regimen, tretinoin will retard healing.

Since tretinoin alters the epidermal actinic damage and TCA frosting is slower in actinically damaged skin, TCA frosting occurs more quickly when the skin has been pretreated with tretinoin. The actual peel depth depends on how much TCA is applied and the degree of rubbing. Less TCA would be necessary to produce the same wound in nonactinically damaged skin. Tretinoin application before and after TCA application does not significantly enhance the efficacy of the peel (31).

Systemic retinoids increase collagen synthesis and decrease collagenase production, thereby inhibiting the enzyme that degrades collagen (32-35). A defect in collagen degradation could allow excess accumulation of collagen and resultant hypertrophic scarring. Fibronectin synthesis is increased by retinoids (36). Retinoids may stimulate fibroblasts and epidermal migration, perhaps by decreasing the tonofilaments and desmosomal attachments, the events that begin re-epithelialization (37-39).

Corticosteroids

Corticosteroids are not the best choice for immediate topical postoperative care. Hydrocortisone seems to neither promote nor retard re-epithelialization rates. Topical fluorinated steroids have a definite effect in retarding the rate of epithelial cell migration and should be avoided. Short-acting systemic corticosteroids in the form of betamethasone are occasionally used to minimize edema in the immediate postoperative period. Although morbidity is decreased clinically, an inhibitory effect of moderate-to-high dose corticosteroids on early wound healing has been reported in the rat model. Cortisone delays the appearance of monocytes and lymphocytes, as well as ground substance, fibroblasts, collagen, regenerating capillaries and epithelial migration in the wound. Corticosteroids prevent the obligatory inflammation that is essential to successive phases and may delay healing. Long-term use of high-dose systemic steroids retards wound healing by interfering with lysosome function in macrophages and inflammatory cells that may predispose some patients to bacterial or fungal infection.

Many systemic medications, corticosteroids, and antineoplastic agents can alter healing times in animal models but do not produce clinically noticeable adverse effects on healing in humans. The use of cortisone after controlled wounding in humans is poorly understood, and its effect on dermal quality is uncertain. The actual time of corticosteroid administration before, during, or immediately after the peel, the dose given, the sustained duration of the drug and the individual's predisposition to infection are all unknown factors at this time (40, 41).

In summary, the skin response in wound healing after a chemical peel obeys most of the same principles as healing after cold steel surgery. The best rule for speeding up wound healing stages, so as to proceed without incident and to provide the best clinical results, indicate soaking the wound to eliminate crusting and applying the proper ointment to maintain the hydration of the healing skin.

CLINICAL AND HISTOLOGIC HEALING OF THE EPIDERMAL AND DERMAL (SUPERFICIAL, MEDIUM, AND DEEP) CHEMICAL PEEL

An understanding of the histology of sun-damaged skin helps to explain the subsequent combined degeneration of the epidermal and dermal systems into the clinical forms of actinic damage familiar to the clinician. As epidermal maturation becomes aberrant, there is a loss of translucency and the appearance of dry, rough, and dull skin with the evolution of keratoses, ephelides (freckles), solar lentigos and comedones. Dermal collagen and elastin degeneration results in the appearance of wrinkles, creases, folds and furrows. As the melanin system becomes disordered, blotching, ephelides, lentigines and pigmented actinic and seborrheic keratoses become evident, and melasma and postinflammatory hyperpigmentation are aggravated. All of these are amplified by irregularities in papillary dermal blood flow and cause telangiectasias and microangiomas with resulting erythema and ecchymosis (42).

After superficial wounding in the epidermis using glycolic acid, Jessner's solution or 15-25% TCA, excellent clinical healing requires minimal postoperative care since dermal wound healing mechanisms are not activated. Without clinical vesiculation, most patients return to their normal daily activities immediately and wear cosmetics to conceal erythema and exfoliation. Restricting water and emollients from the treated skin for 24 to 48 hours after superficial chemical peels to promote epidermal desiccation and separation provides uncertain benefits. Most patients tolerate normal skin washing procedures immediately after a peel. Tretinoin should not be applied for the first 3 to 7 days postoperatively because it may impair healing of wounded skin (24). Sunscreen use may need to be temporarily discontinued for 3 to 7 days after a superficial peel if stinging occurs on application. Consequently, sun exposure should be avoided.

In medium depth wounding that uses combination TCA peels or deep depth wounding that uses phenol, meticulous aftercare is imperative. An hour after the original frost, erythema appears and changes to a brownish hue. Considerable edema is present for the first 48 hours and discomfort is relatively mild to minimal if the patient is applying an emollient. After several days, when the edema partially resolves, a crust forms. Crust separation generally begins between the fourth and the eighth postoperative day and is completed by days 7 to 12, depending on the area and the peel (Fig. 5.2). Patients should be encouraged to minimize

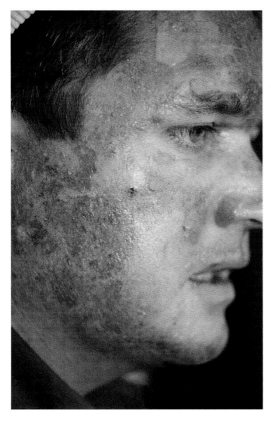

FIGURE 5.2
Clinical healing showing crusting and peeling 5 days after medium depth chemical peeling with 35% trichloroacetic acid (TCA) preceded by a hard 10 second application of solid CO_2.

crusting by washing twice daily with antiseptic compresses and then applying a soothing ointment as detailed earlier in the section on re-epithelialization. For example, a dilute solution of povidone-iodine lathered in the patient's hands in the shower or basin for facial soaking is excellent to begin decrustation. Tap water or dilute 0.25% acetic acid soaks (1 tbsp. of white vinegar in 1 pt of water) are also effective prior to twice or thrice daily bland ointment application. Solar restriction should be imperative until postoperative erythema resolves.

Histologic dermal injury, both upper dermal (medium-depth wounding) and mid-dermal (deep wounding), is sustained by a number of viable wounding agents and combination techniques. The range of injury as defined by the wounding agent 40-60% TCA, for example, is from the lower papillary dermis into the upper reticular dermis. Findings with sun-damaged skin were similar to non-sun-damaged skin in that the elastotic band that occurs in sun-damaged skin did not seem to offer a barrier to wounding (43). The progression or graduation of wound depth was similar when comparing TCA with full-strength phenol or Baker's phenol solution on sun-damaged and non-sun-damaged skin. In medium or deep peels, the epidermis has not returned to normal rete ridge pattern in 30 days (Fig. 5.3).

Ninety days after combination TCA medium depth peeling, a normal-appearing zone of expanded papillary dermis called a Grenz zone is observed. The thickness of this Grenz zone varies with the strength of the wounding agent used and with the depth of the wound produced. A band of thick amorphous brown fibers is present in the middle-to-upper dermis. This band, when stained with both elastic stain and colloidal iron, displays large amounts of elastotic-like fibers and glycosaminoglycans. The thickness and depth of staining of this band increases with the strength of the wounding

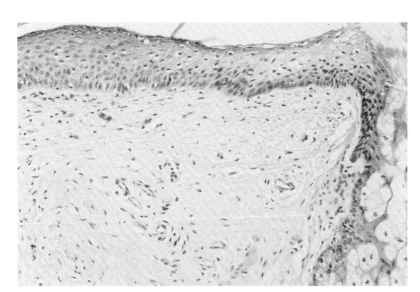

FIGURE 5.3
Histology of newly healed skin 30 days after medium depth peeling with CO_2 hard application followed by 35% TCA showing a hyperplastic epidermis and thickened papillary dermis (Hematoxylin-eosin stain). (Reprinted with permission from Brody H, Hailey CW. Medium depth chemical peeling of the skin: a variation of superficial chemosurgery. J Dermatol Surg Oncol 1986;(12)12:1270-1271.)

FIGURE 5.4

Histology of the skin 90 days after medium depth peeling with CO_2 hard followed by 35% TCA showing a normal epidermal pattern with a papillary dermal Grenz zone and a mid-dermal elastic band (Elastic stain). (Reprinted with permission from Brody H, Hailey CW. Medium depth chemical peeling of the skin: a variation of superficial chemosurgery. J Dermatol Surg Oncol 1986; (12)12:1270-1271.)

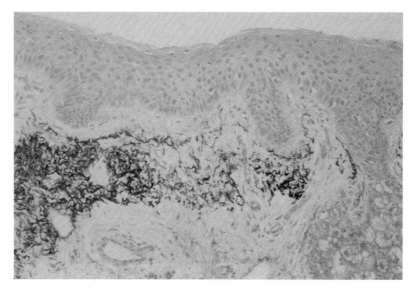

agents, specifically TCA, unoccluded full-strength phenol, Baker's phenol solution, Baker's phenol under occlusion, and dermabrasion. Measurements to quantitate wound depth involve the time to return to normal epidermal thickness, depth of the Grenz zone, and comparison of thickness of the dermal elastotic band. This description of dermal changes at 90 days postoperatively constitutes the essence of the histology of dermal chemical peeling response (Fig 5.4).

GAGs play a major role as the ground substance of the dermal matrix in providing hydration for the skin because of their water-binding capacity. Modalities such as chemical peeling that stimulate the accumulation of GAGs in the skin might maintain normal hydration and counteract fine wrinkling. Although some superficial peeling agents, such as glycolic acid, may produce GAGs without dermal wounding, this accumulation is independent of the clinical appearance of sagging skin associated with altered elastic fibers.

Dermal wounding agent strength is based upon evaluating the reaction at its peak by noting the depth of the wound as opposed to the depth of inflammation. Although the wound may re-epithelialize in 7 to 14 days depending on the residual hair shafts and sebaceous glands, dermal thickening and collagen production does not begin until the inflammatory reaction subsides. Dermal thickening and collagen production begins about 2 weeks after treatment and ends 60 to 90 days later. Dermal elastic-staining fibers do not completely reincorporate at 30 to 60 days, but organize closer to 90 days after peeling (43-53).

The continuum of epidermis and dermis destruction may vary according to pre-peel skin defatting, wounding agent strength or amount applied, and the skin thickness or location. The healing process is similar only in that reformation of less cytologically atypical epidermis is generated from the epidermal appendages. Re-epithelialization may differ and depend on the skin location (e.g., the face vs. the back or neck) and the character of the dermal pathology (e.g., degree of actinic elastotic change or scarring) with ensuing evocation of inflammatory response.

CONCLUSIONS

The clinical appearance following the stages of re-epithelialization and successful collagen remodeling is the hallmark of a successful chemical peel. The wound healing stages can be affected by skin location and thickness because of varying numbers of adnexal structures present for re-epithelialization. The character of dermal pathology—both the degree of histologic elastotic damage and the degree of scarring already present—can also affect the healing phases. Most importantly, the inflammatory response produced during healing depends upon the skin location and the quality of elastotic damage, as well as the inherent properties of the wounding agent. This inflammatory response of varying intensity is an important factor in the clinical appearances of wound healing stages and can be a major factor in the evolution of complications (54-55).

REFERENCES

1. Goslen JB. Wound healing after cosmetic surgery. In: Coleman WP, Hanke CW, Alt TH, et al. eds. Cosmetic Surgery of the Skin. Philadelphia: BC Decker Inc., 1991:47-63.
2. Krawczyk WS. The pattern of epidermal cell migration during wound healing. J Cell Biol 1971;49:247.
3. Martinet N, Harne LA, Grotendorst GR. Identification and characterization of chemoattractants for epidermal cells. J Invest Dermatol 1988;90:122.
4. Hebda PA, Alstadt SP, Hileman WT, et al. Support and stimulation of epidermal cell outgrowth from porcine skin explants by platelet factors. Br J Dermatol 1986;115:529.

5. O'Keefe EJ, Payne RE, Russell N, et al. Spreading and enhanced motility of human keratinocytes on fibronectin. J Invest Dermatol 1985;85:125.

6. Maibach HF, Rovee DT. Epidermal Wound Healing. St. Louis: Mosby Yearbook, 1972.

7. Eaglstein WH, Davis SC, Mehle AL, et al. Optimal use of an occlusive dressing to enhance healing. Effect of delayed application and early removal on wound healing. Arch Dermatol 1988;124:392.

8. Alvarez OM, Mertz PM, and Eaglestein WH. The effect of occlusive dressings on collagen synthesis and re-epithelialization in superficial wounds. J Surg Research 1983;35:142-148.

9. Clark RAF. Cutaneous tissue repair: Basic biologic considerations. J Am Acad Dermatol 1985;13:701.

10. Van Winkle W. The fibroblast in wound healing. Surg Gynecol Obstet 1967;124:369.

11. Folkman J, Klagsbrun M. A family of angiogenic peptides. Nature 1987;329:671.

12. Folkman J, Klagsbrun M. Angiogenic factors. Science 1987;235:442.

13. Folkman J. Angiogenesis: Initiation and control. Ann NY Acad Sci 1982;401:212.

14. Sholley MM, Gimbrone MA Jr, Cotran RS. The effects of leukocyte depletion on corneal neovascularization. Lab Invest 1978;38:32.

15. Doillon CJ, Dunn MG, Bender E, et al. Collagen fiber formation in repair tissue: Development of strength and toughness. Collagen Rel Res 1985;5:481.

16. Eaglstein WH, Mertz PM. "Inert" vehicles do affect wound healing. J Invest Dermatol 1980;74:90.

17. Geronemus RG, Mertz PM, Eaglstein WH. Wound healing: The effects of topical antimicrobial agents. Arch Dermatol 1979;115:1311.

18. Lineaweaver W, McMorris S, Soucy D, et al. Cellular and bacterial toxicities of topical antimicrobials. Plast Reconstr Surg 1985;75:394.

19. Nieder R, Schopf E. Inhibition of wound healing by antiseptics. Br J Dermatol 1986;115(Suppl 31):41.

20. Goodman LS and Gillman AG. The Pharmacological Basis of Therapeutics. New York: MacMillan Publishing Co., Inc., 1980:973.

21. Ghadially R, Halkier-Sorensen L, Elias PM. Effects of petrolatum on stratum corneum structure and function. J Am Acad Dermatol 1992;26:387-396.

22. Elson ML. Effects of petroleum jelly on the healing of skin following cosmetic surgical procedures. Cosmet Dermatol 1993;6:18-22.

23. Smack DP. Bacitracin ointment vs. white petrolatum USP; comparison of post-procedural infection incidence and wound healing in dermatologic surgery patients. Presented at the American Society for Dermatologic Surgery, Palm Springs, CA. May 17, 1996.

24. Fulton JE. The stimulation of postdermabrasion wound healing with stabilized aloe vera gel-polyethylene oxide dressing. J Dermatol Surg Oncol 1990;16:460-466.

25. Weiss JS, Ellis CN, Headington JT, et al. Topical tretinoin improves photoaged skin: A double-blind, vehicle-controlled study. JAMA 1988;259:527-532.

26. Bhawan J, Palko MJ, Lee J, Labadie RR, et al. Reversible histologic effects of tretinoin on photodamaged skin. J Geriatr Dermatol 1995;3(3):62-67.

27. Hevia O, Nemeth AJ, Taylor JR. Tretinoin accelerates healing after trichloroacetic acid chemical peel. Arch Dermatol 1991;127:678-682.

28. Mandy SH. Tretinoin in the preoperative and postoperative management of dermabrasion. J Am Acad Dermatol 1986;15:878-879.

29. Hung VC, Lee JY, Zitelli JA, et al. Topical tretinoin and epithelial wound healing. Arch Dermatol 1989;125:65-69.

30. Vagotis FL, Brundage SR. Histologic study of dermabrasion and chemical peel in an animal model after pretreatment with Retin-A. Aesth Plast Surg 1995;19:243-246.

31. Humphreys TR, Werth V, Dzubow L, et al. Treatment of photodamaged skin with trichloroacetic acid and topical tretinoin. J Am Acad Dermatol 1996;34:638-44.

32. Beach RS, Kenney MC. Vitamin A augments collagen production by corneal endothelial cells. Biochem Biophys Res Commun 1983;114:395.

33. Forest N, Boy-Letevre ML, Duprey P, et al. Collagen synthesis in mouse embryonal carcinoma cells: Effect of retinoic acid. Differentiation 1982;23:153-163.

34. Lee KH. Studies on the mechanism of action of salicylates III: Effect of vitamin A on the wound healing retardation action of aspirin. J Pharm Sci 1968;57:1238-1240.

35. Abergel RP, Meeker CA, Oikarinen H, et al. Retinoid modulation of connective tissue metabolism in keloid fibroblast cultures. Arch Dermatol 1985;121:632-635.

36. Kenney MC, Shih LM, Labermeir U, et al. Modulation of rabbit keratocyte production of collagen, sulfated glycosaminoglycans and fibronectin by retinol and retinoic acid. Biochem Biophys Acta 1986;889:156-162.

37. Jetten MA. Retinoids specifically enhance the number of epidermal growth factor receptors. Nature 1980;284:626-629.

38. Williams ML, Elias PM. Nature of skin fragility in patients receiving retinoids for systemic effect. Arch Dermatol 1981;117:611-619.

39. Clark RAF. Cutaneous tissue repair: Basic biologic considerations I. J Am Acad Dermatol 1985;13:701-725.

40. Bennett RG. Fundamentals of Cutaneous Surgery. St Louis, Mosby-Year Book, 1988:78-87.

41. Ehrlich HP, Hunt TK. Effects of cortisone and vitamin A on wound healing. Ann Surg 1968;167:324.

42. Glogau RG. Chemical peel preparation. American Academy of Dermatology Chemical peel symposium, Dallas, TX. 1991.

43. Stegman SJ. A comparative histologic study of the effects of three peeling agents and dermabrasion on normal and sundamaged skin. Aesthetic Plast Surg 1982;6:123-135.

44. Brody HJ. Variations and comparisons in medium depth chemical peeling. J Dermatol Surg Oncol 1989;15:953-963.

45. Brody HJ, Hailey CW. Medium-depth chemical peeling of the skin: A variation of superficial chemosurgery. J Dermatol Surg Oncol 1986;12:1268-1275.

46. Stegman SJ. A study of dermabrasion and chemical peeling in an animal model. J Dermatol Surg Oncol 1980;6:490-497.

47. Brown AM, Kaplan LM, Brown ME. Cutaneous alterations induced by phenol. A histologic bioassay. J Int Coll Surg 1960;34:602.
48. Spira M, Dahl C, Freeman R, et al. Chemosurgery: A histologic study. Plast Reconstr Surg 1970;45:247.
49. Baker TJ, Gordon HL, Mosienko P, et al. Long-term histological study of skin after chemical face peeling. Plast Reconstr Surg 1974;53:522.
50. Baker TJ, Gordon HL. Chemical face peeling and dermabrasion. Surg Clin North Am 1971;51:387-401.
51. Behin F, Feuerstein SS, Marovitz WF. Comparative histological study of minipig skin after chemical peel and dermabrasion. Arch Otolaryngol 1977;103:271-277.
52. Brown AM, Kaplan LM, Brown ME. Phenol-induced histologic skin changes: hazards, technique and uses. Br J Plast Surg 1960;13:158-169.
53. Litton C. Observations after chemosurgery of the face. Plast Reconstr Surg 1963;32:554-556.
54. Personal communication, Richard G. Glogau, 1991.
55. Brody, HJ. Chemical Peeling and Resurfacing, 2nd Ed. St. Louis: Mosby-Yearbook, 1997:29-38.

CHAPTER 6

Superficial Chemical Peeling

■ Naomi Lawrence
William P. Coleman III

Chemical peels are most simply categorized by the histologic depth of wounding. In a superficial peel, destruction may be limited to the stratum granulosum and stratum spinulosum, or extend through the full thickness of the epidermis to the papillary dermis (1). Moderate to severe actinic damage and acne scarring are not significantly impacted because of the superficial level of biologic action of this type of peel. However, these peels may have an effect on pathologic processes deeper in the skin through a mode of action not related to simple destruction. In acne, comedomolysis can dramatically improve the patient's condition, unplugging sebaceous outflow to facilitate drainage of cysts located in the deep dermis. In melasma, superficial peels may allow improved penetration of medications affecting both epidermal and dermal melanocytes (2).

The agents most commonly used for superficial peeling are listed in Table 6.1. The selection of a particular agent alone does not determine the depth of peel. Almost any of the wounding agents listed can cause a medium depth peel if applied to skin that has been sensitized by physical or chemical abrasion or by overzealous application of tretinoin. Conversely, superficial peeling agents inappropriately applied or used on poor candidates (thick skin, acne scarring) can result in no response. In the early 1990s, patients were enticed by media endorsements of "lunch time peels". In glossy oversimplification, superficial peels were portrayed as treatments with miraculous rejuvenation potential and no morbidity. Application of an agent to the skin that produces cooling and temporary tightening but not peeling, is a facial (3). If there is no erythema and desquamation (small or large flakes) then, there is no peel, (not even a superficial one) and no appreciable clinical change.

INDICATIONS FOR SUPERFICIAL PEELS

Acne

A series of superficial peels is an excellent approach to treating both facial and truncal acne. In acne patients, an abnormal pattern of keratinization results in follicular plugging and forms a comedone (primary acne lesion) (4, 5). As sebum is produced and collects proximal to the keratinous plug, the wall of the follicle thins secondarily to form a papule. Leakage of sebum and generation of free fatty acids by *Propionibacterium acnes* result in inflammatory, pustular acne (6). Superficial chemical peels for acne work primarily through comedomolysis but also epidermolysis as pustules are unroofed (5). After the second peel (and a month of topical therapy) manual acne surgery is a useful adjunct to decrease baseline comedones. A series of superficial peels can give dramatic improvement in active acne over a very short period of time. This has considerable psychological benefit for the patient. They are often much more compliant with topical medications to maintain their improvement than they would be using the same topicals to achieve improvement over a longer time period. Any of the superficial peeling agents can be used successfully to treat acne. An important caveat is that patients with acne tend to have skin very sensitive to peeling (7). It is best to prepare the patient with a minimal peel on the first visit. A very conservative first peel (i.e., one coat of Jessner's

TABLE 6.1

SUPERFICIAL PEELING AGENTS

Very light peels
10-20% Trichloracetic acid (TCA)
Jessner's solution (14 g salicylic acid, 14 g lactic acid,
    14 g resorcinol in 95% ethanol qsad 100 cc)
Neutralized glycolic acid
Tretinoin
Azelaic acid

Light peels
Solid CO_2 slush
35% TCA
70% Glycolic acid unbuffered
Salicylic acid
5 Fluorouracil
Unna's paste
Resorcinol

solution applied with moderate pressure or short contact with 70% glycolic acid) is used to gauge the sensitivity of the skin. The second peel can always be titrated stronger but if the first peel results in significant morbidity, this will discourage the superficial peeling patient from future peels. These patients are committed to no "down" time, (i.e., significant erythema and peeling).

Melasma

Melasma is a disorder of pigmentation which often responds positively to a series of superficial peels (2). Histologically, the pigment in melasma is in the basal layer of the epidermis and/or in the dermis. Superficial peels improve this condition by increasing the penetration of medical therapy, not by "peeling off" the pigment (Fig. 6.1). It is best to pretreat the patient for at least 2 weeks with tretinoin and hydroquinone before the peel series. Either glycolic acid 70% (unbuffered) for 2 to 3 minutes or Jessner's solution (1 to 2 coats) can be used for the peel series. As soon as the patient heals (usually 5 to 7 days), the tretinoin and hydroquinone treatment is resumed. This regimen has been proved to reduce the objective melasma rating by 63% and lighten on colorimeter evaluation in a patient population that was largely resistant to medical therapy alone (2). Most patients respond to this regimen, however responders fall into 2 categories: those with a minimal but positive response, and those with dramatic lightening. Neither depth of pigment (indicated by Wood's lamp exam) nor the patient's Fitzpatrick skin type were good indicators for predicting patient response. Patients who had a deeper peel, due to greater sensitivity to the peel solutions, did not get a better result (and risked post inflammatory hyperpigmentation).

Another peel regimen that can cause significant improvement in melasma is a monthly short contact (30 to 40 seconds) glycolic acid peel combined with a home regimen of tretinoin. Postinflammatory hyperpigmentation (which histologically also shows melanin in the basal epidermis) has been shown to respond to a series of superficial peels in addition to topical therapy with tretinoin, hydroquinone 2%/glycolic acid 10% gel (8).

SKIN REFRESHER, ACTINIC DAMAGE, AND FINE LINES

The use of a series of superficial peels for actinic damage, fine lines and as a skin refresher is controversial. Newman et al compared 50% glycolic acid gel (unbuffered, non neutralized with pH = 1.2) to the vehicle alone for the treatment of actinic damage of 34 patients (9). They performed a series of 4 peels spaced 1 week apart. The patients were evaluated on both clinical and histologic parameters. There was statistically significant improvement in rough texture, fine wrinkling, and a decreased number of actinic keratoses. Solar lentigenes improved only slightly and coarse wrinkling did not improve. Histologic evaluation revealed a decrease in the stratum corneum, and an increase in the stratum granulosum and epidermal thickness. No measurable changes in collagen were seen in this study, although some biopsies appeared to have an increase in collagen thickness.

Moy et al studied the histologic effects of various peeling agents in 2 mini pigs (10). Using a 5 point scale to denote percentage collagen regeneration where (5 = 100%), they saw 2+ dermal growth at 21 days for 50% and 70% glycolic acid. This was the same level of collagen regrowth as generated by 50% trichloroacetic acid (TCA).

Piacquadio et al evaluated the effect of a series of superficial peels on actinic damage in a pilot study of 10 patients (11). Two treatment groups were compared. Both groups had four 70% glycolic acid (NeoStrata Co. Inc., Princeton, NJ) peels, spaced one month apart. One treatment group also used 10% glycolic acid based moisturizer (Aqua glycolic lotion, [Herald Pharmaceuticals, Colonial Heights, VA]). The patients were evaluated by objective clinical scoring, optic profilometry, and histologic parameters. Only mild improvement was seen in pigmentation, fine wrinkling, and roughness. Actinic keratoses counts decreased. Picquadio et al found no statistically significant differences and no appreciable histologic change in either group. Patients using the glycolic lotion in addition to the peels did better than the patients who had the peels alone. Picquadio el al conclude that improvement of actinic damage by superficial peels is minimal and may not be more than

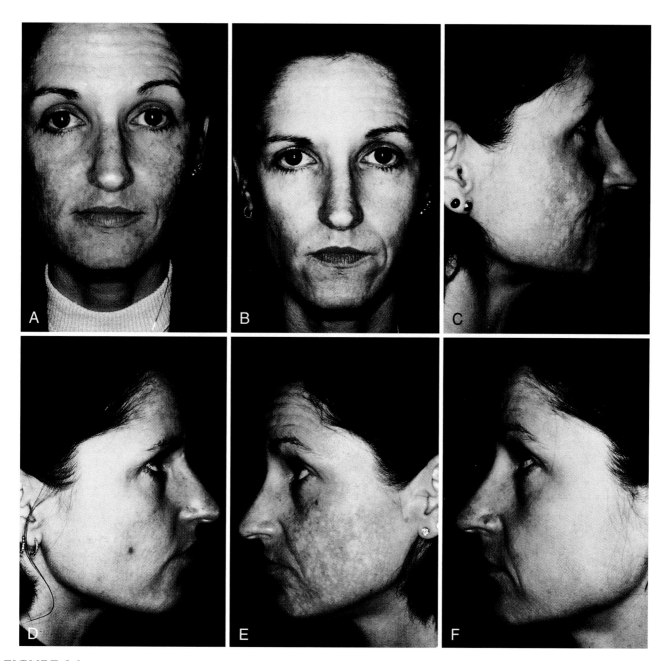

FIGURE 6.1

Widespread Melasma. A, Before peel using glycolic acid on the right and Jessner's on the left. B, One month after 3rd peel (at 1 month intervals). C, Right side view before peel. D, Right side view after 3 70% glycolic acid peels. E, Left side view before peel. F, Left side view after 3 Jessner's peels. (Photographs courtesy of Sue Ellen Cox, MD.)

what can be achieved with low strength topical glycolic products alone.

Most peel experts would agree that medium depth and deep resurfacing give more tangible results in patients with moderate to severe actinic damage. The controversy lies in whether there is benefit to a series of superficial peels in the patient with actinic damage who cannot accept the morbidity of deeper resurfacing. At this point the studies are somewhat contradictory. Statistically, when one is trying to show a small change in a variable, a very large study population is necessary. Additional studies to confirm the efficacy of superficial peels in the treatment of actinic damage are needed. There is a strong clinical impression that a series of superficial peels enhances a home program of tretinoin, glycolic acid, and hydroquinones for treatment of dyschromia (Figs. 6.2, 6.3). However, there are no objective studies to date which verify this.

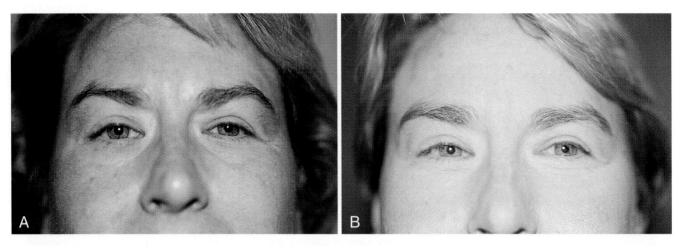

FIGURE 6.2
Facial actinic damage. A, Preoperative appearance of actinic damage and dyspigmentation. B, Significant improvement after 12 monthly 70% glycolic acid peels.

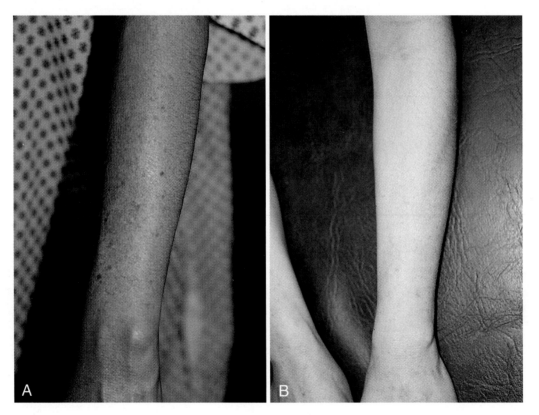

FIGURE 6.3
Non facial actinic damage. A, Preoperative appearance of actinic damage of the arms. B, Appearance after 3 20% TCA peels performed at 3 month intervals.

NONFACIAL CHEMICAL PEELING

A series of superficial peels is the safest way to approach actinic damage and dyschromia in non facial areas (Fig. 6.4) (12). Off the face, a decrease in dermal vasculature and follicular density results in slower and less optimal wound healing (13). Nonfacial areas (e.g., arms, hands, chest, neck, back, legs) have a narrower margin for error than the face. This can be handled by starting with very mild agents for peeling (e.g., 1 coat of Jessner's solution, 12% to 20% TCA) and titrating up on second and third peels (to 70% glycolic acid plus 35% TCA). Another approach is to use test patches to compare the reaction to different agents and different concentrations of agents before proceeding. As with other areas, preparation with tretinoin, glycolic acid lotion and hydroquinone is important.

TECHNIQUE

The application technique as well as pre-peel topical treatment and preparation are as important to results as the agent selection. Most of the light peeling agents can cause an undesired medium depth peel injury with aggressive pre-peel treatment and vigorous skin preparation. The variables that affect peel depth fall into four categories:

1. Patient skin characteristics
2. Pretreatment agents
3. Preparation
4. Method of application

Patient Characteristics

A thoughtful consideration of the patient's skin qualities can maximize efficacy and minimize complications. Classification of Fitzpatrick skin types grade the endogenous melanocytic composition as well as the melanocytic response to sun exposure. (Table 6.2) (14).

Skin types IV, V, and VI are most prone to postinflammatory hyperpigmentation. This can be a significant cosmetic concern in type IV skin where the color differential (between the hyperpigmented area and normal skin color) is often the greatest. Patients with type IV, V,

TABLE 6.2

FITZPATRICK'S CLASSIFICATION OF SUN-REACTIVE SKIN TYPES

Skin Type	Color	Reaction to first summer exposure
I	White	Always burn, never tan
II	White	Usually burn, tan with difficulty
III	White	Sometimes mild burn, tan average
IV	Moderate brown	Rarely burn, tan with ease
V	Dark brown*	Very rarely burn, tan very easily
VI	Black	No burn, tan very easily

*Asian Indian, Oriental, Hispanic, or light African descent, for example.

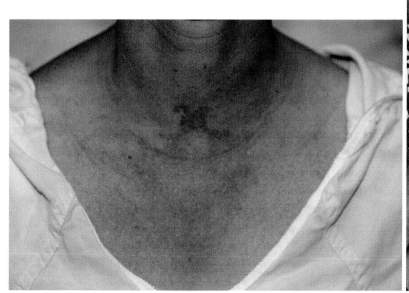
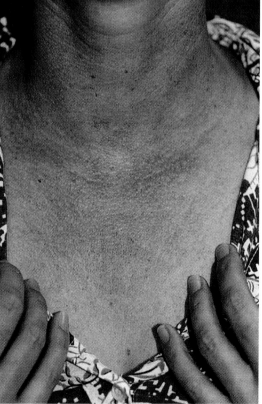

FIGURE 6.4
A, Preoperative appearance of pigmentation and actinic damage of the chest. B, One month after a 20% TCA peel, pigmentation is reduced, but telangiectasia remain.

and VI skin should have a pretreatment and maintenance regimen that includes tretinoin (Retin A [Ortho Pharmaceutical, Raritan, NJ]) and hydroquinone. Superficial peels can be used safely in the darker skin types without significant risk of permanent color change.

The Glogau classification for photoaging groups grades both actinic damage and scarring. (Table 6.3) (15). When considering a series of superficial peels to treat actinic damage, photoaging groups I and II are probably the most appropriate candidates. The hyperkeratosis and parakeratosis seen with advanced to severe photoaging acts as a barrier to peel agent penetration. Also the scarring seen in any of these categories is not improved by an epidermal peel.

Sebaceous gland activity or skin oiliness is another consideration (16). Oily skin can appear clinically thickened or "doughy". It is important to identify these patients because an even, effective superficial peel can be more difficult to obtain. Pretreatment with a higher concentration of tretinoin (0.05% to 0.1%) in combination with topical alpha hydroxy acids (10% to 20%) is often necessary. Also helpful are a more vigorous preparation of the skin and use of light, rather than the "very light," peeling agents. Conversely, skin that appears clinically thin (e.g., translucent, sometimes intrinsically aged,

usually female) can inadvertently progress to a medium depth peel with some of the superficial agents. This skin type must be pretreated and prepared very cautiously. Skin that is inflamed due to seborrhea or over-treatment with topicals can take up more peel solution and result in a deeper than expected peel when using a light peeling agent (17). Patients with rosacea can have persistent erythema although this is more common with deeper resurfacing. Pretreatment is particularly important with superficial peels because results can also be negligible if skin is improperly prepared.

Pretreatment Agents

Tretinoin accelerates healing after partial thickness wounding. For this reason it is commonly used as pretreatment for skin resurfacing of all depths and for most conditions. Hung et al showed an 11 fold increase in the healing rate when tretinoin was compared to vehicle in the porcine model (18). In their study, 0.05% tretinoin was applied to the treatment area daily for 10 days prior to wounding. Continued treatment to the area after wounding had a negative effect. Hevia et al pretreated 16 actinically damaged patients with 0.1% tretinoin for 14 days (19). When compared to the vehicle side, the treated hemiface was twice as likely to be healed 7 days after a 35% TCA peel. They also observed that there was more intense and uniform frosting from the TCA peel on the tretinoin pretreated skin. This is most likely due to a reduction of the layers of the stratum corneum (20). Although this clinically improved frosting might seem to afford a more efficacious peel, a recent study failed to prove this supposition (21). When comparing results after a 40% TCA peel in 7 patients pretreated with 0.1% tretinoin (Retin A) for 6 to 7 weeks to those with no pretreatment, no significant difference in the improvement of moderate photodamage was detected. Perhaps pretreatment plays less of a role when deeper resurfacing is performed.

When pretreating with tretinoin, it is important to look for signs of retinoid dermatitis (20-22). Inflammation can result in deeper, erratic penetration of peeling solution and give a deeper than desired peel (17). The use of other topical agents before peels is more restricted to specific indications. These agents are very important in superficial peels because they maximize results of treatment with minimal morbidity. Similar to tretinoin, topical alpha hydroxy acids have demonstrated both anti-aging and anti-acne therapeutic benefits (23). No studies show that topical alpha hydroxy acids have a similar effect on accelerating wound healing. Effective treatment of melasma with a series of superficial peels is predicated on pre- and postpeel use of tretinoin and hydroquinone (2). If a patient has a history of predilection to post inflammatory pigmentation, hydroquinone should be used for 8 weeks prior to peeling (24). Hydroquinone thereapy should also be resumed once the skin has healed sufficiently to tolerate its use.

TABLE 6.3

GLOGAU'S CLASSIFICATION OF PHOTOAGING GROUPS

Group I-Mild (usually 28-35 years old)
No keratoses
Little wrinkling
No scarring
Little or no makeup

Group II-Moderate (usually 35-50 years old)
Early actinic keratoses-slight yellow skin discoloration
Early wrinkling-parallel smile lines
Mild scarring
Small amount of makeup

Group III-Advanced (usually 50-65 years old)
Actinic keratoses-obvious yellow skin discoloration with telangiectasia
Wrinkling-present at rest
Moderate acne scarring
Wears makeup always

Group IV-Severe (usually 60-75 years old)
Actinic keratoses and skin cancers have occurred
Wrinkling-much cutis laxa of actinic, gravitational, and dynamic origin
Severe acne scarring
Wears makeup that does not cover, but cakes on

Adapted from Glogau RG. Chemical Peel Symposium. American Academy of Dermatology. Atlanta Dec 4 1990; Brody HJ, ed. Chemical Peeling: General Peeling Concepts. St. Louis: Mosby, 1992:38.

Skin Preparation

The skin is often prepared before a peel by applying an agent to remove excess sebaceous secretions as well as built up stratum corneum. This allows for better, more even penetration of the peeling solution. Peikert et al evaluated the effect of four skin degreasers (rubbing alcohol, freon skin degreaser, chlorhexidine glucovate, and acetone) on peel efficacy in 6 patients with androgenetic alopecia (25). They found no difference in the clinical or histologic response to a 35% TCA peel. Most peel experts prefer acetone even though care has to be taken when used with lasers because of its flammability (17).

More important than the choice of a preparation solution is the method of application. A wipe is a unidirectional motion in which the gauze is "passed over" all areas. A scrub is a bidirectional motion which implies friction. The preparation method (wipe or scrub) should be based on several factors: patient skin type, peel indication, and peeling solution. Vigorous scrubbing in preparation for a superficial peel with Jessner's solution or TCA 15% can be used with sebaceous skin, or with advanced photoaging. Vigorous scrubbing in preparation should not be used with a thin skinned patient or for a young acne patient, prior to 70% glycolic acid, unbuffered. An active acne patient often has multiple fresh "wounds" through which solution can penetrate deeper. 70% glycolic acid, unbuffered, can cause a medium depth peel in these patients if the skin preparation is vigorous (2).

Method of Application

The method of application can profoundly affect the peel result. More pressure and rubbing increases the amount of peeling agent applied. The type of applicator also determines the amount of peel solution applied. Brody quantified the solution delivered by commonly used applicators as (from most to least): sable brush, 4×4 wrung out damp gauze, 2 wrung out cotton-tipped applicators (16). With disposable applicators (e.g., cotton tip and gauze), the number of applicators used also helps quantify the amount of solution applied. All of these variables—number and type of applicators, pressure and friction of application—should be documented in any study of chemical peels so that results can be repeatable. Also, if complications occur, knowledge of these variables is helpful in refining peel technique. When considering proper application of peel solutions, the physician must set an end point to the peel application. This is actually more difficult with superficial peels than it is with medium depth or deep peels because of the lack of clear clinical signs.

Matarasso et al developed a fluorescent marker to assess the uniformity of peel applications when viewed with a Wood's lamp (26). They recommend the addition of salicylic acid to the peel solution at a ratio of 1:5 or adding fluorescein sodium at a ratio of 1:15.

To gauge the patient's response to a glycolic acid peel solution, one looks for erythema and vesiculation. A frost with this solution usually indicates a deeper than desired peel. With Jessner's solution and lower concentration TCA, a frost is desirable. It is usually patchy and much less intense than that seen with a medium depth peel.

PEELING SOLUTIONS

Most peel experts have definite solution preferences (5). Each peeling formula has advantages and disadvantages. It is important to become familiar with these and use a solution that gives consistent results. Changing a technique should be done with care until the physician is experienced with the new method.

Trichloracetic Acid (TCA)

Concentrations of 10% to 35% TCA generally lead to destruction in the range of a superficial peel. TCA causes wounding through protein precipitation (27,28). Brodland et al studied depths of necrosis in a porcine model and showed intraepidermal necrosis with 20% TCA and full thickness epidermal and superficial reticular dermal necrosis with 35% TCA. As with all peeling solutions, the extent of actinic damage and thickness of the epidermis affect the penetration of TCA (1). TCA solutions are often compounded by the physician's local pharmacy. A weight to volume preparation (e.g., 35 g of TCA USP crystals, dissolved in a small amount of water then add enough water to make 100 ml) makes a 35% TCA solution (29). When using other methods of preparation the concentration of the 35 g (ml) TCA solution can vary from 29.4% to 48.65%. TCA is stable at room temperature or refrigerated and is not light sensitive, so it can be stored in clear or amber glass bottles (30, 31). An aqueous solution of TCA is stable for at least 6 months (30, 32).

TCA can be used as a very light or light peeling solution. It can be used for all superficial peel indications, including acne, melasma, facial actinic damage, and non facial actinic damage. The frost caused by TCA is more easily identified than that from Jessner's solution or from the erythema produced by glycolic acid. It has a niche as a peel intermediate between light and medium depth approaches. Often one of the very light solutions (glycolic acid or Jessner's solution) is used for the first peel of a superficial peel series, and if the patient's improvement is less than optimal, 25% or 35% TCA is used for the next peel.

Harris et al describe a modification of a low strength TCA peel in which they manually abrade the skin with moistened silicone carbide sand paper before applying 25% trichloracetic acid (see Chapter 12). Although no histology was done in this study, the time course to heal, 7 to 10 days, makes it most likely that this would be classified as a medium to deep resurfacing procedure.

TCA masque is a new cream formulation available in strengths of 11% and 16% (33). The bentonite cream base chelated TCA product causes a much deeper peel at lower TCA percentages than traditional aqueous TCA. Some place the level of peel with the masque alone in the category of 40% TCA. The cream is applied with gloved fingers or a tongue blade. The skin should be checked for frosting at 5 minutes and then 5 minute intervals until the cream sets. Chiarello et al recommends a total of 12 to 15 minutes with this cream for most patients (33). The masque is then washed off with cool water. Exfoliation is complete in 5 to 7 days. This masque has been reportedly used safely in nonfacial areas. However there are no good peer reviewed studies on this approach at the time of this writing.

Jessner's Solution

Jessner's solution was formulated by Dr. Max Jessner in the late 1940s and consists of resorcinol, salicylic acid, and lactic acid (85%) 14 grams each, mixed in 95% ethanol to make a quantity of 100 ml. This combination was developed to take advantage of the keratolytic effects of resorcinol and salicylic acid, while minimizing the side effects that would result from higher concentrations of these two agents (30).

Jessner's solution can be used for all of the superficial peel indications. It is particularly useful in patient's with sensitive skin, such as young acne patients, or thin skinned, elderly patients. It is useful as the first peel in a series to gauge the reactivity of a patient's skin. Although with overaggressive application, one could certainly achieve a deeper peel than desired with Jessner's solution, its margin of safety is greater than TCA or 70% glycolic acid, unbuffered. In a patient with sebaceous skin, a vigorous scrub for 2 minutes is necessary before applying Jessner's solution. Firm pressure with 2 cotton tipped applicators or a 2 × 2 wrung out gauze can be used to apply the solution. Usually in the first peel, only one coat is used, but in subsequent peels 2 to 3 coats can be employed depending on the patient's reaction. The skin will exhibit a faint erythema and a spotty white frost to indicate action of the peel solution.

Glycolic Acid

Although lactic acid and pyruvic acid emulsified in lotions or creams are used in the dermatologic setting, glycolic acid is by far the most commonly used alpha-hydroxy acid for chemical peeling (30). Glycolic acid is a hydrophilic molecule and causes a decrease in corneocyte attachment (34). In vitro studies of human skin fibroblasts have shown that glycolic acid stimulates collagen production (35). Moy et al postulate that this production is due to a direct stimulation of cell protein synthesis and growth without causing cell damage. Because the regrowth of collagen is not related to depth of wounding as it is with TCA, it is possible that the collagen stimulated by glycolic acid is greater than one could predict from the clinical behavior of the peel (10). The choice of glycolic acid solutions can be confusing because a large number of concentrations and pH's are available. The majority of peeling experts use 70% glycolic acid unbuffered and unneutralized (36). This is the most powerful and effective form of this agent.

Becker et al performed a histologic comparison of 50 and 70% glycolic acid solutions with various pH's in two elderly patients with actinic damage. They tested two 70% glycolic acid solutions with pH under 2, two solutions with pH over 2, one 70% esterified glycolic acid solution with a pH of .8, and two 50% glycolic acid solutions with a pH of less than 2. They found that 70% glycolic acid caused more tissue damage than 50% glycolic acid. Also the 70% glycolic acid with the low pH (below 2) caused more tissue damage than the higher pH 70% glycolic acid or the partially neutralized glycolic acid. They left the solutions on the skin for 30 minutes and saw epidermal crusting, epidermal necrosis, and vesiculation in areas treated with the low pH 70% glycolic acid. They felt that there was no clinical advantage in creating the deeper wounding and recommended a higher pH solution (37). On the other hand, low pH solutions are more efficient wounding agents and can be used to obtain a desired effect more rapidly. They are not used for 30 minutes, but rather from 15 seconds to 3 minutes. Dormen (38) maintains that neutralized solutions are in essence inactivated. He feels that it is the amount of bioavailable free acid that determines both therapeutic efficacy and irritation (Table 6.4). Unfortunately most companies do not reveal the free acid concentration of their products. This can be estimated using the Henderson-Hasselblock equation (Table 6.5).

There are several very important technical points to the application of glycolic acid. First, when using the 70% unbuffered, unneutralized solution it is best not to prepare the skin, or only very lightly prepare it. If the area is over-prepared, the solution can penetrate the epidermis causing a dermal wound, in an unpredictable fashion (2). Dermal wounds can occur with any break in the epidermal barrier. One must be cautious in a patient who has erythema from a retinoid dermatitis or from seborrheic dermatitis because the penetration of glycolic acid can cause a dermal wound.

It is important the application of glycolic acid be carefully timed. The effect is immediately reversed by application of water. The time from the initial application of glycolic acid to reversal with water determines the clinical effect. Thus, this agent can be used very precisely, controlled by time on the skin. The peel solution must be applied fairly rapidly so that the time designated is representative of the exposure of the entire face. Because of this timing aspect it is extremely important the solution be washed off completely as a deeper than desired peel can occur if an the acid is not totally re-

TABLE 6.4

ESTIMATED FREE ACID VALUES OF COMMERCIALLY AVAILABLE PRODUCTS BASED ON HENDERSON HASSELBACH EQUATION

Product	Company	Concentration	pH	Free acid value
Skin Removal Peel	NeoStrata	50%	1.3	50.0%
AHA Skin Soothing Cream	NeoStrata	8%	3.67	4.7%
AHA Facial Lotion	NeoStrata	15%	3.7	8.0%
MDF Facial Lotion	Herald Pharmacal	12%	3.3	8.5%
MDF Forte Facial Lotion	Herald Pharmacal	20%	3.4	14.6%
MDF Forte Glycare	Herald Pharmacal	20%	4.3	4.8%
Rejuvenation Peel Pad	Glytone	50%	1.2	50.0%
Non Com Cream 7	Glytone	7%	1.80	6.9%
Emollient Toner 20	Glytone	20%	2.55	18.6%
Glycolic Acid	Delasco	70%	0.5	70%

Table from *Dermatology Times* modified by Naomi Lawrence M.D.

TABLE 6.5

HENDERSON-HASSELBACH EQUATION

$$pH = pKa + \log \frac{[A-]}{[HA]}$$

or

$$HA = \frac{1}{1 + \text{antilog (pH-pKa)}} \times C$$

Where C = original concentration of acid

HA = free acid value

Table from Dermatology Times/Source: Michael A Dorman M.D.

moved. This often occurs on a focal basis when one area is incompletely hydrated. The time also must be carefully titrated with each peel as a patient can have very little reaction with one time period yet extending the time period in that patient 30 to 60 seconds can give a much more intense reaction. In a series of peels, 10 additional seconds for each peel is reasonable. However, additional factors, such as dermatitis or xerosis, may indicate a need to reduce the exposure time rather than increasing in spite of satisfactory prior responses. All glycolic acid peels cause a burning sensation until they are reversed. The endpoint is erythema. If frosting or epi-

dermolysis occurs, this indicates dermal injury. The hydration should begin before these signs occur.

Salicylic Acid

Salicylic acid has been shown to be efficacious in low concentrations (1% to 2% and up to 10%) as an antiaging cream and moisturizer and, in higher concentrations (30% to 50%), as a peeling agent (39). Berger states that an important determinant of the efficacy of the salicylic acid preparation is the pH (39). Salicylic acid is more effective in a low pH vehicle than a neutral one. He also finds that subjective irritation in patients is less common than that experienced with topical alpha hydroxy acid preparations. Kligman recently reported on the use of a 30% salicylic acid solution developed in conjunction with SKIN Inc. (Conshahocken, PA) (40). This preparation has a vehicle that vaporizes rapidly leaving a white precipitate of salicylic acid which is washed off. This salicylic acid preparation produces a superficial anesthesia to light touch 3 to 3.5 minutes after application. The patient is more comfortable with this peel than with glycolic acid peels. There is also less transepidermal water loss (a measure of skin barrier function) than with glycolic acid peels. The clinical reaction is greater, with peeling for 7 to 10 days, 15% of patients peel in sheets of skin, and 20% develop crusting on the lower eyelids. Kligman recommends the use of this new preparation in the treatment of inflammatory and comedomal acne, photodamage, and melasma.

Swinehart recently revisited an earlier approach using a 50% salicylic acid paste (Dermatologic Lab and Supply, Council Bluffs, IA) for photodamage on the dorsa of the hands and forearms in 11 patients (41). Patients were pretreated with 0.1% tretinoin for weeks to months and prepared with septisol, alcohol, and acetone. Actinic keratoses, seborrheic keratoses, and prominent lentigines were first treated with 20% TCA. Then the salicylic acid paste was applied generously with a tongue blade (cotton balls between fingers to prevent migration to palm). The area was occluded with plastic wrap, occlusive tape, and a bulky SOF Kling conforming bandage (Johnson & Johnson Co., Arlington, TX) dressing for 48 hours. During this time, patients can take non-steroidal anti-inflammatory medications for burning discomfort and watch for signs of salicylism (ringing in ears or muffled hearing). If the patient develops salicylism, increased water intake or an early removal of bandages may be necessary depending on the severity of symptoms. Patients can develop maceration, blistering and extensive desquamation which is treated with zinc oxide, and a Vigilon (Bard Co., Murray Hill, NJ), or Duoderm (Convatec, Princeton, NJ) dressing for 4 days. After this, an antibiotic ointment and nonadhesive dressing are used usually for 6 additional days. No histologic data is provided, but because of clinical signs, one must assume that this is at least a full thickness epidermal or superficial dermal peel. No scarring was reported in this group or in an earlier study in which 81 patients were treated (42). This peel preparation should be used cautiously as it has significant morbidity and, certainly because of greater depth of destruction, a higher risk of scarring than more superficial agents.

Resorcinol

Resorcinol (dihydroxy benzene) has been used as a solo peeling agent mostly in Europe. In 1882 the famous German dermatologist, Paul Unna, reported on 10%, 20%, and 30% resorcinol peels (28). Letessier later modified Unna's paste formula to produce a 50% resorcinol paste (Table 6.6) (43). Axurgia is a derivative of pig feet that decreases erythema (30). Ceyassite is a clay bearing soil which acts as a drying agent (44).

TABLE 6.6

LETESSIER MODIFIED UNNA'S PASTE

Resorcinol 40 g
Zinc oxide 10 g
Ceyassite 2 g
Benzoin Axurgia 28 g

Adapted from Letessier SM. Chemical peel with resorcin. In: Roenigk RK, Roenigk HH, eds. Dermatologic Surgery: Principles and Practice. New York: Marcel Dekker, 1989:1017-1024.

Resorcinol is bactericidal and causes keratolysis by breaking the hydrogen bonds of keratin (30). Some authors recommend a test patch of paste be applied, left for 15 minutes, and checked in 4 days for contact sensitivity to resorcinol (43). Others feel that allergic reaction is rare and do not test patch (45). Karam recommends a vigorous scrub with alcohol or acetone as a skin preparation before treatment with resorcinol (45). To facilitate ease of paste application, the plastic container can be immersed in hot water for 2 to 3 minutes.

The paste is applied with a tongue depressor or gloved fingers avoiding the periorbital area and lips. The area of application should be limited. If large areas are to be covered, the treatment should be divided and subsections peeled separately. The interval between peeling sessions can range from a few hours to days. Additional rubbing will increase absorption. The paste is usually left on the face for about 30 minutes and on the trunk or extremities for 1 hour. It is removed with a tongue depressor and cotton balls. The patient will feel a burning sensation or paresthesias 2 to 30 minutes after application. This increases with time and remains even after the paste is removed. Discomfort stops abruptly about 1 hour after removing the paste. This burning response intensifies with subsequent peels. Cold compresses and steroid creams are used to help ameliorate discomfort. After the peel, patients can feel dizzy for 10 to 15 minutes. This is thought to be secondary to cutaneous vasodilation. Patients should be kept supine throughout the peel and immediately after to avoid syncope. Patients develop a thick brown crust at the application site which peels over 10 days. The histology of this peel shows a separation at the granular layer and vasodilatation a few hours after peel, with increased mitosis in the basal layer of the epidermis. There is proliferation of fibroblasts at 1 week, and a thickened epidermis and dermal collagen still evident 4 months after peel (43, 45). Karam recommends this peel for postinflammatory hyperpigmentation, erythema and shallow scars from acne, melasma, and photodamage in skin types I through V.

Solid Carbon Dioxide (CO_2)

Solid CO_2 (dry ice) has a temperature of $-78.5°C$ and can be stored in an ice chest or cooler for 2 to 3 days (28). It can be obtained through ice plants, ice cream manufacturers, dairies, and pharmaceutical supply companies. A 5 or 10 lb block is broken to hand size, wrapped in a towel, and dipped in a solution of acetone, 3:1 with alcohol to facilitate application. Pressure and timing determine the depth of peel. To treat comedomal acne, moderate pressure for 5 to 8 seconds per area is appropriate. Because of its more moderate temperature, it does not cause the hypopigmentation and scarring seen with liquid nitrogen ($-186°C$).

POSTOPERATIVE CARE

Immediate after care can affect the depth of wounding. Most of the studies on postoperative peel care have examined the results of occlusion on deep TCA and phenol peeling. Tape occlusion after TCA lessens the depth of wounding (27). Tegaderm (Astra Co., Westboro, MA) occlusion immediately following the procedure and after 4 hours also reduces the depth of wounding (46). Bacitracin ointment increases the depth of necrosis when applied 4 hours after the peel (46). Immediate after care thus depends on the desired depth of wounding. If the peel seems to have had minimal effect, the reaction could be enhanced by delaying ointment application until 4 hours after the peel. If the patient complains of extreme burning and the peel appears to have had a deeper than desired response, Tegaderm occlusion may lessen necrosis. A topical steroid ointment may also be used if an unintended deeper peel has occurred. Application should begin immediately and continued twice daily until the desired clinical response is obtained.

After the patient heals, a good postoperative care regimen will maintain and even improve results. Because clinical changes are more subtle with superficial peels, this regimen is even more important than with deeper resurfacing. The topicals used in after care are the same as those used in pretreatment. Tretinoin as a single agent reduces rhytides, actinic keratoses and mottling of skin pigment by photodamage when used for at least 6 months (20, 47). After a superficial peel, the patient may have to wait a week for the skin to be able to tolerate tretinoin.

Generally there is no problem with restarting the same strength tretinoin that was used before the peel. This concentration can be increased as the patient tolerates. Similarly, alpha hydroxy acid lotions are started about 1 week after the peel. One can start these at the lower percentage (8%) and increase as tolerated to 15% and 20% lotions. Hydroquinone is used after peels when indicated for treatment of residual pigmentation (e.g., melasma, postinflammatory hyperpigmentation) or to prophylax in patients predisposed to post inflammatory hyperpigmentation (from the peel itself). We do not use the multiproduct packages "systems" that include lotions, cleansers, etc. These are gimmicks that perpetuate the cosmetic myth that women need a myriad of expensive products to look younger. The ethical physician should recommend the least expensive effective preparations.

REFERENCES

1. Brody HJ. Histology and Classification In: Brody HG, ed. Chemical Peeling and Resurfacing (2nd ed). St Louis: Mosby Yearbook, 1997:1-6.
2. Lawrence N, Cox SE, Brody HG. Treatment of melasma with Jessner's solution vs. Glycolic acid: A comparison of clinical efficacy and evaluation of the predictive ability of Wood's light examination. J Am Acad Dermatol 1997; 36(4):589-593.
3. Draelos ZK. Skin Cleansers. In: Barry BK, ed. Cosmetics in Dermatology. New York: Churchill Livingstone, 1990: 153-157.
4. Krutson DD. Ultra Structural Observations in Acne Vulgaris: The normal sebaceous follicle and acne lesions. J Invest Dermatol 1994;62:308.
5. Murad H, Shamban AT, Moy LS, Moy RL. Study shows that acne improves with glycolic acid regimen. Cosmet Dermatol 1992;5(11):32-35.
6. Pusholl SM, Sakamoto M. A reevaluation of fatty acids as inflammatory agents in Acne. J Invest Dermatol 1977;68:93.
7. Moy LS, Murad H, Moy RL. Superficial Chemical Peels. In: Wheeland RG, ed. Cutaneous Surgery. Philadelphia: WB Saunders Co., 1994:463-478.
8. Burns RL, Prevost-Blank PL, Lawry, MA. Glycolic acid peels for postinflammatory hyperpigmentation in black patients. Dermatol Surg 1997;23:171-175.
9. Newman N, Newman A, Moy LS, Babapour R, Harris AG, Moy RL. Clinical improvement of photoaged skin with 50% glycolic acid. A double-blind vehicle-controlled study. Dermatol Surg 1996;22(5):455-460.
10. Moy LS, Peace S, Moy RL. Comparison of the effect of various chemical peeling agents in a mini-pig model. Dermatol Surg 1996;22(5):429-432.
11. Piacquadio D, Dobry M, Hunt S, Andree C, Grove G, Hollenbach KA. Short contact 70% glycolic acid peels as a treatment for photodamaged skin. A pilot study. Dermatol Surg 1996;22(5):449-452.
12. Coleman WP III. Chemical Peels for nonfacial areas. Cosmet Dermatol 1992;5(3):45-46.
13. Bennett RG. Cutaneous structure, function and repair. In: Bennett RG, ed. Fundamentals of Cutaneous Surgery. St. Louis: CV Mosby Co., 1988:17-89.
14. Fitzpatrick TB. The validity and practicality of sun reactive skin types I through VI. Arch Dermatol 1988;124: 869-871.
15. Glogau RG. Chemical peel symposium. American Academy of Dermatology. Atlanta Dec 4, 1990.
16. Brody HJ. General peeling concepts. In: Brody HJ, ed. Chemical Peeling and Resurfacing (2nd ed). St. Louis: Mosby Yearbook 1997:39-70.
17. Lawrence N, Coleman WP III, Brody HJ. Survey of Chemical peeling experts. Chemical peels course. Am Acad Dermatol, Feb 1996 Washington.
18. Hung VC, Lee JYY, Zitelli JA, Hebda PA. Topical tretinoin and epithelial wound healing. Arch Dermatol 1989;125: 65-69.
19. Hevia O, Nemeth AJ, Taylor JR. Tretinoin accelerates healing after trichloracetic acid chemical peel. Arch Dermatol 1991;127:678-682.
20. Kligman AM, Grove GL, Hirose R, Leyden JJ. Topical tretinoin for photoaged skin. J Am Acad Dermatol 1986;15(4 part 2):836-859.
21. Humphreys TR, Werth V, Dzubow L, Kligman A. Treatment of photodamaged skin with trichloracetic acid and topical tretinoin. J Am Acad Dermatol 1996;34(4):638-644.

22. Kaidbey KH, Kligman AM, Yoshida H. Effects of intensive application of retinoic acid in human skin. Br J Dermatol 1975;92:693-701.

23. Stiller MJ, Bartolone J, Stern R, Smith S, Kollias N, Gillies R, Drake LA. Topical 8% glycolic acid and 8% L-lactic acid creams for the treatment of photodamaged skin. A double-blind vehicle-controlled clinical trial. Arch Dermatol 1996;132:631-636.

24. Yi K, Hart LL. Use of hydroquinone as a bleaching cream. Ann Pharmacother 1993;27(5):592-593.

25. Peikert JM, Krywonis NA, Rest EB, Zachary CB. The efficacy of various degreasing agents used in trichloracetic acid peels. J Dermatol Surg Oncol 1994;20:724-728.

26. Matarasso SL, Glogau RG, Markey AC. Wood's lamp for superficial chemical peels, J Am Acad Dermatol 1994; 30(6):988-992.

27. Brodland DG, Cullimore KC, Roenigk RK. Depths of chemexfoliation induced by various concentrations and application of trichloracetic acid in a porcine model. J Dermatol Surg Oncol 1989;15:967-971.

28. Roberts HL. The chloracetic acids: A biochemical study. Br J Dermatol 1926;38:323-391.

29. Bridenstine JB, Dolezal JF. Standardizing chemical peel solution formulations to avoid mishaps. J Dermatol Surg Oncol 1994;20:813-816.

30. Brody HJ. Superficial peeling. In: Brody HJ, ed. Chemical Peeling and Resurfacing (2nd ed). St. Louis: Mosby Year-book 1997:73-108.

31. Dolezal JF. Stability study of trichloracetic acid (letter). J Dermatol Surg Oncol 1990;16:489-490.

32. Spinowitz AL, Rumsfield J. Stability-time profile of trichloracetic acid at various concentrations and storage conditions. J Dermatol Surg Oncol 1989;15:974-975.

33. Chiarello SE, Resnik BI, Resnik SS. The TCA masque. A new cream formulation used alone and in combination with Jessner's solution. Dermatol Surg 1996;22(8):687-90.

34. Van Scott EJ, Yu RJ. Therapeutic potentials. Can J Dermatol 1989;1:108-12.

35. Moy LS, Howe K, Moy RL. Glycolic acid modulation of collagen production in human skin fibroblasts cultures in vitro. Dermatol Surg 1996;22(5):439-441.

36. Brody H, Coleman III WP, Piacquadio D, Perricone NV, Elson ML, Harris D. Round table discussion of alpha hydroxy acids. J Dermatol Surg 1996;22(5):475-477.

37. Becker FF, Langford FP, Rubin MG, Speelman P. A histologic comparison of 50% and 70% glycolic acid peels using solutions with various pHs. Dermatol Surg 1996;22(5): 463-465.

38. Dormen MA. How to deliver good glycolic acid therapy. Dermatol Times 1997;18:50-54.

39. Berger R. Initial studies show salicylic acid promising as antiaging preparation. Cosmet Dermatol 1997;10(1):31-32.

40. Kligman D. Salicylic acid may rival glycolic peel. Skin and Allergy News 1997;28(1):1, 3.

41. Swinehart JM. Salicylic acid ointment peeling of the hands and forearms. J Dermatol Surg Oncol 1992;18:495-498.

42. Aronsohn RB. Hand chemosurgery. Am J Cosmet Surg 1984;1:24-28.

43. Letessier SM. Chemical peel with resorcin. In: Roenigk RK, Roenigk HH, eds. Dermatologic Surgery: Principles and Practice. New York: Marcel Dekker Inc., 1989:1017-1024.

44. Lawrence N, Brody HJ, Alt TH. Chemical peeling. In: Coleman III WP, Hanke W, eds. Cosmetic Surgery of the skin. St. Louis: Mosby 1997:86-112.

45. Karam PG. 50% Resorcinol peel. Intl J Dermatol 1993; 32(8):569-574.

46. Peikert JM, Kaye VN, Zachary CB. A reevaluation of the effect of occlusion on the trichloracetic acid peel. J Dermatol Surg Oncol 1994;20:660-665.

47. Weiss J, Ellis CN, Headington JT, Tincoff T, Hamilton TA. Topical tretinoin improves photoaged skin: A double-blind vehicle controlled study. JAMA 1988;259:527.

CHAPTER 7

Medium Depth Chemical Peeling

■ Gary D. Monheit

A scientific milestone in facial rejuvenation was the objective quantitation of injury depth for each peeling agent used in chemical peeling (1). Thus, the terms superficial, medium and deep chemical peel were developed as a universal gauge for evaluating methods and formulas of chemical peeling. Chemicals such as trichloracetic acid (TCA), phenol, and glycolic acid can now be compared and quantitated as to their efficacy, usefulness and safety. This classification of peeling agents emphasizes depth of penetration as a reflection of activity rather than chemical formulas. Thus labeling a peel as superficial, medium or deep is more meaningful than using chemical or brand names. A new understanding of peeling injury and repair has emerged along with an appreciation of variation in patient skin type, pigmentation and degree of photoaging. Using the Fitzpatrick and Glogau systems of skin pigmentation and sun damage, one can individualize the strength of chemical agents to match the skin pathology (2, 3).

Medium depth peeling is defined as the use of a chemical agent to wound skin to or through the papillary dermis. It creates changes through necrosis of the epidermis and part or all of the papillary dermis with an inflammatory reaction in the upper reticular dermis. This approach is most useful for removing epidermal or superficial lesions and improving skin texture in moderate photodamaged skin (grade II Glogau photoaging skin). The procedure is performed to remove actinic keratoses, mild photoaging of the skin including rhytides, treat pigmentary dyschromia, and improve depressed scars (4) (Table 7.1).

TCA has been the gold standard in quantitating chemical peel strength and depth. Concentrations of 10% to 30% TCA produce superficial wounding while concentrations above 50% cause deep chemical peeling.

Medium depth peeling is achieved with concentrations of 35% to 50% TCA. However, 45% or 50% TCA sometimes produces a wounding level of the mid to deep reticular dermis. This higher concentration of TCA has been found unreliable and is associated with an increased higher incidence of pigmentary dyschromia, textural change, and even scarring (5). However, 35% TCA alone may not produce significant dermal wounding in some patients.

In an attempt to reduce the morbidity of higher concentration TCA but still achieve effective medium depth peeling, combinations of chemical agents have been devised that improve the absorption of the lower TCA concentrations without the associated complications. The current combination peels include:

1. Solid carbon dioxide ice freezing with 35% TCA
2. Jessner's solution with 35% TCA
3. Glycolic acid 70% with 35% TCA

These combinations produce a more even peel with deeper penetration of the wounding agent without the associated complications of higher concentration TCA. This chapter will review the agents available for medium depth peeling, the patients and conditions most commonly treated, the techniques of application, wound healing, and complications.

TRICHLORACETIC ACID AS A SOLO PEELING AGENT

TCA has been used for chemical peeling for at least a century. It is popular for its versatility in peeling, and its chemical stability. TCA is useful in many concentrations because it has no systemic toxicity, can be employed to create superficial, medium or even deep wounds in the skin, and its peel depth in many instances correlates with the intensity of the frosting appearance of the skin. It is naturally found in crystalline form and is mixed with distilled water. It is not light sensitive, does not need refrigeration and is stable on the shelf for over 6 months. The standard concentrations of TCA should be mixed weight-by-volume to accurately assess the concentration. That is, 30 gm of TCA crystals mixed with 100 ml distilled water give an accurate 30% concentration, weight-by-volume. Any other dilutional systems (or volume dilutions weight by weight), are confusing and cannot be compared with the standard weight-by-volume measurements (6).

A typical medium depth TCA peel requires the use of 40% to 50% TCA as a solo wounding agent. Steps in this peel include preparation, cleansing the skin, layered application of acid, and recovery. The technique of application will be reviewed in the next section on the Jessner's TCA Peel, as this is the author's preferred medium depth peel. Skin preparation is of vital importance to encourage correct healing and avoid complica-

tions. Agents used prior to the peel to prepare the skin correctly include (7):

1. Sunscreen
2. Exfoliating agents–abrasive cleansers, 5% to 10% glycolic acid lotion
3. 0.05% to 0.1% Tretinoin used 6 weeks to 3 months in advance of the peel
4. Bleaching agents–hydroquinone 4% to 8% used on patients with pigmentary dyschromia and those with type III-VI Fitzpatrick skin pigmentation
5. Anti-viral agents in selected patients with a history of facial herpetic (HSV I or II) infections (Table 7.2)

The skin is cleansed thoroughly to remove excessive sebum and thickened stratum corneum for a more even peel. The TCA is then layered using cotton tip applicators or with 2 × 2 gauze pads. The endpoint for most medium depth chemical peels is a white frosting with slight erythema showing through. A solid white opaque frosting with TCA may indicate a deeper level of penetration. Care must be taken in the application of 45% to 50% TCA because high concentration TCA has a very quick reaction time on skin and frosts rapidly. Higher concentrations of TCA are much more difficult to control than the lower concentrations. TCA has a cumulative effect and the more applied, the deeper the penetration. With stronger concentrations one can easily overshoot the margin of safety and penetrate to the deeper reticular dermis causing unwanted side effects. If deeper dermal resurfacing is indicated, phenol peeling, dermabrasion, or lasers are more predictable at this depth. It is for this reason that most authorities have abandoned the use of 45% to 50% TCA as a medium depth or deep depth peeling agent. The

TABLE 7.1

MEDIUM DEPTH CHEMICAL PEELING AGENTS

1. 50% TCA
2. Brody version, solid CO_2 + 35% TCA
3. Monheit version, solid Jessner's solution + 35% TCA
4. Coleman version, Glycolic acid 70% + 35% TCA
5. 88% phenol
6. Jessner's solution + glycolic acid 70%
7. Pyruvic acid

TABLE 7.2

ADJUNCTIVE AGENTS IN CHEMICAL PEELING

Agent	Formula	Mechanism	Treatment Program
Tretinoin	Retin-A, retinoic acid .05%–0.1%	Decrease corneocyte adhesion, decrease stratum corneum thickness, increase epidermal, growth kinetic, affect new collagen production	Begin a QHS dosage 6 weeks prior to peeling and continue after re-epithelialization
Sunscreens	UVA and UVB block	Decrease pigmentation, darkening stimulation, decrease UV damage allowing the skin to rest prior to the peel	Begin 3 months prior to peel and continue thereafter
Bleach	Hydroquinone 4%–8%	Blocks production of new melanin	Begin 6 weeks prior to resurfacing and continue after re-epithelialization
Exfoliation	Abrasive scrubs for sloughing stratum corneum–glycolic acid, lactic acid, tartaric acid	Disrupts the stratum corneum to stimulate new epidermal growth. Decreased corneocyte adhesion.	Epidermabrasion begun 6 weeks prior to peeling, moisturization with glycolic acid lotions 6 weeks prior to peel.

author prefers a combination TCA peel for medium depth wounding.

COMBINATION PEELS

A combination chemical peel is the use of two peeling agents in conjunction to create a deeper peel than if only one of the agents was used. Because TCA concentrations above 40% have a higher incidence of complications, the use of combination peeling allows the physician to use a lower concentration of TCA (e.g., 35%) but have it penetrate as deeply as 50% TCA with few side effects.

The Brody Combination: Solid Carbon Dioxide Ice plus 35% TCA

Brody et al in 1986 first published the results of a combination procedure using a refrigerant that would injure the epidermal surface prior to the application of 35% TCA (8). Of the cryosurgical agents available, solid carbon dioxide ice (CO_2) was felt to be the safest and most reliable to use. This is because the temperature of the CO_2 block creates an epidermal injury without risk of a deeper dermal freeze. Liquid nitrogen and the aerosol refrigerants used for dermabrasion can create a freeze injury deep enough to induce hypopigmentation, textural change and scarring even without application of TCA (9).

Preoperative preparation for this peel is performed in the following manner. The patient may require preoperative sedation with sublingual diazepam and regional nerve blocks. After the skin is adequately cleansed with a povidone iodine solution, an alcohol wipe and an acetone scrub for 3 minutes, the areas of treatment are outlined. Deeper rhytides and thicker epidermal growths that will require a heavier CO_2 freeze are outlined for icing. The block of solid CO_2 is broken to hand size and then continually dipped in a 3:1 solution of acetone in alcohol so that the dry ice moves freely over the skin. Varying pressure is applied to induce micro-epidermal vesiculobullous formation over areas that require a deeper freeze. Manual pressure over the ice block and time of application determine the depth of freeze injury. Mild pressure is 3 to 5 seconds, moderate pressure is 5 to 8 seconds, and hard pressure is 8 to 15 seconds. Rhagades around the mouth, the shoulders of deeper furrows in the melolabial grooves, glabellar furrows, crow's feet, and the rims of acne scars are treated with hard pressure prior to the application of 35% TCA (9).

The skin is then wiped dry so that the TCA is not diluted, and then with dry gauze or cotton tip applicators, the 35% TCA is applied in a sequential fashion over the face. With the Brody technique, the most sensitive areas such as the eyelids, are treated first and then the nose, cheeks, and perioral area are treated in rapid succession followed by the least sensitive areas of the forehead.

TCA peeling with this concentration creates a burning and stinging which subsides at the conclusion of the peel. When the patient is ready to leave, he or she is usually comfortable with no further pain. Dr. Brody applies cool ice packs wrapped in paper towels after the frosting has occurred. After 5 minutes, a soothing emollient is applied. This peel will typically heal in 7-10 days using open occlusive wound healing techniques with frequent soaks and bland ointments.

The solid CO_2–35% TCA peel has a long history of usage and safety by Brody. Over 4,000 combination peels using this technique confirm the safety and efficacy of this combination peel (4). Histologic correlation has documented wound injury to the upper reticular dermis, the same as found with a 50% TCA peel. The destruction of elastotic material and the appearance of a Grenz zone of new collagen has confirmed the histologic appearance of a mid dermal injury pattern (8).

Though this technique has been proven safe, effective, and objectively accurate as a mid to deep dermal peel, its popularity has not caught on because of the materials and technique. Solid CO_2 is difficult to maintain and store and is technique sensitive in its usage. Those who do use this technique as their medium depth peel, however, feel that it reliably can produce better results than other combinations currently available, especially for acne scars and thicker epidermal growths such as hypertrophic actinic keratoses and seborrheic keratoses.

The Monheit Combination: Jessner's Solution plus 35% TCA

The use of Jessner's solution before a 35% TCA peel has been found to be an efficacious method of producing medium depth wounding similar to the Brody peel (10). The Jessner's solution, a superficial peeling agent employed for many decades, disrupts the barrier function of the skin allowing more rapid and uniform TCA penetration than if it were applied to untreated skin. Jessner's solution is made up of the following ingredients:

1. Resorcinol (14 gm)
2. Salicylic acid (14 gm)
3. 85% Lactic acid (14 gm)
4. Ethanol to make 100 ml

Jessner's solution maintains its strength and stability on the shelf for over one year but is light and air sensitive and may develop a yellow color. It is important that Jessner's solution be compounded correctly in both percentages and ingredients. Fresh resorcinol should be used along with light-protected salicylic acid. The ingredients are solids; thus computation should be weight-in-volume (wv) in ethanol USP. Ethanol should be used in place of denatured alcohol as the latter product has an unreliable interaction with the solid compounds. It is best to advise one's pharmacy or pharmaceutical house as to the specifics of compounding

Jessner's solution to obtain a stable and reliable wounding agent.

The Jessner's–TCA peel has superior results for the following indications:

1. Removal of epidermal lesions–actinic keratoses, lentigines, seborrheic keratoses
2. Treatment of moderate photoaging skin–Glogau level II
3. Pigmentary dyschromia
4. Blending facial areas in conjunction with deep peeling or laser resurfacing

The technique for each of these indications is similar as to preparation, cleansing, application of acids, and postoperative care and produces similar results.

Preparation

The use of sunscreens, exfoliative preparations, tretinoin, and bleaching agents as needed (pigmentary dyschromia or Fitzpatrick type III-VI skin) is similar to other medium depth peels (11). Moderate sedation is used during the peel and can consist of diazepam 5 to 10 mg orally or sublingually, meperidine 25 mg (Demerol [Sanofi Winthrop Pharmaceuticals, New York, NY]), or hydroxyzine 25 mg intramuscularly (Vistaril [Pfizer Laboratories, Inc., New York, NY]). Concurrently, acetyl salicylic aspirin (aspirin or Bufferin [Bristol-Myers Squibb, Princeton, NJ]) grains ten are given prior to the peel and then every 4 hours after the peel for relief of discomfort. As with other medium depth TCA peels, the patient is comfortable after the peel is concluded and the aspirin is all that is needed postoperatively in most cases as an anti-inflammatory.

Cleansing

Vigorous cleansing and degreasing is necessary for an even penetration of the Jessner's solution. The face is scrubbed gently with Ingasam (Septisol [Vestal Laboratories, St. Louis, MO]), 4 × 4 gauze pads and water, then rinsed, dried and repeated twice. Next, acetone is applied to remove residual oils and debris. The skin is essentially debrided of stratum corneum and excessive scale. Care must be taken to thoroughly degrease oilier areas such as the hair line, the temples, nose, and upper lip for an even, fully penetrant peel.

Application of Acids

After cleansing is complete, Jessner's solution is applied with either cotton tip applicators or 2 × 2 gauze pads. The Jessner's solution is applied evenly with usually one or two coats to achieve a light but even frosting. The frosting achieved with Jessner's solution is much lighter than that produced by TCA and the patient is usually comfortable, experiencing only heat and mild stinging. The endpoint visually is a fairly uniform erythema with areas of splotchy white frosting

(Fig. 7.1). An even coating of Jessner's solution is necessary to enhance an even penetration of the TCA (12). A Wood's light can be used to further visualize how complete the application of Jessner's solution is. The salicylic acid in Jessner's solution fluoresces under Wood's light, giving the physician an additional method to ensure even coverage with the Jessner's solution (13). One must wait 5 minutes after the application of Jessner's solution to allow full penetration before applying the TCA.

The TCA is then applied evenly with either cotton tip applicators or saturated 2 × 2 gauze pads. The author prefers using cotton tip applicators because the amount of TCA applied can be quantitated. Four heavily saturated cotton tip applicators are used over broad, expansive surfaces such as the forehead and cheeks. Two or three are used on the temples, chin and upper lips, one or two on the nose, and one damp cotton tip applicator is used on the eyelids and periorbital skin. Broad strokes are used to evenly apply the first coating of TCA over the unit area. Anatomic areas of the face are peeled sequentially from the forehead to temple to cheeks, finally to the lips, nose and eyelids. One must then wait one or two minutes for the reaction of frosting to be complete. The time it takes for the frosting to achieve its maximal reaction is dependent upon intrinsic skin sensitivity, degree of photodamage (the greater the photodamage, the longer the reaction time and thus the more TCA needed), the degree of preparation (prepared skin frosts quicker and more evenly), and the amount and strength of TCA applied. After the reaction is completed, a second layer of TCA may be applied to unfrosted or poorly frosted areas. The physician should look for a consistent degree of frosting over a pink background to achieve medium depth results (Fig. 7.2). Areas of poor frosting should be retreated carefully with a thin application of TCA. The white frosting indicates protein coagulation and at this point, the reaction is complete. For this reason, TCA cannot be neutralized once the reaction has occurred. It can only be diluted prior to keratocoagulation, usually within the first 30 seconds after application (11).

Careful feathering of the solution into the hairline, brows and around the rim of the jaw conceals the line of demarcation between peeled and non-peeled areas. The perioral area often has rhytides that require a complete and even application of solution over the lip skin on to the vermilion. This is accomplished best with the help of an assistant who stretches and fixates the upper lip and lower lip while the peel solution is applied with the wooden tip of the applicator.

Certain areas and skin lesions require special attention. Thick keratoses do not frost evenly and thus do not pick up enough peel solution. Additional applications rubbed vigorously into the lesions with a cotton-tip ap-

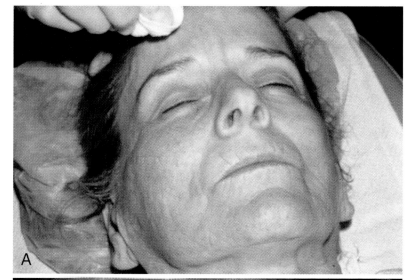
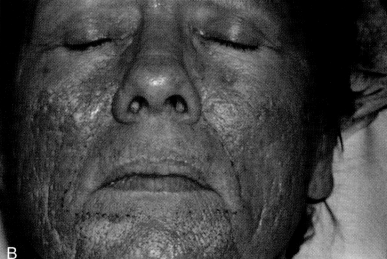

FIGURE 7.1
A, Jessner's solution applied with 2 × 2 gauze sponges.
B, End point of Jessner's solution is erythema with
blotchy frosting.

plicator may be needed for peel solution penetration. Wrinkled skin should be stretched to allow an even coating of solution into the folds and troughs. Deeper furrows, such as expression lines, will not be eradicated by the peel solution and should be treated like the remaining skin.

Eyelid skin must be treated delicately and carefully. A semi-dry applicator should be used to carry the solution within 2 to 3 mm of the lid margin. The patient should be positioned with the head elevated at a 30° angle and told to look upward, stretching the lower eyelid to its maximum. Excess peel solution on the cotton tip should be drained and the applicator then rolled gently on the lower lid in a clockwise movement which will push the lid upward. Never leave excessive peel solution on the lids because the solution can leak into the eyes. Two dry cotton tip applicators are used to blot both canthi, preventing tears to form which can pull peel solution hygroscopically into the eye. The upper lid is treated with the eye closed and a damp cotton tip

applicator rolled in a counterclockwise fashion, pushing the lid downward (Fig. 7.3).

There is an immediate burning sensation as the peel solution is applied, but this subsides as frosting is completed. After the peel is completed, cool saline compresses are placed over the areas for symptomatic relief. It is important to complete the peel prior to the application of the saline compresses as further application of TCA is diluted by the saline absorbed in the stratum corneum (14). After 5 to 6 minutes, the patient is comfortable and most of the frosting has faded into a brawny, shiny appearance.

Postoperative Care

Postoperatively, edema, erythema and desquamation are expected. Eyelid edema can occur as well as significant perioral edema. For the first 24 hours, the patient is instructed to soak four times a day with a 0.25% solution acetic acid compress made of one tablespoon of white vinegar in one pint of warm

FIGURE 7.2
The intensity of the frost correlates to the evenness of peel penetration. A, Thin, pale white. B, White to grey white. C, Solid white.

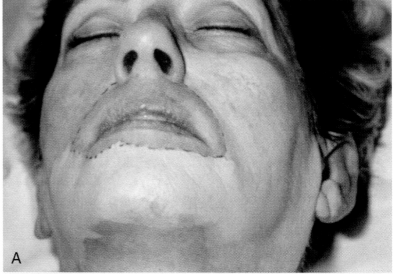

A

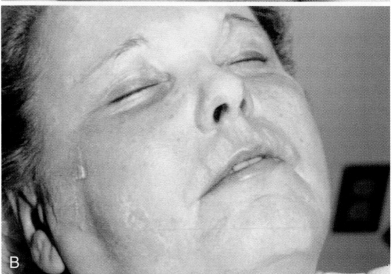

B

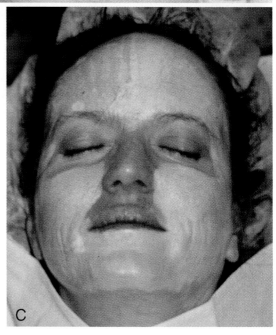

C

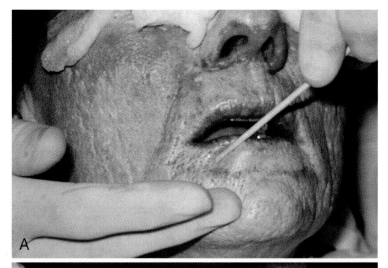

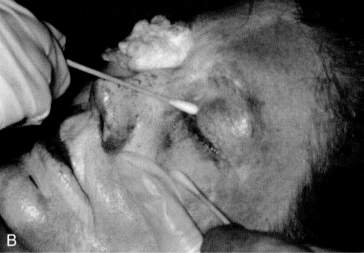

FIGURE 7.3

A, Perioral rhagades are stretched and peel solution is applied with a cotton tip applicator. B, Dry cotton tip applicators are used around the eyes to prevent tearing.

water. A bland emollient is applied to the desquamating areas after soaks. This emollient can be Eucerin cream (Beiersdorf Inc., S. Norwalk, CT), Aquaphor ointment (Beiersdorf Inc.), or Vaseline petrolatum jelly (Chesebrough-Ponds, Inc., Greenwich, CT). After 24 hours, the patient can shower and clean gently with a mild, nondetergent cleanser. The erythema intensifies as desquamation becomes complete within 4 to 5 days. Most healing is completed within 7 to 10 days. At the end of 1 week, the bright red color fades to pink and has the appearance of a sunburn. This can be covered by cosmetics and will fade fully within 2 to 3 weeks.

Results

This medium depth peel usually produces superior results for the conditions listed (Table 7.3). Removal of actinic keratoses, both present and incipient, affords the patient a single procedure with a healing time of 7 to 10 days as a preventive therapeutic modality for removing precancerous growths over the face (Fig. 7.4). A com-

TABLE 7.3

INDICATIONS FOR MEDIUM DEPTH CHEMICAL PEELING

1. Epidermal growths
2. Moderate Photoaging Skin–Glogau grade II
3. Pigmentary Dyschromias
4. Mild to Moderate Acne Scars
5. Blending Photoaging Skin with Laser Resurfacing and Deep Chemical Peeling

parison study of the efficacy of Jessner's solution with 35% TCA and 5-fluorouracil documented superior effectiveness of this single procedure with a significant reduction in morbidity (15). It is, thus, an effective, safe and simple single procedure that can be used to remove actinic keratoses and epidermal growths as both a therapeutic and cosmetic procedure.

Glogau grade II photoaging skin can be effectively treated for improvement in both texture, color change, and epidermal growths with a medium depth Jessner's–TCA peel. Of equal importance to the procedure is choosing the correct patient for the procedure. Patients with superficial textural changes and those with epidermal growths seem to respond best to this peel. Fine wrinkles, cross-hatched lines, sallow color changes of photoaging along with the crinkly appearance are the textural changes that will respond to this peel. Additionally, epidermal growths such as freckles, lentigines, actinic keratoses, and seborrheic keratoses will also re-

FIGURE 7.4
A, Preoperative patient undergoing a Jessner's–35% TCA peel for the removal of actinic keratoses. B, Appearance after Jessner's solution. C, Frosting after TCA.

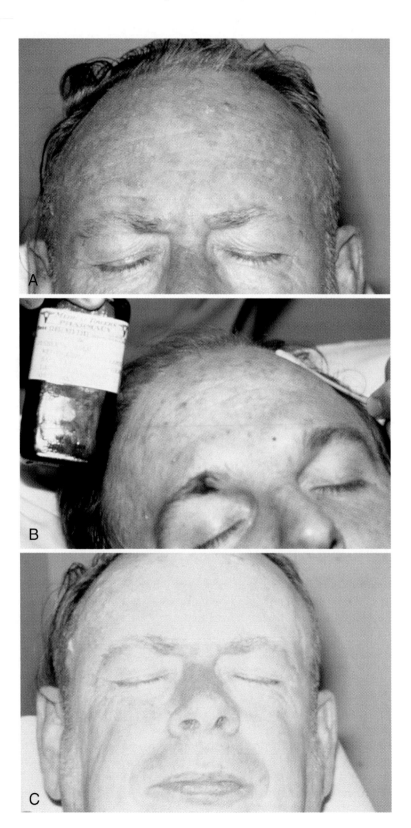

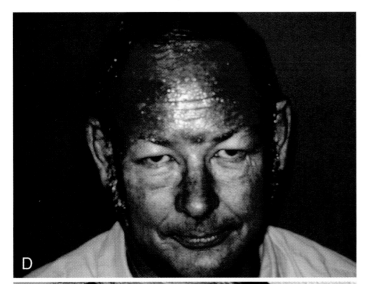

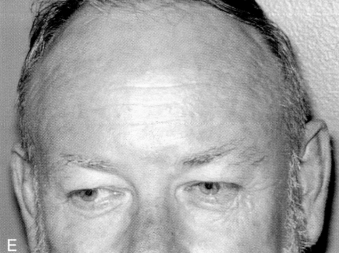

FIGURE 7.4 (continued)
D, Appearance 3 days postoperatively. E, Appearance 3 weeks postoperative.

spond well (Fig. 7.5). The more advanced changes seen with deeper grooves and wrinkles, pebbly appearance of the skin and more pronounced gravitational changes of Glogau III and IV photoaging skin require either deep chemical peeling, dermabrasion, or laser resurfacing. Use of TCA or any of its combinations as a deep chemical peel for these more advanced indications will only risk potential side effects and complications.

Pigmentary dyschromia such as melasma, blotchy hyperpigmentation, and pigmentary growths do respond well to medium depth chemical peeling. This peel is especially suited for those problems that have not resolved optimally with medical treatment or repeated light chemical peeling. Epidermal pigment seems to respond the best and this can be identified with Wood's light examination. Dermal pigment will show some response but not as predictably as epidermal pigment. This combination peel is effective in that it fully removes the epidermis as well as affects melanocytes in the pilar appa-

ratus during re-epithelialization. It is important that these patients be prepared correctly with 4% to 8% hydroquinone, tretinoin and sunscreen application begun at least 6 weeks prior to the peeling procedure. The bleaching agent is reinstituted after re-epithelialization and tretinoin 6 weeks later. It should be continued for up to 3 months after the chemical peel and sunscreen used indefinitely to ensure that dyschromia does not return. There are many bleaching agents on the market today that have some lightening effect, but hydroquinone is the most effective.

When localized areas of the face have advanced or severe photoaging such as deeper wrinkles around the eyelids and rhagades on the lips, the combination Jessner's–TCA peel can be used to blend the remaining areas of the face if they have only moderate photoaging of the skin. The eyelids and lips can be resurfaced with a pulsed CO_2 laser and the remainder of the face treated with the Jessner's–TCA peel. In this instance, the peel should be performed first in the manner described above

FIGURE 7.5
Jessner's–TCA peel for moderate photoaging skin,
Glogau level II. A, Preoperative photo demonstrating
rhytides, lentigines, keratoses and sallow skin. B, Jessner's
solution applied to face. C, Full application of 35% TCA
with solid white frosting.

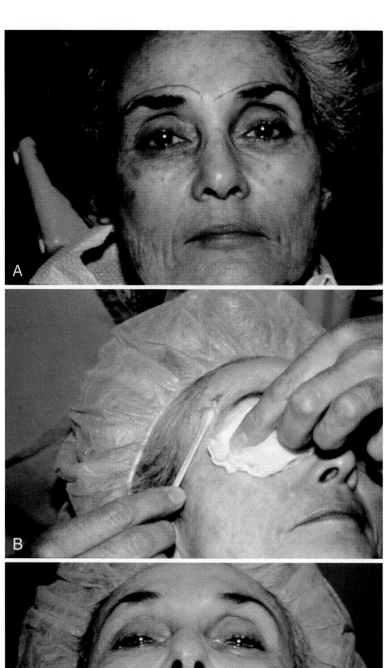

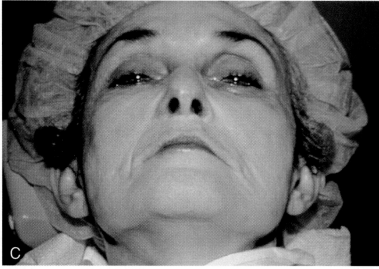

and then using appropriate anesthesia, eye protection
and preparation, laser the designated areas. Healing occurs in the usual manner for either laser or peel procedures with soaks and occlusive ointments. This combined approach is an effective method of reducing morbidity with deeper agents to areas that do not need them.
It will also blend the photoaging skin, texture, color and
appearance to that of the laser treated skin (16) (Fig. 7.6).

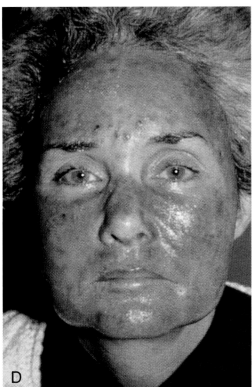 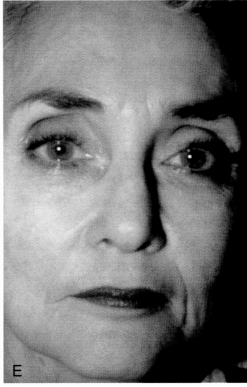

FIGURE 7.5
(continued)
D, Appearance 4 days postoperatively. E, Appearance 6 months postoperatively.

The Coleman Combination: Glycolic Acid plus 35% TCA

The combination of 70% glycolic acid and 35% TCA is another combined peel designed to improve the efficacy of 35% TCA without the risks and complications of higher strength TCA (17). Chemicals, methodology and techniques are different so that one must have a thorough understanding of this peel and not use the methods of the preceding combination peel or TCA alone. This combination peel produces a similar wounding depth to the Jessner's–TCA combination peel as demonstrated in histologic studies, but a significantly greater wound level than 35% TCA alone (18). It has also demonstrated the ability to stimulate new collagen production with a comparable Grenz zone to the other medium depth peels. Application of the glycolic acid prior to the TCA peel allows for an even debridement of the stratum corneum similar to that obtained with a degreasing procedure and the Jessner's solution (18).

In this procedure, no cleansing or degreasing procedure is done. After washing the face with soap and water, unbuffered 70% glycolic acid is applied directly to the patient's facial skin with a rectal swab and, after a strict 2 minute contact period, the solution is removed with tap water. Next, the 35% TCA is applied in a sequential pattern with either cotton tip applicators or 4 × 4 gauze pads to the entire face. The usual frosting is obtained and cool compresses are placed to alleviate the stinging and burning.

This combination peel has also been found effective in the treatment of actinic keratoses and epidermal growths, Glogau grade II photoaging skin, and pigmentary dyschromia. The same skin preparations are used with the other combination peels in a similar postoperative wound care regimen. Advantages of this peel are that most physicians are already familiar with the use of glycolic acid and its time-dependent action. It is a fairly simple learning curve to add the 35% TCA onto this already established chemical peel. Drawbacks can include the uneven nature of glycolic acid peeling and the possibility of accentuating "TCA hot spots." In addition, the use of water to neutralize the glycolic acid may theoretically inhibit some TCA absorption for the second part of this combination peel, but this can be prevented by thorough drying of the skin before TCA application (19). Although these are theoretical points, in practicality, Dr. Coleman has demonstrated excellent results with this combination medium depth peel.

Other medium depth peels include:

1. Full strength unoccluded phenol peel
2. Pyruvic acid (alphaketo acid)
3. Jessner's–Glycolic acid peel

Eighty-eight percent phenol has the ability to wound through the papillary dermis similar to other peeling strengths discussed. Its disadvantage is inherent in the absorption of phenol with potential for significant cardiac and hepato renal toxicity. For this reason, the other peels discussed have significant advantages.

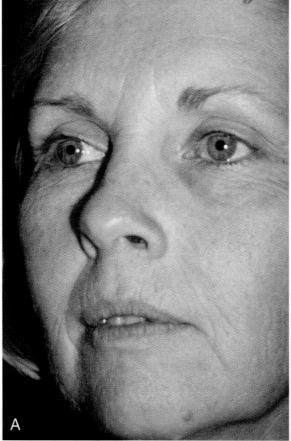

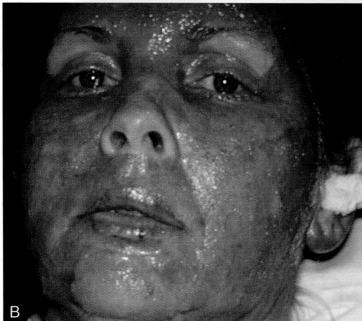

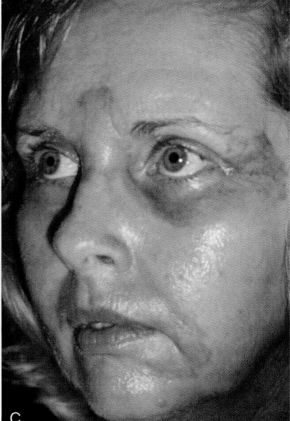

FIGURE 7.6
Combination laser resurfacing and Jessner's–35% TCA peel. A, Preoperative areas for laser (perioral and periorbital) and peel over the remainder of the face. B, Immediate appearance postoperatively. C, Appearance 3 months postoperatively.

Pyruvic acid is an alpha keto acid that is a very potent chemical peeling agent and has been used experimentally for photoaging skin. The rapid dermal penetration has the potential for scarring and side effects and though some results have been demonstrated by Griffin

to be excellent, its safety and efficacy has not been well established (20).

The Jessner's solution and glycolic acid combination peel has two theoretical advantages: 1) Jessner's solution allows for deeper penetration of the glycolic acid, and 2)

The glycolic acid will be a greater stimulant for collagen regeneration without further exfoliation. Since this technique is both time-dependent and restricted to visual endpoints, the chances for over treating are great which may create potential side effects and complications.

POSTOPERATIVE CARE AND COMPLICATIONS

The four stages of wound healing are apparent after a medium depth chemical peel (21). They include:

1. Inflammation
2. Coagulation
3. Re-epithelialization
4. Fibroplasia

At the conclusion of the chemical peel, the inflammatory phase has already begun with a brawny, dusky erythema that will progress over the first 12 hours. The epidermis begins to separate with the medium depth peels, creating a leathery, dry, cracking appearance to the epidermis. There is an accentuation of pigmented lesions on the skin as the coagulation phase separates the epidermis, producing serum exudation, crusting and pyoderma. It is during this phase that it is important to use debriding soaks and compresses as well as occlusive salves. These will remove the sloughed necrotic epidermis and prevent the serum exudate from hardening as a crust and scab. I prefer the use of 1/4% acetic acid soaks found in the vinegar water preparation (1 tsp. white vinegar, 1 pt. warm water), as it is antibacterial, especially against pseudomonas and gram negative bacteria. In addition, the mildly acidic nature of the solution is physiologic for the healing granulation tissue, mildly debriding, as it will dissolve and cleanse the necrotic material and serum. Occlusive dressings include bland emollients and salves and semipermeable biosynthetic membranes. For medium depth peeling, I prefer the occlusive salves since healing can be visually monitored carefully day by day for potential complications.

Re-epithelialization begins on day three and continues until day seven to ten. Occlusive salves promote faster re-epithelialization and lessen the tendency of delayed healing (22). The final stage of fibroplasia continues well beyond the initial closure of the peeled wound and continues with neoangiogenesis and new collagen formation for 3 or 4 months. Prolonged erythema may last 2 to 4 months in unusual cases of sensitive skin or with contact dermatitis. New collagen formation can continue to improve texture and rhytides for a period up to 4 months during this last phase of fibroplasia.

Many of the complications seen in peeling can be recognized early during healing stages. The cosmetic surgeon should be well acquainted with the normal appearance of a healing wound in its time frame for medium depth peeling. Prolongation of the granulation tissue phase beyond 1 week may indicate delayed wound healing. This could be the result of viral, bacterial or fungal infection, contact irritants interfering with wound healing, or other systemic factors. This "red flag" should alert the physician that careful investigation and prompt treatment should be instituted to forestall potential irreparable damage that may result in scarring. Thus, it is vitally important to understand the stages of wound healing in reference to medium depth peeling. The physician then can avoid, recognize and treat any and all complications early. Specific complications are discussed in Chapter 26.

Long term care of peeled skin includes sunscreen protection for up to 6 months along with reinstitution of medical treatment such as low strength hydroxy acid lotions and tretinoin. Repeat peels should not be performed for 6 months from the previous peel. If any erythema or edema persists, the peel should not be performed since reinjury may create complications. Medium depth peels should not be performed on undermined skin such as facelift or flap surgery performed up to 6 months prior to the peel (11).

The evolution of medium depth chemical peeling has changed the face of cosmetic surgery. Medium depth peeling is a new technique in the cosmetic surgeon's armamentaria that treats skin problems that were previously approached with inadequate tools and obtains positive results for moderate photoaging skin while avoiding overly-aggressive treatment using deep peeling agents. The combination peels have provided some of the more popular tools needed to approach a burgeoning population with photoaging skin.

REFERENCES

1. Stegman SJ. A comparative histologic study of the effects of three peeling agents and dermabrasion on normal and sundamaged skin. Aesthetic Plast Surg 1982;6:123-135.
2. Fitzpatrick TB. The validity and practicality of sun-reactive skin types I through VI. Archiv Dermatol 1988;124:869-871.
3. Glogau RG. Chemical peeling and aging skin. J Geriatr Dermatol 1994;2(1):30-35.
4. Brody HJ. Chemical peeling and resurfacing. Mosby, 1997:109-110.
5. Brody HJ. Trichloracetic acid application in chemical peeling, operative techniques. Plast Reconstr Surg 1995;2(2):127-128.
6. Dolezal J. Trichloracetic acid solutions and basic pharmacy. In: Manual of Chemical Peels. Rubin M, ed. Philadelphia: J.B. Lippincott, 1995:112-114.
7. Monheit GD. Skin preparation: an essential step before chemical peeling or laser resurfacing. Cosmet Dermatol 1996;9:9-14.
8. Brody HJ, Hailey CW. Medium depth chemical peeling of the skin: a variation of superficial chemosurgery. J Dermatol Surg Oncol 1986;12:1268-1275.
9. Brody HJ. Variations and comparisons in medium depth chemical peeling. J Dermatol Surg Oncol 1989;15:953-963.

10. Monheit GD. The Jessner's + TCA peel: a medium depth chemical peel. J Dermatol Surg Oncol 1989;15:945-950.
11. Monheit GD. Advances in chemical peeling. Facial Plast Surg Clin North Am 1994;2:5-9.
12. Monheit GD. The Jessner's-trichloracetic acid peel. Dermatol Clin 1995;13(2):277-283.
13. Matarasso SL, Glogau RG. Chemical face peels. Dermatol Clin 1991;9:131-150.
14. Rubin M. Manual of chemical peels. Philadelphia: J.B. Lippincott, 1995:120-121.
15. Lawrence N, Cox SE, Cockerell CJ, et.al. A comparison of efficacy and safety of Jessner's solution and 35% trichloracetic acid vs. 5% fluorouracil in the treatment of widespread facial actinic keratoses. Arch Dermatol 1995;131:176-181.
16. Monheit GD. Skin resurfacing for photoaging: laser resurfacing vs. chemical peeling. Cosmet Dermatol 1997;10:11-22.
17. Coleman WP, Futrell JM. The glycolic acid and trichloracetic acid peel. J Dermatol Surg Oncol 1994;20:76-80.
18. Brody HJ. Chemical peeling and resurfacing. St Louis: Mosby, 1997:21-22.
19. Rubin M. Manual of chemical peels. Philadelphia: Lippincott Co, 1995; p 129.
20. Griffin TD, Van Scott EJ, Madden S. The use of pyruvic acid in the treatment of actinic keratoses: a clinical and histopathologic study. Cutis 1991;47:325-329.
21. Fazio MJ, Zitelli JB, Goslen JB. Wound healing. In: Coleman WP, Hanke CW, Alt TH, et al. eds. Cosmetic Surgery of the Skin. 2nd ed. St. Louis: Mosby, 1997:18-38.
22. Maibach HF, Rovec DT. Epidermal wound healing. St. Louis: Mosby, 1972:72-95.

Facial Rejuvenation: Phenol-based Chemexfoliation

■ William H. Beeson

The concept of cutaneous rejuvenation is not a contemporary idea. For centuries, people have strived to aesthetically improve the skin. Reports of chemexfoliation date back to the ancient Egyptians (1, 2). At the beginning of the 20th century, Unna, a German dermatologist, documented the use of phenol peels (3). In the early 1900s another dermatologist, Mackee, further advanced these chemical exfoliation techniques (4). At the midpoint of this century, chemical face peeling took a new dimension when Urkov (1946), and Gillies reported on chemical exfoliation using phenol (5, 6). However, peels were primarily confined to clandestine procedures performed by cosmetologists until Litton, Baker, and Gordon advocated the use of phenol-based peels in facial cosmetic surgery (7–9). Throughout the 1970s and even today, the phenol-based peel remains the gold standard for cutaneous rejuvenation and the standard to which other treatment modalities are compared; even though the potential problems of cutaneous scarring and hypopigmentation associated with phenol-based peels does occur (10).

Traditionally, chemical peels are used to treat photodamaged skin. However, there are a variety of indications for chemical peels. Many laymen and physicians have the misconception that a facelift is the panacea for treatment of the aging face. In reality, a chemical face peel alone or in combination with a facelift may be the most appropriate form of treatment. Chemical face peeling for deep facial rhytides, actinic keratoses, hyperpigmentation and some specific acne scarring conditions has long been an accepted modality (11). Surgery alone cannot eliminate deep facial rhytides; chemexfoliation can. In addition, chemical face peeling may provide more "tightening" of facial tissues, thus making it an important primary and adjunctive procedure for the facial cosmetic surgeon.

INDICATIONS

To obtain the best and most consistent results with chemical face peeling, the surgeon must know the limitations of the procedure and the expectation of each patient who seeks help. There is no substitute for experience when selecting the patient for this procedure, but there are helpful guidelines. Ideally, patients are thin-skinned women with fair complexions and fine generalized wrinkling. These individuals are less likely to have pigmentary contrasts at the margins of the peeled area and less spotty pigmentation that can occur in darker olive skinned patients. Men are not generally as favorable candidates for chemical face peeling as are women, due to potential problems with hypopigmentation. The following are conditions in which chemical face peeling have produced favorable results:

1. Fine facial wrinkles, particularly in the perioral and periorbital regions
2. Pigmentary dyschromia
3. Actinic keratoses
4. Superficial acne scarring

The aging process is dynamic, not static. As we age, the skin loses its elasticity, the muscles atrophy, and there is a redistribution of adipose tissue. The rate of the aging process is influenced by many factors such as stress, nutrition, and general health. However, primary influences on skin aging are the environmental factors of wind and sun.

Understanding the histology of photoaging is important because it has such a significant influence on the aging process. In this process, the epidermis is variably thinned, the cells have pyknotic nuclei, and there is a loss of vertical polarity to cells in the epidermis. The basement membrane is thickened, and there is an uneven distribution of melanocytes. In the dermis, elastosis is the hallmark of sun damaged skin. The dermis consists of thickened, coiled, and tangled masses of ultra-elastic fibers. As we age, the dermis is almost completely replaced by damaged elastic fibers that normally make up less than 5% of the dermis by weight. As elastosis deepens, collagen disappears proportionally. Thus, skin has little resistance to stretching.

As with any surgical procedure, caution must be exercised in regard to patient selection. Determining the patient's skin type is of paramount importance in determining which type of chemexfoliation (superficial, medium, or deep) may provide the patient with the most satisfactory results. Fitzpatrick's classification provides a measure of pigmentary responsiveness of the skin to ultraviolet light (Table 8.1) (12). When skin type is combined with eye color in the patient evaluation process, one is better able to predict which chemexfoliation agent will produce the most favorable response. In general terms, patients who are types I-III are ideal for phenol-based chemexfoliation. Patients who are types IV-VI can undergo phenol-based chemexfoliation, but are at greater risk for pigmentary changes.

Glogau also developed a classification system that can aid patient selection for chemexfoliation (Table 8.2) (13). One cannot generalize and treat all groups with a specific treatment modality. For example, groups I and II cannot always be treated with superficial or medium depth peels and groups III and IV cannot always be treated with deep chemexfoliation. As Brody has pointed out, every cosmetic unit of the skin, from the perioral, periorbital, and cheek area to the forehead and nasal area, should be individually assessed to determine which peeling agent or procedure is necessary for the best correction of the area without undue risk (Tables 8.3 and 8.4) (13).

The treatment for premalignant lesions and severe epithelial dysplasia following actinic exposure has long been recognized as a principal indication for chemical face peeling (14). Roenigk noted that treatment of actinic keratoses may decrease the incidence of basal and squamous cell carcinoma (15). Although modalities such as cryotherapy are effective, in many cases, the number of actinic keratoses is such that a more complete facial treatment, such as full face phenol-based chemexfoliation, is more appropriate. Phenol-based chemexfoliation has been shown to be an appropriate modality for treating a variety of skin pigmentation disorders, melasma being the most frequent.

Melasma is a relatively common acquired systemic hypermelanosis characterized by irregular light to grey-brown maculas involving sun-exposed areas. Grimes has pointed out that there is a predilection for involve-

TABLE 8.1

FITZPATRICK'S CLASSIFICATION FOR SUN-REACTIVE SKIN TYPES

Skin Type	Color	Reaction to First Summer Exposure
I	White	Always burn, never tan
II	White	Usually burn, tan with difficulty
III	White	Sometimes mild burn, tan average
IV	Moderate brown	Rarely burn, tan with ease
V	Dark brown	Very rarely burn, tan very easily
VI	Black	Tan very easily

TABLE 8.2

GLOGAU'S CLASSIFICATION OF PHOTOAGING GROUPS

Group I-Mild (usually 28-35 years old)
No keratoses
Little wrinkling
No scarring
Little or no makeup

Group II-Moderate (usually age 35-50 years old)
Early actinic keratoses-slight yellow skin discoloration
Early wrinkling
Parallel smile lines
Mild scarring
Little makeup

Group III-Advanced (usually 50-60 years old)
Actinic keratoses, obvious yellow skin discoloration with telangiectasias
Wrinkling-present at rest
Moderate acne scarring
Wears makeup always

Group IV-Severe (usually 60-75 years old)
Actinic keratoses and skin cancers have occurred
Wrinkling-much cutis laxa of actinic gravitational and dynamic origin
Severe acne scarring-wears makeup that is caked on

Adapted from Glogau RG. Chemical peeling and aging skin. J Geriatr Dermatol 1994;2(2)30-35.

TABLE 8.3

INDICATIONS AND PEEL DEPTH

Indications	Peel Depth for Best Response
Actinic keratoses	Medium or Deep
Facial rhytides Very mild	Superficial or Medium
Mild	Medium
Moderate	Medium or Deep
Severe	Deep

Adapted from Brody HJ. Chemical peeling and resurfacing. St. Louis: C.V. Mosby, 1997.

TABLE 8.4

PIGMENTARY DYSCHROMIAS

Indications	Peel Depth for Best Response
Melasma-Superficial	Superficial or Medium
Melasma-Combined	Superficial, Medium, or Deep
Post-inflammatory hyperpigmentation	Superficial, Medium, or Deep
Ephelides (Freckles)-Basal cell layer	Superficial or Medium
Lentigenes-Basal cell layer and upper dermis	Superficial or Medium

ment of the cheeks, forehead, upper lip, nose, and chin (16). The disease is most commonly observed in women with men representing only 10% of cases. Melasma affects all racial groups, but is most prevalent in darker-complexioned individuals (skin types IV–VI). Although the precise cause of melasma is unknown, multiple factors are implicated in its ideology. These factors include the use of oral contraceptives, estrogen-progesterone therapies, pregnancy, exposure to UV radiation, thyroid disfunction, cosmetics, phototoxic and antiseizure drugs, as well as genetic influences.

Three clinical patterns of hyperpigmentation are recognized in patients with melasma. These include centrofacial, malar, and mandibular patterns. Based on a Wood's light examination of the skin, melasma can be divided into three types (epidermal, dermal, and mixed) (17). The epidermal variety is characterized by increased melanin in the basal, suprabasal, and stratum corneum layers. The pigmentation is intensified by Wood's light examination. Dermal melasma has a predominance of melanin in the superficial dermis and in the deep dermis; pigmentation with dermal melasma is not intensified by Wood's light examination. The mixed variety exhibits both epidermal and dermal pigment alterations. Because of its ability to inhibit the production of melanin and melanocytes, the phenol-based chemical peel is an important modality for the treatment of melasma (Table 8.5).

Temporary and permanent alterations in color remain the most significant limiting factors in deep chemical peeling and are the major driving forces behind the preoperative classification schemes. It is relatively easy to select the peeling regimen on the basis of rhytides that one wishes to correct. It is much more difficult to successfully manage the pigmentary alterations that are a predictable sequence of peeling (13).

TABLE 8.5

CLASSIFICATION OF PEELING AGENTS

Class	Type of Peeling Agent	Depth of Penetration
Superficial	10%-25% Trichloracetic acid Jessner's solution Alphahydroxy acids (30%-70% glycolic acid) Carbon dioxide Snow	0.06 mm (stratum granulosum to superficial papillary dermis)
Medium	88% Phenol (full strength) 35%-50% Trichloracetic acid	0.45 mm (papillary to upper reticular dermis)
Deep	Baker-Gordon phenol formula (occluded, nonoccluded)	0.6 mm mid reticular dermis

Adapted from Glogau, Matarasso. Dermatol Clin 1995 Apr;13(2):263.

RELATIVE CONTRAINDICATIONS

There are relative contraindications to deep phenol peels, depending upon the patient's skin type and medical history. Since phenol is cardiotoxic and may predispose the patient to arrhythmias, those individuals with cardiac disease may not be appropriate candidates. Likewise, the phenol is cleared through the renal and hepatic system. Thus, individuals with hepatic or renal disease may not adequately metabolize the peel solution.

Active herpes simplex infections, should be allowed to heal prior to chemexfoliation. If there is a history of recurrent herpes simplex, pretreatment with oral acyclovir is advantageous. Supplemental estrogen and birth control medication may predispose individuals to post inflammatory pigmentary disturbances. Patients who are at the greatest risk of developing pigmentary problems are those individuals who continue to have extraordinary occupational exposure or recreational exposure to sunlight following chemexfoliation. Scarring is probably the most feared complication associated with chemical peeling. Those individuals with a history of hypertrophic scarring should be viewed as increased risks and may not be appropriate candidates.

Since the pilosebaceous apparatus is of critical importance for adequate re-epithelialization following phenol-based chemexfoliation, those individuals who have had recent treatment for acne using cys-13 retinoic acid (Accutane, Roche Laboratories, Nutley, NJ) are usually not appropriate candidates. It is recommended that at least 9 months and preferably 12 months elapse before a patient who has been on Accutane undergoes chemexfoliation. If the physical examination reveals normal cutaneous topography including the presence of appropriate numbers of vellus hairs, treatment can be undertaken. If there is any question as to the appropriateness and acceptability of treatment, it is recommended that histologic evaluation via a small biopsy be pursued.

One needs to be extremely careful to fully evaluate patients who have a history of facial radiation as a treatment for acne. If the result of the physical examination is satisfactory, they can be acceptable candidates for chemexfoliation (Table 8.6). The absence of significant vellus hair formation on the face as well as the presence of numerous telangiectasias, would indicate an increased risk for facial scarring (18).

Phenol-based chemical peeling is often performed in conjunction with facelift surgery. However, one needs to avoid chemical peeling over areas that have recently been undermined, as this may result in delayed healing. Thus, chemical peeling over undermined areas of a facelift is not recommended. In general, it is recommended to delay 6 to 9 months before peeling these ar-

TABLE 8.6

FACTORS IN PATIENT EVALUATION FOR PHENOL-BASED CHEMEXFOLIATION

General	General state of physical and mental health
	Medications
	Pregnancy history
	History of herpes simplex
	Skin pigmentation classification evaluation
	History of hypertrophic scarring
	History of facial radiation or use of Accutane
	Realistic expectations
Relative Contraindications	Cardiac disease
	Renal disease
	Hepatic disease
	Hormonal replacement therapy
	Continued exposure to Ultraviolet light
	History of radiation exposure or use of Accutane
Contraindications	History of hypertrophic scarring or keloid formation
	Fitzpatrick skin classification of IV-VI
	Recent facelift (deep chemical peeling in areas of recently undermined skin may result in vascular compromise and resultant scar formation)

eas. Medium depth peeling over undermined areas may be undertaken simultaneously (19, 20). It is also important to realize that phenol-based chemical peel solutions should not be used to peel cervical tissues due to the propensity for scar formation secondary to the paucity of pilosebaceous apparati compared with the face.

PHARMACOLOGY

There are a variety of chemical caustics that can be used by the cosmetic surgeon. Different chemical peel solutions vary significantly in their depth of penetration and ultimately in the aesthetic result they produce. Stegman and others have shown that occlusion of the wound surface following phenol chemexfoliation results in deeper wounding (21).

The chemical peel solution that penetrates the deepest into the reticular dermis to correct the most severe actinic damage uses a formula containing phenol (Figs. 8.1, 8.2). In strengths up to 1%, phenol is clinically bacteriostatic and above 1% is bacteriocidal. The compound also serves as a local anesthetic to cutaneous nerve endings. When the solution is initially applied to the skin, a burning sensation occurs, but after 1 to 2 minutes an anesthesia develops which persists for 20 to 30 minutes in the average individual. Phenol is soluble in oil and fats and the addition of salt increases its activity by reducing its solubility in water. The solution can be rapidly removed from the skin with glycerin or alcohol.

The absorption of phenol is very rapid with 70% of it absorbed by the body within 30 minutes. It is metabolized in the liver and cleared through the renal system with 75% of phenol being excreted unchanged in the urine and 25% being metabolized to CO_2 and water (22).

Baker's chemical peel solution (which is an emulsion) is probably the most widely used formula for phenol-based chemexfoliation. Some experts feel that to ensure proper concentration, the solution should be mixed fresh before each application. Storage for a short period of time is possible if the solution is sealed in an amber glass bottle, but each bottle should be carefully dated and agitated before use to ensure proper mixing.

The major active ingredient in the phenol solution is phenol (carbolic acid). In its concentrated form (greater than 88%), phenol is thought to be a keratocoagulant, precipitating the surface protein and thus preventing extension of the peel solution into the deeper layers of the skin. Reducing the concentration of the phenol to 50%, however, significantly changes its activity so that it becomes a keratolytic agent, disrupting the sulfur bridges in the keratin layer and producing greater destruction than is desired. The specific formula proposed by Baker and Gordon dilutes the concentration to approximately 50% to 55% and the resulting keratolysis promotes further penetration into the dermis (10).

TABLE 8.7

PHENOL PEEL FORMULA

Ingredients	Amount
Phenol (88%, USP)	3 ml
Croton oil	3 drops
Septisol (liquid hexachlorophene soap in alcohol-Septisol-Calgon Vestal Laboratories, St. Louis, Mo.)	8 drops
Distilled water	2 ml

The theoretical explanation given by Rothman regarding the coagulation-keratolytic properties of the phenol-based chemical solution has never been proven (23). Brody has stated that below 30%, lesser phenol concentrations are progressively more dilute and weak (3). A variety of Baker-Gordon formulas using solutions between 25% and 50% and less than 2 drops of croton oil may produce good clinical results for lesser degrees of photoaging and certain types of skin. However, Brody points out that trichloracetic acid (TCA) peels can produce the same results without the need for systemic precautions that are required with milder forms of phenol-based chemical peeling.

Croton oil is expressed from the seed of the Croton Tiglium shrub and is composed of the glycerides of several acids and a very phytotoxic substance called croton. When applied to the skin in a concentrated form, croton oil generally causes pustular eruptions and skin destruction. Thus, it is an epidermolytic vesicant that enhances absorption of the phenol and increases inflammation. A liquid soap solution, usually Septisol (Vestal Laboratories, St Louis, MO), is added to the formula to reduce the interface surface tension. This enhances penetration of the phenol and croton oil to the deeper keratin layers.

Water is used only as a diluent in the phenol solution, but the amount used is crucial for producing the proper emulsion concentration. The freshly prepared emulsion is not miscible and must be stirred constantly in the bottle, both before and during patient application, to ensure proper mixing and to achieve a more even peel (Table 8.7).

HISTOPATHOLOGY

After chemical cauterance with the phenol solution, a series of histopathologic changes begin to occur to the skin. The epidermis regenerates, nearly to normal. The papillary dermis, appears thickened, but is normal. In the mid dermis, a band of irregular collagen fibers develops with an increase in aminoglycans. Stegman, in his study comparing the histologic effects of various peeling agents, showed that with Baker's phenol mixture, occluded specimens were wounded more extensively than nonoccluded specimens (21). Dermabrasion produced wounding very similar to that of occluded Baker's phenol peel mixture, but the edema did not extend as deeply into the dermis.

Stegman's studies showed that the depth of wound penetration progressed gradually as the strength of the escharotic agent increased. The phenol-based solutions penetrated the greatest. This progression was noted to be the same on both non-photodamaged and photodamaged skin and both occluded and nonoccluded specimens. Results after 60 days show that the epidermis returned to normal thickness in nonoccluded specimens and in 120 days, the epidermis returned to its normal thickness when a taping technique was used. An expanded papillary dermis was noted which Stegman referred to as a Grenz zone. This band developed in the middle to upper dermis during the later stages of healing and exhibited large amounts of glycosaminoglycans. This band was generally thicker in occluded specimens as compared with unoccluded specimens.

Kligman demonstrated that with phenol peels, the dominant event is the formation of a wide band of new dermis in which thin, straight, parallel bundles of compacted collagen are arranged horizontally to the surface (24). He also noted that elastin fibers abundantly regenerated, forming a network of branched, fine fibers often paralleling the distribution of the collagen bundles. These fibers were of sufficient density and quality to at least partially serve the function of elastin by keeping the skin under tension and snapping it back after deformation. However, Kligman noted that the vertical subdermal candelabra-like pattern of fibers seen in normal skin did not reform.

Kligman also noted that the dermal reconstruction persisted for at least 2 decades. In another study, he reviewed patients who had previously undergone a Baker's chemical peel and 1.5 to 20 years later underwent a facelift procedure. Strips of removed skin were analyzed to compare peeled with nonpeeled specimens. In contrast to the markedly abnormal elastotic appearance of the un-peeled skin, a new band of connective tissue 2 to 3 mm in width was noted in the subepidermal areas with fine elastic fibers forming a dense network in the band of regenerated collagen. While the epidermal changes were also notable, they probably contributed less to the gross benefits of the phenol peel than did the dermal alterations. Histologic studies have also shown that melanocytes are present following phenol-based chemexfoliation. It is believed that the hypopigmentation, which can occur following phenol-based chemical peeling, is not due to destruc-tion of the melanocytes, but rather to some impairment of melanin synthesis.

TAPED VERSUS OPEN TECHNIQUE

As stated previously, Stegman and others have shown that occlusion of the wound surface following chemexfoliation with a phenol-based solution results in a deeper wounding (21). Baker and Gordon originally described the application of waterproof tape after the peel to increase the penetration, presumably through a mechanism of maceration. In recent years, others have advocated an open technique by which more aggressive defatting of the skin and aggressive removal of the epidermal barrier are achieved with acetone before a heavier application of the peel formula so that the need for taping is eliminated along with the discomfort associated with tape removal. Taping is replaced with application of petrolatum or other ointment that prevents surface dehydration.

Wound healing occurs more rapidly in covered wounds (3). A covering over the wound keeps the tissue fluid on the wound surface in liquid state rather than allowing a deep crust to form as happens in uncovered wounds. The crusting represents a mechanical barrier to epidermal migration.

When hydration of the wound surface is maintained by topical ointments, no mechanical barrier is present and the migration of epithelial cells occurs on a plane with the uninvolved dermis. The rate of re-epithelialization of these nonhydrated wounds appears to be increased by 40%. A variety of topical ointments have been advocated for use with the non-taping technique (Table 8.8).

TABLE 8.8

TOPICAL AGENTS THAT AFFECT EPIDERMAL MIGRATION

Agent	Relative Healing Rate
Neosporin ointment	+25
Silvadene cream	+28
Eucerin cream	+5
Petrolatum, USP	−8
Triamcinolone acetonide ointment, 0.1%	−34

Adapted from Geronemus, RG, Mertz PM, Eaglestein WH. Wound healing. The effects of topical antimicrobial agents. Arch of Dermatol 1979;115: 1311-1314.

PREOPERATIVE PREPARATION

One of the most important facets of chemexfoliation is adequate cleansing of the face and removal of deep facial oils. This is even more critical when a nontaping technique is used. It is extremely important for patients to wash their face 4 to 5 times with Septisol (hexachlorophene and alcohol) before peeling. The Septisol acts as an astringent and helps to remove the stratum corneum. This washing promotes the penetration of the phenol solution. While other facial soaps can be used, they may not possess the keratolytic properties of Septisol. Soaps that are oilier may actually interfere with the penetration of the peel solution.

Tretinoin compounds (retinoic acid) can be an important adjunct in skin preparation prior to chemexfoliation. Since Weiss and Ellis published their findings, tretinoin has been used to eliminate actinic keratoses and for the treatment of fine facial rhytides (25). Tretinoin increases epidermal turnover by increasing the rate of mitosis and stimulates collagen synthesis. Use of tretinoin has also been shown to reduce desmesomal attachments of compact corneocytes and increases epidermolysis. Thus, retinoic acid appears to facilitate peel penetration and facilitate epidermal regeneration. Kligman and Hung recommend using retinoic acid 3 to 4 weeks prior to chemical face peeling or dermabrasion in order to "prime" the skin (26, 27). Mandy reported that skin pretreated with tretinoin healed more quickly following dermabrasion (28). However, the cosmetic outcome was not influenced by pretreatment techniques.

Following adequate facial cleansing, the areas to be peeled are gently cleansed with 2×2 gauze pads soaked in acetone. This further helps to remove the deep facial oils and facilitate the penetration of the peel solution. Care must be taken to protect the eyes, nose, and mouth while using acetone since it is extremely aromatic and is an irritant to the mucus membranes. In addition, avoid rubbing too vigorously and possibly creating microabrasion of the skin which would result in deeper local peel penetration than what is desired.

The application of phenol-based chemical peel solutions can be uncomfortable and usually requires some type of sedation. If a regional peel such as a perioral or periorbital peel is being performed, little, if any, sedation is required. However, with full face phenol-based chemexfoliation, intravenous sedation is usually required. Patients are commonly given 20 mg of diazepam and 200 mg of dimenhydrinate orally 2 hours before and scopolamine 0.4 mg sublingually 1 hour prior to the procedure. The oral medications are supplemented with intravenous diazepam given in increments until the desired level of sedation is achieved prior to the peel solution being applied.

In the past, it was thought that lidocaine injections produced delayed healing or increased the penetration of the chemical peel solution (29). This was based on the fact that phenol activity is increased in an acid environment. It was also theorized that, if epinephrine was used in combination with lidocaine, the vasoconstrictive effects of the epinephrine could allow for greater penetration of the phenol. I have found that lidocaine injections in combination with a 1:10 sodium bicarbonate solution with or without epinephrine to be an effective anesthetic regimen for both regional blocks and local infiltration prior to phenol or Baker-Gordon chemexfoliation. Despite the theoretical potential for increased penetration of peel solution, I have not found this to be true and have not encountered any complications using this technique for over 8 years. The lack of complications could be due to the fact that most injections are actually into the subdermal tissues and therefore the anesthetic solution probably has little, if any, effect on the pH of the dermis.

When full face chemical peels are performed, regional blocks can be obtained with a 1% lidocaine and 1:100,000 adrenaline solution diluted with 1 ml of sodium bicarbonate per 10 ml of lidocaine and injected with a 27-gauge needle. The mental, infraorbital, supratrochlear and supraorbital nerves are blocked near their foramina. Local subdermal infiltration may be used along the mandible, over the malar eminence, or in the area of regional peels such as the periorbital and perioral tissues.

Adequate hydration is important in order to avoid potential complications, especially since phenol is excreted by the renal system. While the toxic dose of phenol is estimated at 7 to 15 mg per 100 ml, the toxicity has been shown to relate very closely to the rate of excretion. Hemal recommends that the peel solution be applied for short periods of time to limited areas (150 cm^2 area or less) and at the same time increase the output of an alkaline urine (22). As a measure to avoid toxicity associated with phenol, it is recommended that the patient be hydrated with 500 ml of Ringer's lactate before applying the chemical peel solution followed by an additional 1,000 ml of fluid given during the operation and during the immediate postoperative period. As the face is commonly divided into 5 aesthetic units (forehead, perioral, malar, nasal, and periorbital areas), it is advised that these aesthetic units be peeled sequentially with 10 to 15 minutes allowed to lapse between treatment of each unit in order to reduce toxicity and allow for adequate excretion of phenol. Thus, the entire facial peel will take between 60 and 90 minutes.

Phenol is known to be cardiotoxic. Cardiac arrhythmias including paroxysmal atrial contractions, premature ventricular contractions, and bigeminal and trigeminal rhythms may occur within minutes of the peel solution being applied to more than one-third of the face. For that reason, it is recommended that the sequential peeling technique at proper time intervals be used and that each patient undergoing full face phenol-based

FIGURE 8.1
A, B, C. 67-year-old female with facial rhytides pre-peel.

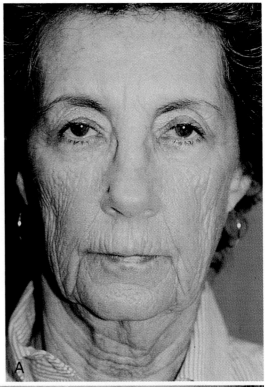

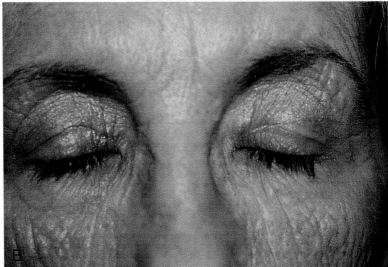

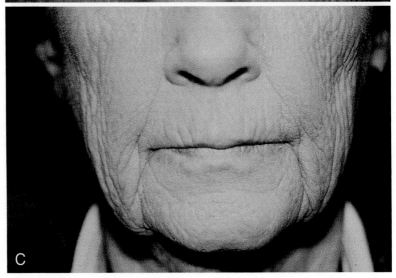

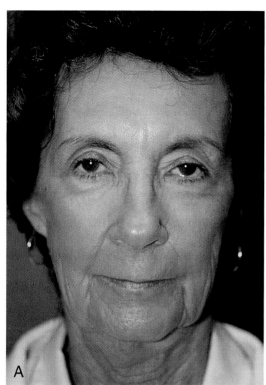

FIGURE 8.2
A, B, C. Same patient 2 years after Baker-Gorden full face chemical peel using the "non-taping" technique.

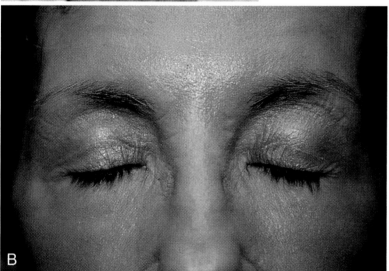

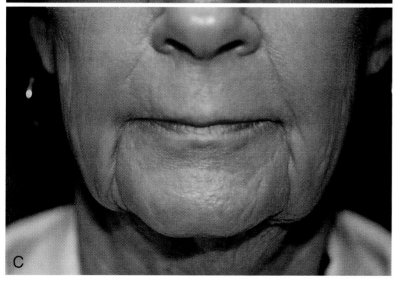

chemexfoliation be monitored with a cardiac monitor during and after the procedure. If a small single aesthetic unit is being peeled, such monitoring may not be necessary.

It is important that the chemical peel solution be mixed precisely. In order to avoid any errors in the compilation of the peeling solution, it is recommended that it be formulated with 2 individuals verifying the accuracy of the formulation process. The peel solution is stored in an amber bottle which is then dated and initialed by the individuals that observed the peel solution being mixed. For additional quality control purposes it is recommended that a log of the patients treated be maintained along with a lot number. Thus, if an untoward event occurs and an individual develops scarring, the log may help verify that previous or subsequent patients had healed without difficulty with that same phenol-based chemical peel mixture which would substantiate that the peel solution was mixed correctly.

It is important to remember that the peel solution is an emulsion and needs to be kept in solution. For that reason, if the peel solutions are not mixed for each individual patient, the bottle must be vigorously agitated prior to and during the procedure to ensure adequate mixing of components. While there are many phenol-based chemical peel formulas, the one developed by Baker and Gordon in the 1960s is the most widely employed (9).

CHEMICAL PEEL PROCEDURE

After the face has been properly cleansed with Septisol, copiously irrigated with water, and cleansed using acetone-soaked 2×2 gauze pads, the peeling procedure may begin. The peel solution is applied using a cotton-tipped applicator that has been dipped into the solution and pressed against the rim of the bottle to remove any excess. The solution is then systematically applied to the facial aesthetic units, allowing 10 to 15 minutes to elapse between regions in order to reduce the likelihood of increased blood levels which could produce cardiac arrhythmias.

The solution is applied first to the forehead area using the applicator to spread the solution smoothly and evenly over the forehead tissues. The peel solution should be feathered into the hairline in order to avoid potential lines of demarcation between peeled and unpeeled areas. It is noted that hair follicles are not affected by the peel solution and that alopecia does not occur. The solution is also feathered into the eyebrows in order to provide a more homogeneous appearance.

When the peel solution is initially applied, the patient commonly complains of an intense burning sensation that lasts for 10 to 20 seconds. The pain quickly subsides due to the anesthetic effects of phenol, but then recurs in approximately 20 minutes. This pain frequently persists for 6 to 8 hours postoperatively and then spontaneously resolves. The discomfort can be prevented with the anesthetic infiltration technique previously discussed.

A thick white frost appears on areas where the peel solution is applied. If this is not seen, one must suspect that the skin has not adequately been prepared and one might elect to repeat the pretreatment process with acetone cleansing to areas undergoing peeling. The white frost dissipates over a matter of minutes into a red, and then amber color. After waiting approximately 10 to 15 minutes, the next area is peeled. The process is repeated for other areas that are to be peeled.

Deep vertical rhytides are often noted in the perioral area which extend to and across the vermilion border. To ensure complete and even application, the upper and lower lip areas should be firmly stretched and fixed using a thumb and index finger while the peel solution is evenly applied with a cotton tipped applicator. Tension must be maintained until the white frost has appeared. In areas containing the deepest facial rhytides, a broken wooden applicator stick can be used to apply more peel solution into deep crevices. The peel solution should be applied across the vermilion border and approximately 2 to 3 mm onto the lip in order to adequately treat the deep rhytides that extend to the vermilion margin.

When peeling the periorbital region, special care must be exercised to ensure that none of the peel solution enters the eye and that the peel solution is not diluted by tears, as this alters the concentration of the peel solution and could lead to streaking, secondary to uneven peel penetration. During application to the periorbital areas, an eye irrigation solution should be readily available in the event that the peel solution inadvertently contacts the cornea or conjunctiva. Should this occur, prompt and copious irrigation should be instituted and the condition of the eye followed closely postoperatively. In most cases, such chemical irritation to the eye completely resolves with conservative management.

When the peel solution is applied to the periorbital area, the cotton applicator should be pressed firmly against the lip of the bottle to remove any excess solution and then blotted in a gauze pad to further remove excess solution. The solution is applied to the upper eyelid area to within 3 to 4 mm of the ciliary margin with the peel being carried down to the superior tarsal fold, but no lower. Peeling below the superior tarsal fold results in significant periorbital edema that can persist for a number of weeks. Satisfactory results in the periorbital area can be obtained without peeling below the superior tarsal fold. In the lower eyelid area, the peel solution is applied with the patient gazing in an upward direction. An assistant must carefully observe the medial and lateral canthi for any accumulation of tears. If tears appear, they should be blotted with a dry, cotton-tipped applicator. The peel solution is then carried into the lateral canthal area. A broken applicator stick may be used to further direct peel solution into the deeper rhytides in the lateral canthal area. If only a regional periorbital peel is being performed, a feathering technique can be used at the margins to avoid a frank demarcation between peeled and unpeeled areas. It must be pointed out that the periorbital tissues are extremely delicate and even a very small amount of chemical peel solution can produce significant reaction. One must avoid the temptation to "over peel" the periorbital tissues.

POST-PEEL MANAGEMENT

With phenol-based chemexfoliation using a Baker's chemical peel solution an initial frosting is noted which gradually progresses to an amber color. At this point, cold compresses or a moist dressing consisting of a variety of ointments can be safely applied without fear of altering the peel concentration. I do not use the taping technique following Baker's chemical and I feel that the results are equally aesthetically pleasing as those obtained with a taping technique. This observation has been confirmed by others (30). The advantage to the nontaping technique is that it is safer, there is less penetration of the peel solution as compared with the taping technique and therefore a reduced chance of scarring. In addition, patients are more comfortable. With the taping technique, many patients complain of significant discomfort and significant sedation may be required when tape removal is required at the appropriate time. This can be avoided with the nontaping (moist dressing) technique. Finally, the moist dressing technique with associated frequent showering markedly decreases the chance of localized infection postoperatively and facilitates re-epithelialization (31).

However, it should be pointed out that some of the deepest rhytides in the perioral area may not be completely removed with one application of the Baker's chemical peel solution. "Touch up" peels are usually not required. However, in the case of persistent rhytides, additional phenol-based chemexfoliation can be applied after approximately 9 to 12 months following initial treatment in order to achieve more significant eradication of such rhytides. Brody and others recommend regional taping to treat such areas, stating that the combination of one peel and taping results in eradication of these most persistent rhytides (3). I however, elect for a more conservative approach that employs an open technique and the potential for repeat treatment at a later date, because it significantly reduces the risk for potential scarring.

Petrolatum should be liberally applied to the peeled areas and the patient released with oral pain medication and seen the following morning. At that time, the patient is instructed to liberally apply the petrolatum to the peeled areas to avoid dehydration that would result

in crust or scab formation. Gentle washing, either in the shower or with a spray nozzle at a kitchen sink, is recommended to gently hydrodebride peeled areas and remove any petrolatum. The face is then gently blotted with a clean towel or wash cloth and a thick layer of petrolatum is again applied. This process should be repeated at least 4 to 6 times a day until the area is completely re-epithelialized. Re-epithelialization usually occurs within 7 days.

After 1 week, most of the crusting disappears and peeled areas heal, revealing a sensitive new pink skin. Most individuals are able to begin wearing makeup within 10 days after a peel procedure. A nonfluorinated steroid cream (2.5% hydrocortisone) can be applied once a day for 3 weeks after re-epithelialization is complete. This cream helps to reduce the erythema as well as reduce the chance for irritation from application of makeup and topical cover ups.

Prolonged exposure to sunlight should be avoided in order to prevent blistering and splotchy hyperpigmentation of the new immature skin. If sun exposure is expected, special sunscreen preparations are advocated for up to 6 months following chemical peel. Most patients are able to return to work the end of the first week after chemical peeling, providing their work does not necessitate exposure to the sun.

At 1 month postoperatively, patients are usually started on topical applications of Vitamin C lotion in the morning and evening applications of tretinoin. These ointments are continued indefinitely and provide an additional subjective degree of aesthetic improvement. In addition, they may help to decrease milia formation that can be noted in the first 1 to 2 months following chemexfoliation.

PHENOL-BASED CHEMEXFOLIATION VERSUS LASER RESURFACING

Laser resurfacing using the CO_2 laser has become increasingly popular in recent years, challenging phenol-based chemexfoliation as the mainstay for skin rejuvenation. There are distinct advantages and disadvantages inherent with each of these treatment modalities. The cost of CO_2 lasers used in skin resurfacing as well as the ancillary supplies used for each procedure can be significant. These costs can range from $25,000 to $150,000. In addition, there are yearly maintenance costs which can easily exceed 10% of the purchase price of the laser on an annual basis. In contrast, the cost for the chemical components for phenol-based chemical peel solutions is minuscule and the shelf life long.

The intraoperative time required for full face rejuvenation significantly differs between the two techniques. Phenol-based peels take between 60 and 90 minutes to complete in contrast to full face laser resurfacing which can be completed in as little as 20 to 30 minutes. The development of the fourth generation of laser scanners may reduce this time interval even further. However, with phenol peeling, the office-based surgeon can attend to other patients after each segment is peeled. A total of 10 to 15 minutes of treatment time is required.

Both laser resurfaced areas and phenol treated areas can be treated with a moist dressing technique that facilitates re-epithelialization. Re-epithelialization is slightly more expeditious with the CO_2 laser than with phenol peels; however, this can vary with the type of equipment used and closely approximates the re-epithelialization time required for full face phenol chemexfoliation. While the persistence of erythema (on average 6 to 8 weeks) with the phenol peel is slightly less than with the CO_2 laser, both treatment modalities can result in some persistence of erythema in selected cases, which can last as long as 2 to 3 months.

The most prominent differences between the two techniques lie in the effects on pigmentation and contour changes. While both treatment modalities can result in transient hyperpigmentation, only the phenol-based peel more predictably produces hypopigmentation. In some isolated cases, hypopigmentation can be advantageous, such as with periorbital peeling. In most cases, hypopigmentation is a negative factor and a relative contraindication to using this peel in male and in younger individuals who do not desire to wear make up.

An additional area where there is a divergence between the two techniques lies in the uniformity of surface contouring. The laser more predictably produces a uniform depth of penetration that is not as dependent upon the preoperative skin preparation as is the phenol peel technique. In addition, the laser can be used to vaporize wound margins and provide saucerization of acne scars that further improves the final aesthetic result. While mild acne scars can be treated with both treatment modalities, I have found laser resurfacing to be far more efficacious when dealing with acne scarring.

When histologic studies were performed comparing a high-energy, direct current CO_2 laser (SurgiPulse XJ-150, Sharplan Laser Inc, Allendale, NJ) to occluded Baker-Gordon phenol peel at 90 days postoperatively, it was noted that the depth of injury of the laser resurfacing approximated that of a medium depth peel. However, the wound healing that occurred after laser treatment was much more rapid and inflammatory infiltrates cleared more quickly than after phenol peeling. It appeared that the subdermal repair zone of fibrosis accounted for the improved clinical appearance following laser treatment.

In a clinical comparison between laser resurfacing and phenol-based chemical peeling, patients were noted to have less discomfort during and after laser resurfacing. Re-epithelialization was expedited with the laser resurfacing, with most individuals achieving re-epithelialization in 3 to 5 days as opposed to 7 to 10 days for the phenol peel patients. In addition, there was a quicker resolution of erythema as well as noted dyschromia following laser resurfacing. However, the laser resurfacing seemed less effective in eradicating deep rhytides with a single treatment as compared with the phenol peel. Two to three laser resurfacing procedures at 3 month intervals subjectively provided 80% reduction of perioral rhytides as compared with one phenol chemexfoliation treatment (32).

Brody noted similar findings in a preliminary clinical comparison between the laser and Baker-Gordon chemexfoliation which revealed that the laser improves severe photodamaged skin by approximately 50%. In the treatment of Glogau, photoaging Type III perioral skin, the laser can eliminate mild rhytides in one treatment with little risk of pigmentary change. The peel does the same, but may be more likely to result in slight hypopigmentation of the skin. In contrast, photoaging Type IV skin with severe rhytides may require multiple touch ups by the laser for adequate treatment. The Baker's peel, however, can eliminate the vast majority of rhytides in one treatment.

It is interesting to compare the histopathology of laser resurfacing versus phenol-based chemexfoliation. At the present time, phenol-based chemexfoliation remains the gold standard for facial rejuvenation. However, the development of the new generation of high-energy CO_2 laser scanners and the advent of the erbium lasers may well advance laser resurfacing into a new realm. Ongoing research in the role of tissue growth factors and their manipulation to stimulated accelerated wound healing may hold the key for future advances and needs to be monitored closely.

I frequently use a combination of techniques for facial rejuvenation. A phenol peel of the periorbital tissues in combination with full face CO_2 laser resurfacing is often employed in patients of all ages. I feel that the phenol peel provides more efficacious management of deep rhytides in the periorbital tissues with a quicker resolution of erythema than is obtained with laser resurfacing. In addition, the hypopigmentation that can occur with the phenol-based peel effectively manages the mild dyschromia frequently seen in the periorbital tissues, especially in the lower lid.

A light 100% phenol peel can be used to rejuvenate the lower eyelid in conjunction with transconjunctival blepharoplasty. This can result in a tightening of the lower lid tissues and often negates the need for a skin excision.

COMPLICATIONS

Chemexfoliation has proved to be a useful technique with an extremely low complication rate. However, it is important to remember that complications can occur with any surgical procedure.

Pigmentation Changes

A line of demarcation usually exists between peeled and nonpeeled areas. This can be minimized by feathering the peel at the lateral margins. This is especially important when peeling the regional areas such as the perioral or periorbital areas. Rarely is the neck peeled. However, the application of the peel solution is carried 1 to 2 cm below the mandibular margin and chin using the feathering technique.

Spotty hyperpigmentation in peeled areas can occur if the patient is exposed to sun, becomes pregnant or takes estrogens during the first 6 months following the peel. Patients are encouraged to avoid sunlight for prolonged periods of time. The use of sunscreens is advocated. The appropriate use of sunscreen agents with a sun protection factor (SPF) of 15 to 30 applied daily to the peel areas, avoidance of direct sun exposure for 3 to 6 months postoperatively, the avoidance of oral contraceptives (2 months preoperatively and postoperatively), exogenous estrogens, and photosensitizing drugs (1 month preoperatively and postoperatively); and strict post operative wound care to minimize crust formation can dramatically reduce the incidence of pigmentary changes.

Bleaching agents are unpredictable in reducing hyperpigmentation. If hyperpigmentation is a result of an unequal application of the peel solution, the under-peeled areas may be touched up within 6 to 9 months of the initial peel procedure. Permanent redness of the peeled areas has not occurred with the moist dressing technique advocated by the author. However, in almost every case, peeled skin will have color and texture changes that contrast with the adjacent, unpeeled skin. Some patients may develop a contact dermatitis in the treated areas due to the increased sensitivity of the new skin. If dermatitis occurs, it should be treated by identifying and eliminating the offending agent. Lipsticks, nail care products, hair spray and cologne are common irritants. In some cases, 0.5% hydrocortisone is helpful. Fluorinated steroids should be avoided for more than a few days.

It is important that patients be aware that some pigmentation changes are inevitable. Most often the peeled areas are lighter and smoother than contrasting areas. As a general rule, superficial peeling tends to lead to hyperpigmentation, whereas deeper peeling tends to produce hypopigmentation. These pigmentation problems can usually be handled with proper makeup applications. However, it is essential that the patient understands that there is a tradeoff for smoother, more youthful skin.

Infection

Infections in association with phenol-based chemexfoliation are unusual. This is due partly to the fact that phe-nol is bactericidal and the fact that the moist dressing technique using frequent showering greatly reduces the chance of secondary infections with Staphylococcus or Streptococcus. When poor wound hygiene is noted and a foul odor is detected along with significant crusting and drainage, one must suspect Pseudomonas infection. When infection is suspected, cultures should be taken and treatment immediately started with ciprofloxacin along with acetic acid soaks (5% acetic acid or white vinegar diluted 1:1 with tap water).

Toxic shock syndrome has been reported in association with phenol-based chemical peels (33). Such patients would be noted to have fever, vomiting or diarrhea, hypotension and a rash within the first several days following chemexfoliation. Prompt medical treatment in such cases is required.

Herpes Simplex Type I is a cytopathic DNA virus frequently associated with microcutaneous labial infections. Between 16% and 45% of all adults have experienced at least one episode of herpes simplex. Herpetic infections often follow face peeling without resultant scarring. This is probably because a larger and clinically more significant subdermal vascular has not been surgically manipulated with the chemical damage. However, the vascular endothelium is susceptible to herpetic viral infections. For this reason, it is advisable to use a prophylactic dose of acyclovir (Zovirax, Glaxo Wellcome, Triangle Park, NC) in patients prone to herpetic lesions. It is important to note that acyclovir is poorly absorbed. For that reason, significant doses are required in order to obtain proper blood levels. Zovirax administration at 800 mg twice a day has been shown to be as effective as the previously recommended dose of 200 mg, five times a day in treating the acute infection. In addition, some feel that applications of topical acyclovir ointment (Zovirax) 4 to 6 times a day in combination with the oral therapy is helpful.

Because the herpetic virus does not activate until re-epithelialization, it is recommended that treatment be initiated immediately before the chemical peel procedure and extend for 12 to 14 days following the procedure in order to provide proper coverage during the re-epithelialization process and in the early re-epithelialized state. Recent studies have shown valacyclovir (Valtrex, Glaxo Wellcome, Triangle Park, NC) to be very effective in inhibiting human Herpes simplex virus types I and II. Valacyclovir is readily absorbed from the gastrointestinal tract. Bioavailability of acyclovir after administration of valacyclovir is approximately 3 to 5 times greater than from high oral doses of Zovirax and coverage comparable to that obtained from intravenous acyclovir. For this reason, I prophylactically treat chemical peel patients with Valtrex 500 mg 2 times daily the day before chemical exfoliation and for 14 days postoperatively. If a herpetic infection did develop, doses would be increased to valacyclovir 1000 mg every 8 hours in combination with topical Zovirax ointment until the lesion resolved.

Milia

Milia, or small epidermal inclusion cysts, occasionally occur following chemical peels. If they develop, it is usually within the first 1 to 3 months. They are usually self-limiting. Should they persist, they can be unroofed with an 18-gauge needle.

Prolonged Erythema and/or Pruritis

Erythema is common following phenol-based chemical peeling and usually resolves within 6 to 8 weeks. When erythema in a localized area persists, one must be concerned for the potential of scar formation or the possibility of contact dermatitis. The latter is usually treated by eliminating the irritating agent and using a topical nonfluorinated steroid such as 2.5% hydrocortisone cream twice daily. In some rare cases, erythema may persist for a prolonged period of time. In such cases, fluorinated steroid creams or tape can be used. Intralesional triamcinolone (3 to 10 mg) may be necessary. In some cases, oral antihistamines or short term systemic steroids may be of benefit.

Pruritis is associated with re-epithelialization and is a normal consequence of the healing process. This is usually self limiting and easily controlled with aspirin or possibly propranolol in low doses. If the pruritis is intense, a contact dermatitis should be suspected. In such cases, topical steroids, as noted above, independently or in combination with oral antihistamines and possibly low dose short term systemic steroids can be of assistance in eliminating these symptoms.

Textural Changes

At times, a grainy, peau d'orange texture can occur following chemical peel. According to Brody, this appearance is due to use of an agent that is too weak to peel evenly below the defect, that lacks the surfactant to provide an even depth of wounding, or has too high a surface tension resulting in a textural change (3). Ideally the wounding agent should penetrate just below the photodamaged tissue. Often this can be corrected by repeat peeling giving attention toward proper prepeeling preparation.

Cardiac Arrhythmias

Litton, Gross and others have all reported cardiac arrhythmias occurring with phenol peels. There has been no reported predictable relationship between serum phenol levels and the appearance of cardiac arrhythmias. However, there is suggestive evidence that peeling segments and intervals allow the metabolism of the absorbed phenol and thus decrease the chance of arrhythmias. For that reason, cardiac monitoring is extremely important. In general, it is recommended that certain precautions be taken when performing phenol chemexfoliation. Hydrating the patient to produce an alkaline urine is recommended. Patient should receive approximately 1500 ml of hydration before, during and after chemical peeling. In addition, one should limit peeling to a 150 cm² area with 10 to 15 minutes allowed to elapse between peeling of each segment in order to allow for proper clearance and metabolism of the phenol. It is extremely important to employ cardiac monitoring and to have appropriate cardiac resuscitation equipment when full face phenol chemexfoliation is being performed.

Scarring

While there are numerous complications associated with chemical peeling, the most significant is scarring. Many authors have reported scarring associated with peeling the perioral area. The most common area for scar formation is the perioral area (34). Scarring develops as late as 3 months after perioral chemical peels. Baker and Gordon reported scarring developing 2 to 3 months after peeling the midportion of the upper lip in 6 patients who had facelifts and perioral peels (30). They state that the problem was upper lip edema secondary to the facelift and that taping the lip postoperatively compounded the problem. Spira theorized that interference with the lymphatic drainage or subclinical cellular necrosis secondary to undermining adjacent to, but not under, the peel area could encourage scar formation (35). For this reason, most experts do not recommend peeling directly over recently undermined areas, such as chemical peel in association with facelift procedure or after a skin muscle flap blepharoplasty procedure. There are many possible ideologies for scar development. These include excessive depth of the peel penetration, delayed healing complicated by infection, digital manipulation, or iatrogenic causes.

Anti-inflammatory agents may be very beneficial in a prophylactic sense, because they modify the inflammatory phase of wound healing following chemexfoliation. System steroids are effective if they are given within the first 48 hours. Many surgeons use systemic steroids during surgery as well as steroid dose packs following chemical face peeling in order to help modify or reduce the inflammatory response. Topical steroid ointments can be of benefit in the early stages of wound healing. A nonfluorinated steroid is recommended to help eliminate or reduce the possibility of thinning of the dermis.

When persistent inflammation with associated induration is seen following chemical face peeling, one must be very suspicious of a developing scar formation. It is very important to treat these areas vigorously with topical steroids, intralesional triamcinolone, or possibly a homeopathic dose of steroids such as prednisone 4 to 5 mg daily for a period of 30 days.

Certain deep phenol injuries of the facial skin might activate wound healing mechanisms similar to those seen in deep freeze induced injuries. In both forms of injury, the cellular element of the epidermis and the upper layers of the dermis are destroyed. However, the dermal collagen connective tissue matrix remains intact. The dermal collagen matrix stimulates the effect of a full thickness skin graft to an open wound by inhibiting myofibroblast formation and therefore, an apparent scar may result. Thus, a conservative approach to scars associated with phenol chemical face peeling may be very appropriate and the acute use of skin grafting and other vigorous forms of treatment might well be suspect.

If induration persists, one may consider the use of intralesional injections of triamcinolone (10 mg/ml to 20 mg/ml at 6 to 8 week intervals). In addition, silicone gel dressings may provide beneficial effects. Silicone gel may be useful in the treatment of hypertrophic scars. This action may be due to either a physical effect such as pressure, temperature, oxygen tension, hydration, occlusion, or by means of a chemical effect. It is possible that a relatively impermeable silicone gel acts in the same way as the stratum corneum does and therefore restores homeostasis to the scar reducing capillary hyperemia, secondary fibrosis and hypertrophic scar formation.

Alster has shown the pulsed-dye laser to be an effective treatment modality in treating hypertrophic scars (36). Seven J/cm² energy levels can be used to serially treat areas of facial scarring following chemexfoliation. A moist dressing technique using a topical antibiotic ointment is used for the first 4 to 5 days following treatment. Treatment is usually performed at 4 to 6 week intervals (Table 8.9).

Persistent Wrinkles

Deep furrowing and wrinkling, especially in the periorbital and perioral regions, may not be completely eradicated by a single peel. Such defects may require a second application of peel solution 9 to 12 months following the initial procedure. Often times, the persistence of wrinkles is secondary to failure to properly remove facial oils and to properly apply the peel solution in each of the furrows.

TABLE 8.9

MANAGEMENT OF SCARRING

Topical nonfluorinated steroids
Topical silastic sheeting
Possible low dose oral steroids (4 mg Medrol dose pack)
Intralesional steroid injection (Kenalog 10 mg to 20 mg/ml at 6 week intervals)
Pulsed-dye laser treatment (7 J/cm² at 4 to 6 week intervals)

SUMMARY

Phenol-based chemical peeling is a technically simple surgical procedure that usually provides dramatic results. Since the potential for serious complications does exist, cautious assessment, attention to details, and meticulous management after the procedure are essential.

Aesthetically pleasing long-term results can be obtained by using phenol-based chemexfoliation without taping when the moist dressing technique is employed. This technique eliminates the need for a second anesthesia and reduces the need for an additional postoperative visit to remove facial taping. Meticulous cleansing and the constant application of nonirritating ointments provide an atmosphere for accelerated wound healing and reduced recovery.

REFERENCES

1. Bryan CP. Ancient Egyptian medicine: the papyrus Ebers (translation). Chicago: Ares Publishers, 1974:158-61.
2. Ebbell B. Papyrus ebers (translation). Copenhagen: Ejmar Munksgaard, 1937.
3. Brody HJ. Chemical peeling. St. Louis; C.V. Mosby, 1997.
4. Mackee GM, Karp FL. Treatment of post acne scars with phenol. Br J Dermatol 1952;64:456-459.
5. Urkov JC. Surface defects of skin: treatment by controlled exfoliation. Ill Med J 1946;89:75.
6. Gilles HD, Millard DR. The principles and art of plastic surgery. Boston: Little Brown & Co., 1957:403.
7. Litton C. Chemical face peeling. Plast Reconstr Surg 1962;29:371.
8. Baker TC. Chemical face peeling and rhytidectomy. Plast Reconstr Surg 1962;29:199.
9. Baker TJ, Gordon HL. The ablation of rhytides by chemical means: a preliminary report. J Fla Med Assoc 1961;48:541.
10. Beeson WH, McCollough EG. Aesthetic surgery of the aging face. St. Louis: C.V. Mosby, 1986.
11. McCollough EG, Hillman RA. Chemical face peel. Otolaryngol Clin North Am 1980;13:353-365.
12. Fitzpatrick TB. The validity and practicality of sun-reactive skin types I-IV. Arch Dermatol 1988;124:869-871.
13. Glogau RG. Chemical peeling and aging skin. J Geriat Dermatol 1994;2(1):30-35.
14. Brodland DJ, Roenignk RK. Trichloracetic acid chemexfoliation for extensive premalignant actinic damage of the face and scalp. Mayo Clin Proc 1988;63:887.
15. Roenigk RK. A primer of facial chemical peel. Dermatol Clin 1993;11(2):349-359.
16. Grimes PE. Melasma-ideology and therapeutic considerations. Arch Dermatol 1995;131:1453-1457.
17. Sanchez PN, et al. Melasma. J Am Acad Dermatol 1981;4:698-710.
18. Goldman PM, Freed MI. Aesthetic problems in chemical peeling. J Dermatol Surg Oncol 1989;15:1020-1024.
19. Dingman DL, Hartog J, Siemionow M. Simultaneous deep-plane facelift and trichloracetic acid peel. Plast Reconstr Surg 1994;93:86-93.
20. Gaughan RN, Otto RA, Renner GJ, et al. The effect of sterile inflammation on skin flap survival. Otolaryngol Head Neck Surg 1986;95:90-93.

21. Stegman SJ. A comparative histologic study of the effects of three peeling agents and dermabrasion on normal and sun damaged skin. Aesthetic Plast Surg 1988;6;123-135.

22. Hemel HG. Percutaneous absorption and distribution of 2-naphthol in man. Br J Dermatol 1972;87:614.

23. Rothman S. The principles of percutaneous absorption. J Lab Clin Med 1945;28:1305-1321.

24. Kligman AM, Baker TJ, Gordon HL. Long-term histologic follow up on phenol face peels. Plast Reconstr Surg 1985;75(5):652-659.

25. Weiss JS, Ellis CN, Headington JT, et al. Topical tretinoin improves photo aged skin: a double-blind vehicle controlled study. JAMA 1988;259:527-532.

26. Kligman AM, Grove GL, Hiroser R, Leyden JJ. Topical tretinoin for photo aged skin. J Am Acad Dermatol 1986;15:836-859.

27. Hung VC. Topical tretinoin and epithelial wound healing. Arch Dermatol 1989;125:65-69.

28. Mandy SH. Tretinoin and the Preoperative and postoperative management of dermabrasion. J Am Acad Dermatol 1986;15:878-879.

29. Davies B, Guyuron B, Husami T. The role of lidocaine, epinephrine, and flap elevation in wound healing after chemical peel. Ann Plast Surg 1991;26:273-278.

30. Baker TJ, Gordon HL. Chemical peel with phenol. In: Epstein E, Epstein E Jr, eds. Skin Surgery, 6th Ed. Philadelphia: WB Saunders, 1987:423-438.

31. Lindsay WK, Birch JR. Thin skin healing. Can J Surg 1964;7:297.

32. Fitzpatrick RE, Goldman MP, Sauter NM, et al. Pulsed carbon dioxide laser resurfacing of photo aged facial skin. Arch Dermatol 1996;132:395-402.

33. Resnik SS. Complications of chemical peeling. Cosmet Dermatol 1995;13(2):309.

34. Litton C, Trinidad G. Complications of chemical peeling as evaluated by a questionnaire. Plast Reconstr Surg 1981; 67:738.

35. Spira M, Gerow FJ, Hardy SB. Complications of chemical face peeling. Plast Reconstr Surg 1974;54:397.

36. Alster TS. Improvement of erythematous and hypertrophic scars by the 585-nm flashlamp pumped pulsed dye laser. Ann Plast Surg 1993;31:1-5.

Dermabrasion

CHAPTER 9

Skin Response to Abrasive Resurfacing

■ Christopher B. Harmon

The science of cutaneous wound healing is rapidly expanding as greater insight into the biology of cell-cell interactions and cell-matrix intercourse is gained. On a molecular level soluble growth factors, extracellular matrix proteins, and extravascular peptides all influence the role of keratinocytes and fibroblasts in regenerating and repairing injured skin. Conventionally, the dynamic processes by which wounds heal are categorized according to first and second intention mechanisms. The reparative steps of first intention healing apply to wounds that have been primarily closed or approximated. Conversely, wounds heal by second intention without any primary closure, approximation or intervention.

Both first and second intention wound healing are frequently divided into four stages even though they are a continuous process: (1) a vascular and inflammatory response, (2) granulation tissue formation, (3) re-epithelialization, and (4) connective tissue remodeling. Anatomically, second intention wounds may be classified according to the width, depth or degree of tissue loss. Superficial wounds are those that involve the epidermis and papillary dermis but preserve the adnexal structures and deeper dermal tissues. These wounds typically heal without visible scarring. Deep wounds extend into or beneath the reticular dermis with a loss of adnexal structures and surrounding tissue, and these injuries are much more likely to produce a visible cicatrix.

VASCULAR AND INFLAMMATORY RESPONSE

Surgical planing of the skin creates a superficial wound and initiates a second intention wound healing process.

Superficial abrasions heal faster than deeper abrasions. If the abrasion does not extend deeply into the reticular dermis, the skin heals without any visible evidence of scar formation. Because of the preservation of adnexal structures and their role in re-epithelialization, dermabrasion of facial skin heals more reliably than nonfacial skin. Likewise dermabrasion of previously radiated skin or skin grafts from nonfacial donor sites may heal more slowly with a higher incidence of scarring because of the paucity of skin appendages.

The anatomy and architecture of the skin illustrate the relationship of the papillary-reticular interface to the vessels of the dermal papillae (Fig. 9.1). As the level of planing passes through the epidermis, fine corn rows of bleeding herald the entry into the papillary dermis. Deeper abrasion into the reticular dermis is signified by yellow dots that represent sebaceous glands in the mid-dermis. Herniations of fat through the collagen fibers can be seen if the subcutaneous tissue is violated (1).

Clinically, the postoperative changes observed closely parallel the cellular and molecular events of cutaneous tissue repair. Active bleeding stops after 1 to 2 minutes and the abraded surface becomes a glistening bright red (Fig. 9.2). This appearance represents the vascular phase of tissue repair in which the early response of vasoconstriction is followed by vasodilation. Blood components covering the wound form a coagulum of platelets, inflammatory cells, clotting factors, a fibrin mesh, chemoattractant factors, and growth factors. The platelet clot initiates complement and coagulation cascades. A fibrin-fibronectin matrix is laid down as a scaffold upon which the subsequent phases of neovascularization, re-epithelialization and fibroplasia take place.

Cross-section of the skin

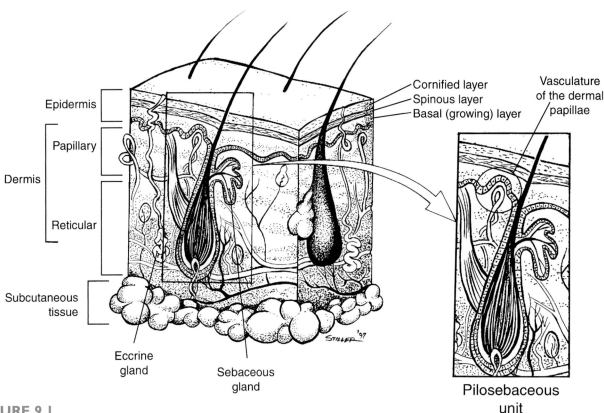

Epidermis

Papillary

Dermis

Reticular

Subcutaneous tissue

Eccrine gland

Sebaceous gland

Cornified layer
Spinous layer
Basal (growing) layer

Vasculature of the dermal papillae

Pilosebaceous unit

FIGURE 9.1

A schematic illustration of normal skin anatomy.

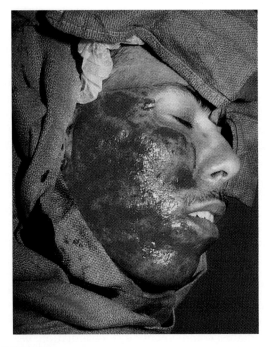

FIGURE 9.2

Appearance immediately following wire brush dermabrasion.

Within 48 hours, fibroplasia and capillary proliferation can be seen beneath the coagulum (2).

The inflammatory phase of the healing process is seen histologically as an eosinophilic exudate containing neutrophils and lymphocytes that develop over the dermis immediately following abrasion (3). Polymorphonuclear leukocytes and macrophages enhance the wound environment by phagocytizing foreign body debris and bacteria. Consequently, the risk of secondary bacterial infection is exceedingly low following abrasive procedures. Furthermore, macrophages stimulate granulation tissue formation, fibroplasia, and further collagen deposition through the release of cytokines, interleukin-1, and macrophage derived growth factor (2).

GRANULATION TISSUE FORMATION

Much of the skin's glistening red surface becomes covered with a yellow film and some areas of pink new epidermis can be seen 24 and 48 hours after abrasion (Figs. 9.3 and 9.4). Within 24 hours of injury, epithelial cells begin to migrate from the adnexal structures and wound edges. Cell-cell and cell-matrix interactions via cell surface proteins and their receptors direct the process of re-epithelialization. Reconstitution of the basement membrane zone occurs as cell-substratum adherence is re-established with the adhesion molecule complex (4).

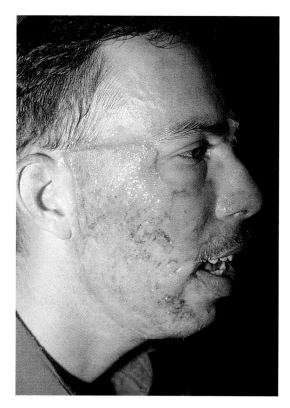

FIGURE 9.3
Appearance 24 hours following wire brush dermabrasion.

Hemidesmosomes are disassembled before keratinocyte movement, and are then reestablished along the basal surface of the cells upon completion of migration. This process is thought to involve the integrins, a family of transmembrane adhesion receptors recognized as extracellular matrix receptors and part of the hemidesmosome (5). Specifically the alpha-6/beta-4 heterodimer is expressed along the dermal pole of the basal keratinocyte at the leading edge of re-epithelialization (6-8). Rabbit corneum models have shown increased alpha-6 expression on basolateral and apical surfaces of actively migrating epithelial cells (9). The integrin subunits, alpha V/beta 3, are vascular cell receptors for the adhesive proteins of fibronectin, fibrin, and vitronectin and have demonstrated a role during invasive angiogenesis and granulation tissue formation (10). Furthermore, transforming growth factor beta one (TGF-beta 1) may induce epidermal keratinocytes to express integrins that facilitate the migratory component of re-epithelialization (11).

RE-EPITHELIALIZATION

Another critical molecule along with TGF-beta 1 that is involved with re-epithelialization is tenascin, an extracellular matrix glycoprotein associated with epithelial-mesenchymal interfaces during wound healing and embryogenesis (12). In healing mouse skin, tenascin appears along the wound edge 24 hours after injury and stains intensely within granulation tissue for 5 to 7 days. It is expressed before epithelial cell and fibroblast migration in fetal wounds and interferes with the integrin-mediated fibroblast attachment to fibronectin. Subsequently, it is thought to play an active role in promoting re-epithelialization (13).

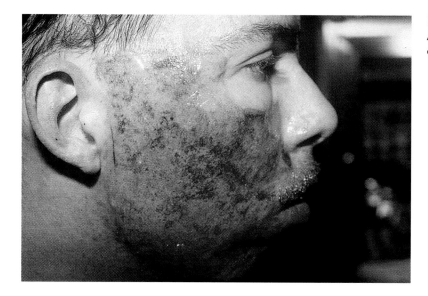

FIGURE 9.4
Appearance 48 hours following wire brush dermabrasion.

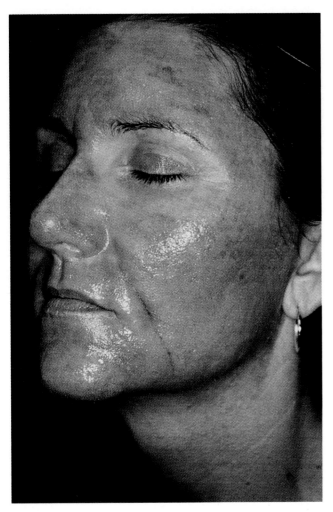

FIGURE 9.5
Appearance 5 days following wire brush dermabrasion.

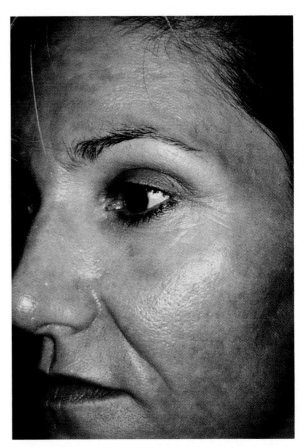

FIGURE 9.6
Appearance 1 month following wire brush dermabrasion.

Re-epithelialization is usually complete 5 to 6 days postoperatively, and the face is bright pink in color with very few areas of red or yellow buildup (Fig. 9.5). Histologically, the new epidermis may be only 2 to 3 cells thick with poorly developed rete ridges. A newly formed subepidermal zone of type III collagen appears more dense than the preexisting type I collagen of un-injured skin (2). Collagen synthesis (primarily types I and III) begins 3 to 4 days after injury as fibroblasts migrate and proliferate along the fibronectin matrix to form granulation tissue. Fibroblast migration appears to occur preferentially in fibronectin rich regions that have small amounts of collagen. As the wound matures and more collagen is deposited, fewer fibroblasts migrate into the maturing scar (14, 15). As part of the provisional matrix and granulation tissue, hyaluronic acid and proteoglycans (chondroitin-4-sulfate, dermatan sulfate, and heparan sulfate) further serve to regulate

fibroblast and epidermal cell migration. Early in tissue regeneration, production of nonsulfated hyaluronic acid facilitates fibroblast migration and proliferation. During later stages, a transition in the matrix toward sulfated proteoglycan components occurs which promote epidermal cell migration over fibroblast migration (16-18).

CONNECTIVE TISSUE REMODELING

The later phases of wound maturation are seen clinically as the pinkness fades and normal skin tone returns (Fig. 9.6). It is thought that a regression of vasculature and the re-establishment of basal melanocytes contribute to the restoration of natural skin color. During the time when new melanocytes are being formed (1 to 3 months postoperatively), any amount of sun exposure may produce uneven pigmentation. Therefore patients should avoid sun exposure until all the postoperative pinkness has faded.

At 3 months postoperatively, acne scars and wrinkles may appear more prominent than they did earlier in the postoperative course because the surgically induced edema has been completely resorbed. However the healing process is not yet complete, and connective tissue remodeling proceeds with the sequential deposition of fibronectin, type III collagen, and then type I collagen (19). Stromal reorganization occurs as fibronectin disappears and type III collagen is replaced by type I collagen (20). In addition to structural influences, collagen also acts as a chemoattractant for fibroblasts and alters epithelial cell functions (21, 22). During the 6-month period following abrasion, continuous collagen remodeling contributes to improved aesthetics by elevating the base of acne scars and softening the shoulders of wrinkles and pits. The smoother contours cast less shadow and appear less visible (Fig. 9.7). Consequently, any decision regarding subsequent resurfacing should be deferred until at least 6 months after the initial surgery.

SKIN RESPONSE TO SCAR REVISION

In contrast to dermabrasive resurfacing, scar revision by dermabrasion interrupts the first intention wound healing process and superimposes second intention mechanisms on the remodeling phase of the first wound. When dermabrasion is performed 6 to 8 weeks following injury, this approach to scar revision may yield a complete elimination of any visible evidence of primary scar formation. While clinically reproducible, the

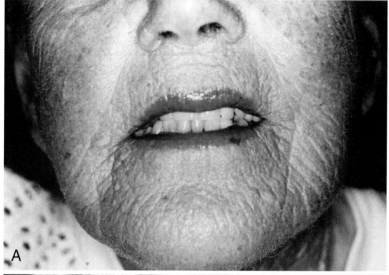
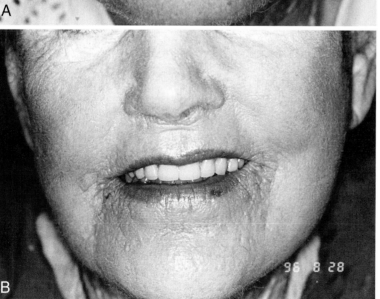

FIGURE 9.7
A, Photoaging and perioral rhytides prior to dermabrasion. B, Appearance 6 months following wire brush dermabrasion.

cellular mechanisms of revising scars by this method are incompletely understood.

Theories about the mechanisms of this type of scar revision include a collagen restructuring and layering parallel to lines of tension to provide smoother wound contours and epidermal defect elimination by the upward and horizontal migration of epithelial cells from viable adnexal appendages; however, these findings were difficult to demonstrate with the light microscope (23). Other reports suggest that a macroscopic blending or diffusing effect may create a less perceptible scar. On a biochemical and cellular level, rewounding during fibrillogenesis (i.e., abrading 4 to 8 weeks after injury) may cause a reaccumulation of hyaluronic acid in the wound matrix thereby stimulating more epidermal cells to migrate and proliferate in the wound (24). This concept is reasonable because fetal wounds, which heal without scarring, have in-creased amounts of hyaluronic acid in the collagen wound matrix (25).

Comparative electron microscopic and immunohistochemical studies on punch biopsy specimens taken from the primary scar site before and after dermabrasion have revealed post-abrasive changes in collagen patterns and extracellular matrix proteins. An increase in collagen bundle density and size with a tendency toward unidirectional orientation of fibers parallel to the epidermal surface was observed in the post abrasion specimens (Fig. 9.8). This alteration in collagen fibers may contribute to the proposed smoother wound contours.

Furthermore, the revised scars exhibited a more diffuse expression of alpha-6/beta-4 integrin subunits in the stratum spinosum (Figs. 9.9 and 9.10). The role of these integrin subunits in promoting keratinocyte migration suggests that the postabrasive alteration of

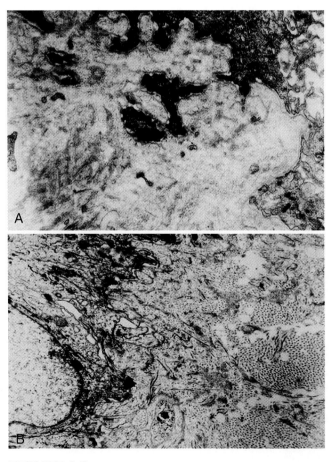

FIGURE 9.8
Electron micrograph. A, Specimen taken 7 days after primary closure shows disorganized fibers sparsely occupying the papillary dermis (×15,000). B, Specimen taken 7 days after dermabrasion shows a comparative increase in the number of more oriented collagen fibers (×15,000).

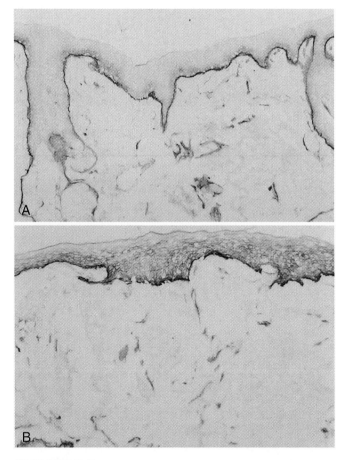

FIGURE 9.9
A, Specimen taken 5 weeks 5 days after primary closure shows linear basement membrane zone staining of alpha-6 integrin subunit (×100). B, Specimen taken 6 weeks after dermabrasive scar revision shows staining throughout the epidermis with alpha-6 integrin subunit (×100).

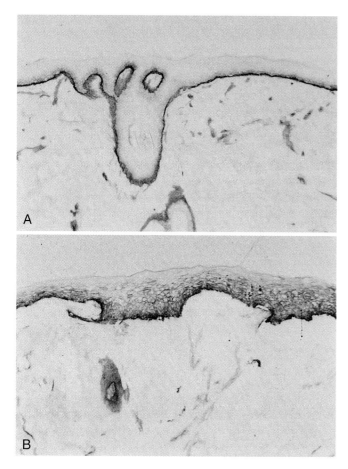

FIGURE 9.10

A, Specimen taken 5 weeks 5 days after primary closure shows linear basement membrane zone staining of beta-4 integrin subunit (×100). B, Specimen taken 6 weeks after dermabrasive scar revision shows staining throughout the epidermis with beta-4 integrin subunit (×100).

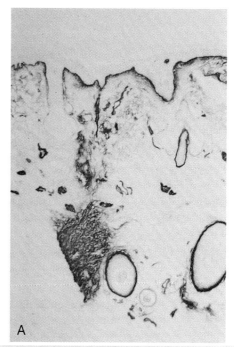

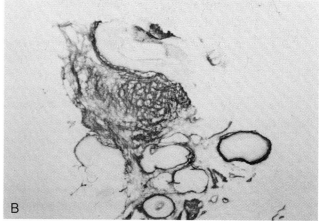

FIGURE 9.11

A, Specimen taken 5 weeks 5 days after primary closure shows tenascin staining localized along the basement membrane zone and the primary incision site (×100). B, Specimen taken 6 weeks after dermabrasive scar revision shows staining of tenascin throughout the papillary dermis (×100).

alpha-6/beta-4 expression may enhance cellular movement across the initial scar boundaries to provide a less perceptible epidermal defect. Likewise, an upregulation of tenascin was seen throughout the papillary dermis following dermabrasive scar revision (Fig. 9.11). As an extracellular matrix glycoprotein thought to promote epithelial cell and fibroblast migration, tenascin may allow fibroblasts and keratinocytes to cross the cicatrix and restore a more normal dermis and epidermis. Collectively, these observations suggest that dermabrasive scar revision reorganizes the primary cicatrix by altering extracellular ligand expression which influences the cell-cell and cell-matrix interactions of the wound healing process (26).

As the basic science of wound healing expands our understanding of cutaneous tissue repair, improved surgical results will be afforded to the patients undergoing these procedures. Whether dermabrasive resurfacing or scar revision by dermabrasion, the skin's healing response to this surgically controlled injury offers the potential for facial rejuvenation and the benefit of less perceptible scars and wrinkles.

REFERENCES

1. Stegman SJ, Tromovitch TA, Glogau RG. Cosmetic dermatologic surgery. Chicago: Year Book Medical Publishers, 1990:68.
2. Clark RA. Cutaneous tissue repair: Basic biologic considerations. J Am Acad Dermatol 1985;13:701-725.

3. Burks JW. Dermabrasion and chemical peeling in the treatment of certain cosmetic defects and diseases of the skin. Springfield, Ill: Charles C. Thomas, 1979:34.

4. Woodley DT, O'Keefe EJ, Prunieras M. Cutaneous wound healing: a model for cell-matrix interactions. J Am Acad Dermatol 1985;12:420-433.

5. Clark RA. Fibronectin matrix deposition and fibronectin receptor expression in healing and normal skin. J Invest Dermatol 1990;94:1288-1348.

6. Stepp MA, Spurr-Michaud S, Tisdale S, Elwell J, Gipson IK. Alpha six beta four integrin heterodimer is a component of hemidesmosomes. Proc Natl Acad Sci USA 1990; 87:8970-8974.

7. Sonnenberg A, Calafat J, Janssen H, Daams H, van der Raaij-Helmer LM. Integrin alpha six/beta four integrin heterodimer is located in hemidesmosomes, suggesting a major role in epidermal cell-basement membrane adhesion. J Cell Biol 1991;113:907-917.

8. Cavani A, Zambruno G, Marconi A, Manca V, Marchetti M, Giannetti A. Distinctive integrin expression in the newly forming epidermis during wound healing in humans. J Invest Dermatol 1993;101:600-604.

9. Paallysaho T, Tervo K, Tervo T, van Setten GB, Virtanen I. Distribution of integrins alpha six and beta four in the rabbit corneal epithelium after anterior keratectomy. Cornea 1992;11:523-528.

10. Clark RA, Tonnesen MG, Gailit J, Cheresh DA. Transient functional expression of alpha V beta three on vascular cells during wound repair. Am J Pathol 1996;148:1407-1421.

11. Gailit J, Welch MP, Clark RA. TGF-beta 1 stimulates expression of keratinocyte integrins during re-epithelialization of cutaneous wounds. J Invest Dermatol 1994;103:221-227.

12. Whitby DJ, Longaker MT, Harrison MR, Adzick NS, Ferguson MW. Rapid epithelialization of fetal wounds is associated with the early deposition of tenascin. J Cell Science 1991;99:583-586.

13. Murakami R, Yamaoka I, Sakukura T. Appearance of tenascin in healing skin of the mouse: possible involvement in seaming of wounded tissues. Int J Dev Biol 1989;33(4):439-444.

14. Demarchez M, Hartmann DJ, Herbage D, Ville G, Drunieras M. Wound healing of human skin transplanted onto the nude mouse. II. An immunohistological and ultrastructural study of the epidermal basement membrane zone reconstruction and connective tissue reorganization. Dev Biol 1987;121:119-129.

15. Gabbiani G, Lelous M, Bailey AJ, et al. Collagen and myofibroblasts of granulation tissue: A chemical, ultrastructural, and immunologic study. J Cell Pathol 1976;21: 133-145.

16. Silbert JE. Structure and metabolism of proteoglycans and glycosaminoglucans. J Invest Dermatol 1982; 79(Suppl): 31S-37S.

17. Bently JP. Rate of chondroitin sulfate formation in wound healing. Ann Surg 1967;165:186-191.

18. Trabucchi E, Preis-Baruffaldi F, Baratti C, Montorsi W. Topical treatment of experimental skin lesions in rats: macroscopic, microscopic, and scanning electron-microscopic evaluation of the healing process. Int J Tissue React 1986;8:533-544.

19. Suzuki M, Choi BH. The behavior of the extracellular matrix and the basal lamina during the repair of cryogenic injury in the adult rat cerebral cortex. Acta Neuropathol (Berl) 1990;80(4):355-361.

20. Kurkinen M, Vaheri A, Roberts PJ, Stenman S. Sequential appearance of fibronectin and collagen in experimental granulation tissue. Lab Invest 1980;43:47-51.

21. Postlethwaite AE, Seyer JM, Kang AH. Chemotactic attraction of human fibroblasts to type I, II, and III collagens and collagen-derived peptides. Proc Natl Acad Sci USA 1978;75:871-875.

22. Sugrue SP, Hay ED. Response of basal epithelial cell surface and cytoskeleton to solubilized extracellular matrix molecules. J Cell Biol 1981;91:45-54.

23. Yarborough JM. Ablation of facial scars by programmed dermabrasion. J Dermatol Surg Oncol 1988;14:292-294.

24. Katz BE, Oca AG. A controlled study of the effectiveness of spot dermabrasion ("scarabrasion") on the appearance of surgical scars. J Am Acad Dermatol 1991;24:462-466.

25. Siebert JW, Burd DAR, McCarthy JG, Weinzweig J, Ehrlich HP. Fetal wound healing: a biochemical study of scarless healing. Plast Reconstr Surg 1990;85:495-502.

26. Harmon CB, et al. Dermabrasive scar revision—immunohistochemical and ultrastructural evaluation. Dermatol Surg 1995;21:503-508.

CHAPTER 10

Wire Brush Dermabrasion

■ John M. Yarborough
William P. Coleman III
Naomi Lawrence

In 1953, when Kurtin published his first studies on wire brush dermabrasion, he ushered in a new phase in the history of resurfacing (1). But his work was neither original nor unique as Kromayer had published a number of papers on motorized dermabrasion in the early 1900s (2, 3). Kurtin became interested in dermabrasion as a method for removing tattoos from the thousands of victims from concentration camps who lived in New York after World War II. He was aware of manual dermasanding techniques that had become popular again in the 1940s (4). However, Kurtin was looking for a more efficient and reliable method for deep dermal abrasion to remove pigment fragments. He settled on modifying existing dental equipment. His technical collaborator was Noel Robbins, who played an important role for over 40 years developing equipment for dermabrasion and later hair transplantation. His company, Robbins Instrument Co., became the prime supplier of instruments and disposables for dermabrasion procedures.

With the large volume of patients eagerly hoping to have their tattoos removed, Kurtin was able to quickly amass a great deal of experience in dermabrasion. Physicians quickly became interested in this procedure, and techniques improved rapidly. By 1953, Lowenthal and Burks were removing pitted scars with dermal punches and replacing them with postauricular grafts, followed by dermabrasion (5). The fluorinated hydrocarbon refrigerants crucial to freezing the skin were well understood by the mid 1950s (6). Fluor Ethyl (Gebauer Co., Cleveland, OH) and Frigiderm (Frigiderm Corp., Costa Mesa, CA) became the refrigerants of choice and have continued in this role ever since. Burk's textbook

Wirebrush Surgery, published in 1955, is as relevant today as it was nearly a half century ago (7).

CLINICAL PRINCIPLES OF WIRE BRUSH DERMABRASION

Dermabrasion is a surgical procedure in which physical abrasion is employed to remove skin to a desired depth. When motorized instruments are used, a fraise, serrated wheel, or a wire brush is rapidly rotated by a fixed hand piece. The power of the hand piece motor determines the number of revolutions generated per minute (rpm). The higher the rpm, the more aggressive the instrument and the easier it is to penetrate human skin. The wire brush is less aggressive in removing tissue than the serrated wheel, but more aggressive than the diamond fraise. Using the now-standard Bell hand engine (Bell International, Burlingame, CA), skin can easily be abraded using a wire brush without exertion by the operator.

The torque created by this instrument requires firm manual control by the surgeon. Lifting the end piece at an angle away from the skin, creates a tendency for the instrument to "run" much like an electric floor polisher. Instead, steady strokes across the skin surface with the hand piece parallel to the skin provide the most control.

Abrasive injury to the skin is only feasible down to the reticular dermis; deeper penetration causes entry to the subcutaneous tissue and a permanent scar. The follicular structures that remain in the deep dermis allow re-epithelialization without scarring. The goal of dermabrasion is to remove skin to the depth necessary to achieve the desired clinical result. To achieve this goal, a superficial dermabrasion for superficial disorders such as hyperpigmentation to deep dermabrasion for acne scars may be required. Some scars penetrate through the reticular dermis and thus are beyond the reach of dermabrasion. However, in these cases it is not necessary for the surgeon to abrade to the bottom of the scar. Reticular dermal abrasion sets into motion the re-contouring and tightening of the skin such that even deeper scars will be at least improved. When the bottom of the depressed scar is not skin, but scar tissue, ancillary techniques such as punch grafting, punch elevation, or scar excision and repair may be needed prior to dermabrasion.

After dermabrasion, the treated skin heals through re-epithelialization from the residual appendageal structures. Deep dermabrasion may require 10 to 14 days for satisfactory re-epithelialization, but modern wound healing techniques, including the use of biologic dressings, have reduced healing time and permit patients to return to work and social life more rapidly than in the past.

SKIN CONDITIONS AMENABLE TO DERMABRASION

Dermatologic disorders improved by dermabrasion are listed in Table 10.1. However, the main indications for dermabrasive resurfacing include rhytides, actinic damage, scars secondary to disease or trauma, and pigmentary disorders.

TABLE 10.1

INDICATIONS FOR DERMABRASION

Rhytides
Actinic damage
Scars (from disease, surgery, or injury)
Pigmentary Disorders
Tattoos (decorative and traumatic)
Active acne
Rhinophyma
Syringomas
Trichoepitheliomas
Neurofibromas
Verrucous nevi
Linear epithelial nevi
Congenital nevi (at birth)
Angiofibromas
Xanthelasma
Lentigines
Darier's disease
Actinic keratoses
Seborrheic keratoses
Ephelides

Rhytides

Rhytides result from intrinsic aging of the skin as well as from extrinsic exposures to physical agents. Intrinsically, even skin that is covered throughout a lifetime eventually wrinkles and sags. However, the major causes of wrinkles are extrinsic forces, particularly sun exposure (Fig. 10.1). Rhytides are also due to facial expressions formed by the repeated action of underlying muscles. Dermabrasion has limited benefits on these types of expression lines. The use of filler substances (e.g., fat, collagen, Gore-Tex [W.L. Gore & Associates, Flagstaff, AZ], Fibrel [Mentor Corp., Irving, TX], hyalin gel) is more helpful than resurfacing for these muscle induced wrinkles. More recently, Botulinum toxin (BOTOX [Allergan, Inc., Irvine, CA]) denervation of facial muscles has also proved successful in smoothing lines of expression.

Actinic Damage

Actinic Damage results from chronic sun exposure. Repeated sun burning and tanning gradually causes deterioration of the dermal collagen leading to the classic physical signs of actinic damage: variegated pigmentation, wrinkling, and focal areas of inflammation (Fig. 10.2). This can progress into the development of actinic and seborrheic keratoses. Actinic keratoses are precancerous and may gradually evolve into squamous cell carcinomas. Actinic damage is most apparent where the person has had the most sun exposure. Although many people falsely believe that these changes are due to aging alone, most older individuals in fact have very smooth, even-toned skin in nonexposed areas, such as the buttocks.

Scars

Scars result from either disease or trauma. The most common skin disorder which leads to scarring is acne vulgaris. Cystic acne results in chronic inflammation of sebaceous glands and ducts in the dermis leading to a breakdown of the supporting collagen fibers. This results in a variety of types of scars (Fig. 10.3). Some scars are slightly depressed, but pliable, while others are deeply atrophic and may be firm. Others are pitted as in "ice pick" scars. Still, others have frank scar tissue at the base demonstrating full thickness loss of skin. These scars, as well as ice pick scars, often need to be pretreated with punch grafting or excision prior to dermabrasion to achieve significant benefits. However, sloped and atrophic scars are quite amenable to dermabrasion alone. The generation of new collagen that results from abrasive injury causes scar elevation and general skin tightening. Dermabrasion of scars is not a sculpting technique as with carpentry, but rather the entire skin surface is abraded to a given depth and left to re-epithelialize as a more even surface. New collagen generation causes skin tightening further improving scars.

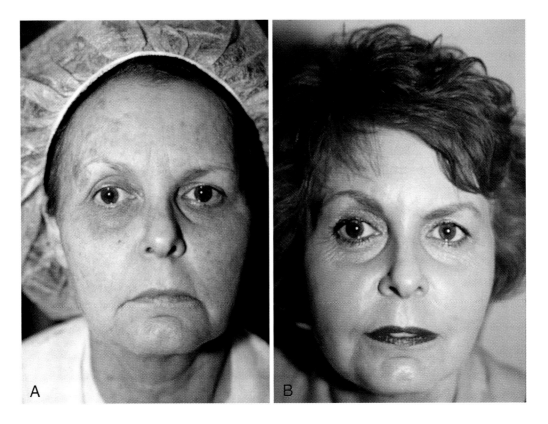

FIGURE 10.1
A, Photoaging with rhytides, lentigines, actinic keratoses and sallow coloration of facial skin in 53-year-old female. B, Four months post wire brush abrasion.

FIGURE 10.2
A, Elastotic degeneration and extensive formation of actinic keratoses over the face of a 76-year-old female. B, Seven months post wire brush abrasion.

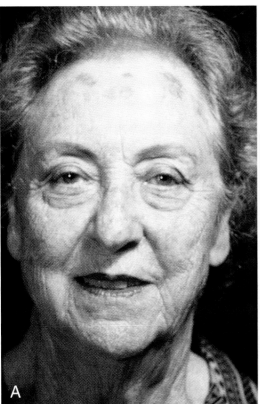

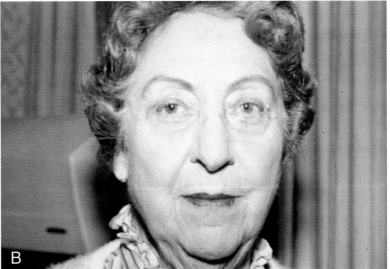

Traumatic or surgical scars can also be improved by dermabrasion. Whether these scars were sutured at the time of the initial injury or not, dermabrasion approximately 6 weeks postoperatively is quite effective in remodeling the scar tissue and smoothing the appearance of the wound. This can be a valuable adjunct to excisional and flap surgery and full thickness skin grafting. It is also highly effective in improving lacerations. Studies have shown that a window of opportunity exists between 4 and 8 weeks postoperatively, during which the tensile strength of the wound is sufficient to not be disrupted by dermabrasion while the collagen fibers are not yet so rigid that they cannot be realigned by abrasive wounding (8) (Fig. 10.4).

Pigmentary Disorders

Pigmentary disorders can also be improved by dermabrasion, which is often successful in creating a more uniform color to the skin. In postinflammatory hyperpigmentation, melanophores are trapped in the dermis. Abrading down to the deep dermis and permitting reepithelialization to occur will remove many of these pigmented foci allowing the skin to assume a more even color. In melasma, the pigmentation is more superficial and thus more superficial dermabrasion is sufficient to achieve improvement of the condition. In both disorders, there is a strong tendency for hyperpigmentation to recur so that postoperative use of bleaching agents, such as hydroquinones, is mandatory to achieve long term success.

Although decorative and traumatic tattoos are increasingly treated with lasers, dermabrasion remains an effective alternative. Dermabrasion is less costly and avoids the need for lasers of multiple wavelengths when tattoos contain several colors of pigment. The resulting scar is usually minimal (Fig. 10.5).

PATIENT CONSULTATION

Patients who present for dermabrasion should be evaluated for the entire spectrum of resurfacing procedures. Often, a patient will schedule a consultation thinking that dermabrasion is the most appropriate treatment for their condition when laser resurfacing or chemical peeling may be more appropriate. In many other cases, soft tissue fillers or BOTOX may also be more appropriate or should be used in conjunction with dermabrasion. The physician must first determine the patient's chief complaint and gauge the rest of the consultation based on the patient's desires. In some cases, pointing out additional problems that might benefit from resurfacing or ancillary procedures may also be appropriate, particularly if the problems could be treated in conjunction with the patient's primary problem.

It is convenient for the physician and patient to observe the problem area together using a mirror. In most

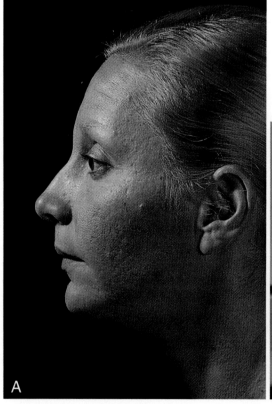

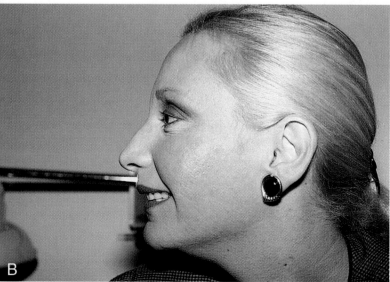

FIGURE 10.3
A, Extensive, deep acne scars over the face of a 34-year-old female. B, Improved facial contour four months after wire brush abrasion.

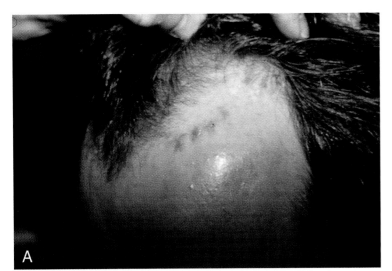

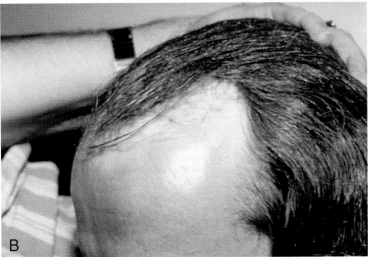

FIGURE 10.4
A, Surgical sites 6 weeks after punch removal of hair transplant autografts. B, Near complete ablation of surgical scars post wire brush abrasion.

cases, the pathology will be on the facial skin. The extent of actinic damage, pigmentary disorders, rhytides, and scarring should be noted. The types and depth of wrinkles and scars should also be discussed. A history of previous surgical procedures on the facial skin should be elicited as well as the degree of patient satisfaction from these treatments. Evidence of radiation treatments should also be noted.

The physician should also question patients as to their general physical condition. This includes at least a peripheral medical history, concentrating on active disorders and medications currently taken. Any history of allergies to medications should also be determined. If the patient is on any psychiatric medication, it is important to focus on the stability of their psychological disorder. Social history is also important as many patients seek cosmetic improvement after major disruptions in their lives such as divorce.

Any problems with healing or excessive scarring tendencies (hypertrophic scars or keloids) should also be noted. Resurfacing is not absolutely contraindicated in

patients who have keloids as the face is often spared this tendency, however it may indicate the need for a test site. The physician must also elicit whether or not the patient has been on isotretinoin (Accutane, [Roche Laboratories, Nutley, NJ]) within the last year as there is evidence that recent treatment with this drug may impair healing after surgery (9). There is some disagreement as to how long the patient should be off Accutane prior to dermabrasion, but most experienced dermabrasion surgeons recommend between 6 and 12 months (10).

A history of recurrent herpes simplex is also important since resurfacing may trigger a flare of this viral disorder leading to herpetic spread across the newly wounded skin. Although some physicians refuse to abrade patients with recurrent herpes simplex, the newer antiviral agents such as valacyclovir may be effective in preventing herpetic flares after dermabrasion. A conservative option is to abrade the entire face except for the recurrent "trigger" zone. After the rest of the face is re-epithelialized, this zone can then be abraded without fear of spread of the lesions. Prophylaxis with

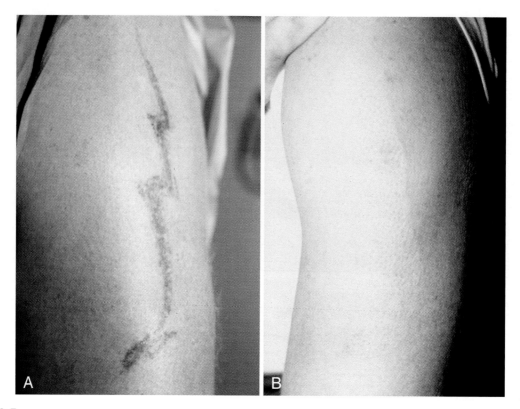

FIGURE 10.5
A, Decorative tattoo on lateral aspect of upper left arm. B, Complete ablation of tattoo and minimal scar formation 4 months after wire brush abrasion.

antiviral agents for all patients is debatable, but these drugs have minimal side effects and can be used without exposing the patient to significant risk.

HIV status is an important issue in bloody surgery. Wenzell et al have shown that there is potential for viral contamination in the ambient air after dermabrasion (11). This condition could potentially create risks for the operating surgeon and staff and perhaps other office personnel. In spite of this theoretical possibility, there is no evidence that any patient or assistant has ever developed AIDS from abrasion of an HIV-positive patient. Obviously protective gowns and masks are important in reducing contamination and every patient should be treated as though they may have an infectious disease. This will provide the ultimate safety for the physician and staff. Patients with advanced AIDS are poor candidates for any surgical procedure and should be discouraged from dermabrasion or any other elective procedure.

Darker skin patients are often good candidates for dermabrasion, but they must be aware that the area abraded will temporarily lose its color and that they may be more prone to post operative hyperpigmentation. Hyperpigmentation is more common in Fitzpatrick type IV and V skin (orientals, East Indians) than in type VI skin (dark blacks).

INFORMED CONSENT

Proper informed consent is not only a legal, but a moral responsibility of the physician. Patients should not be "talked into" surgery at any time. The decision to undergo abrasive resurfacing should be a joint one by the patient and physician. Both should feel comfortable with each other as individuals and ready to shoulder the benefits and the potential risks for this procedure. A patient who is educated in the possible side effects of dermabrasion will be much more comfortable working with the physician postoperatively if any complications occur.

The potential complications of dermabrasion are listed in Table 10.2. Sequelae are naturally occurring events that are commonly expected but vary from patient to patient (Table 10.3). Complications, however, are uncommon and although anticipated, are not expected to occur. Patients should be informed that each of these sequelae and complications have potential for treatment and that the physician is prepared to institute effective measures as required. Most complications of dermabrasion, if they do occur, can be ameliorated by prompt action. The most feared complication is scarring.

By 30 days postoperatively, the patient should be clearly recovering from dermabrasion. Although there may still be erythema, focal areas of red or possibly thickened skin should be a warning of an incipient scar. Prompt treatment (see Postoperative Care) can eliminate the eventuation of this area into a permanent scar.

After a thorough discussion of the potential for complications, the physician should review any consent forms that the patient is expected to sign prior to surgery. It is better if the consent forms are signed during a preoperative visit rather than on the day of surgery. On the day of surgery, patients are often presedated and may also be anxious and not as able to make rational decisions. A preoperative visit also gives the physician another opportunity to educate the patient in the pre- and postoperative care of dermabrasion. A checklist for the physician to review is helpful so that nothing is overlooked. The preoperative visit also provides an opportunity to write any necessary prescriptions and to review the medications the patient is currently taking, so that those that would interfere with dermabrasion can be discontinued. Nonprescriptive medications must also be reviewed since Vitamin E, many analgesics, and alcohol can increase bleeding.

PREOPERATIVE PREPARATIONS

Patients are naturally apprehensive prior to dermabrasion. A prescription or sample of a minor tranquilizer taken before bed the night before surgery and 1 hour prior to arriving at the office is helpful in allaying anxiety. This makes the entire procedure more comfortable for both the patient and physician. A driver is required to both drop off and pick up the patient after surgery. Male patients should arrive at the office cleanly shaven. All patients should shampoo their hair prior to arrival and remove any jewelry. Antibiotic prophylaxis is probably unnecessary in dermabrasion since an abrasive

TABLE 10.2

COMPLICATIONS OF DERMABRASION

Infection (viral or bacterial)	Hypopigmentation
Persistent erythema	Hyperpigmentation
Scarring	

TABLE 10.3

VARIABLE SEQUELAE OF DERMABRASION

Swelling	Acne Flares
Pain	Milia
Pruritus	Erythema
Petechia	Pigmentary Disorders

wound is quite clean as opposed to laser resurfacing. If antibiotic prophylaxis is selected, a wide spectrum of topical antibiotics can be applied intranasally and in the ear canals beginning the day prior to surgery. Most maintenance medicines used for systemic disorders such as antihypertensives should be continued unless they have anticoagulant effects.

The patient should be instructed to wear comfortable clothing that buttons up the front or back and thus does not have to be pulled over the head for removal. Old, easily cleaned clothing is recommended since it may become stained with blood. Shirts or blouses should be removed in the operating room and replaced with a clean surgical gown. The entire face is then prepped with a surgical scrub such as chlorhexidine gluconate.

The degree of sedation required for dermabrasion varies considerably from patient to patient. Patients who are premedicated with oral diazepam the night before and 1 hour prior to surgery are usually not apprehensive prior to the procedure. Gentle soothing words from the surgeon and staff help to maintain the impression that all is going well and the patient can relax. Most patients inherently fear the concept of abrasion. Although topical approaches to skin anesthesia are effective, additional systemic sedation is usually appreciated by the patient. Fifty mg to 100 mg of Demerol (Sanofi-Winthrop Pharmaceuticals, New York, NY) administered with 50 mg of an antihistamine, such as Vistaril (Pfizer Laboratories, Inc., New York, NY), adjusted to weight, is an effective sedative combination for dermabrasion. This intramuscular approach has proved quite safe and usually does not impair the patient's reflexes. It does however allow a sense of tranquility and well being while enabling the patient to still cooperate with the surgeon.

Deeper sedation can be employed using intravenous or inhalant agents preferably under the supervision of a nurse anesthetist or anesthesiologist. Legal opinion holds that the operating surgeon is the "captain of the ship" and is responsible for those working under him (12). This would include nurse anesthetists. Therefore, any physician who employs these personnel must act in conformity with the community standard required for an anesthesiologist. Anyone uncomfortable with this legal doctrine should consider the services of an anesthesiologist if deeper anesthesia is chosen.

Not only does deep sedation require more supervision and extensive monitoring of respiratory and cardiovascular status, but it also makes it more difficult for the patient to recover postoperatively. A recovery room may be needed and the patient may need several hours before they can take care of themselves. Using intramuscular Demerol and Vistaril, most patients are ambulatory immediately after the dermabrasion and can return to the comfort of their homes where they can begin postoperative care without assistance.

TOPICAL ANESTHESIA FOR DERMABRASION

For nearly a half century Fluor Ethyl (freon 114-ethyl chloride) has been the standard for freezing skin prior to dermabrasion. Freezing the skin allows temporary anesthesia and renders the tissue into a solid state so that it can be more easily abraded. Dermabrasion works best on a firm, nonmobile surface. There is however, the potential to injure the skin using these freezing agents. Over freezing the skin creates cryosurgical wounding that can lead to pigmentary problems or even scarring. Colder cryogens have been developed that have been rejected by surgeons because of their potential to cause scarring (13). Fluro Ethyl has stood the test of time as a reliable freezing agent without exerting significant negative effects. However, even with this safe agent, over freezing can occur and cause injury to the skin.

In recent years, fluorinated hydrocarbons have come under fire as a partial cause of the thinning ozone layer in the atmosphere. There has been some discussion of discontinuing the availability of these compounds and the development of alternative cryogens. However to date, Fluro Ethyl and Frigiderm remain available. It could be argued that if such small amounts of this product are employed on a daily basis, it would have a minimal effect on the atmosphere.

In the past, some hospital-based surgeons have attempted to perform dermabrasion under general anesthesia without prior freezing of the skin or infiltration of local anesthetics. The soft, moveable natural state of human skin reacts poorly to the rapidly rotating brush. This results in less control and the potential for uneven wounding or even scars.

In the 1990s, there has been some interest in using the tumescent technique for performing dermabrasion (14). This approach, adopted from "tumescent liposuction," involves the infiltration of large quantities of very dilute lidocaine and epinephrine. Enough of this dilute tumescent fluid must be injected that the skin becomes firm. This results in anesthesia and effective vasoconstriction. Thus, there is less bleeding and splatter with potential for reducing contamination for the surgeon and staff. Furthermore, the firm surface created by the tumescence allows dermabrasion to be performed on a firm surface similar to that created by the use of cryogens. An effective approach is to inject 250 to 300 ml of 0.1% lidocaine and 1:500,000 of epinephrine into the subcutaneous tissue of the face. Local blocks of the key facial sensory nerves with 2% lidocaine and 1:100,000 epinephrine are also employed. This degree of anesthesia falls well within the acceptable safe range of 500 mg for lidocaine injected into facial tissue. Although vastly larger doses can be safely used for liposuction in the fatty tissue, there are no studies clearly demonstrating that the 500 mg dose can be safely exceeded for facial infiltration. Nevertheless, 250 to 300 ml of 0.1% tumescent solution is usually sufficient for performing facial dermabrasion. Some patients experience "hot spots" in focal areas and require supplementary cryoanesthesia with Fluro Ethyl to give maximum comfort. However, it is possible to dermabrade an entire face using only the tumescent anesthetic approach. Goodman has suggested preoperative topical EMLA anesthesia (Astra USA Inc., Westboro, MA) to further augment the local anesthetic effect (15).

OPERATING ROOM SETUP

The patient should be dressed in a gown that protects their clothes from blood splatter. The head should be secured tightly and covered with an elastic cap. The skin should be prepped with chlorhexidine gluconate soap. The operating room should be sufficiently air conditioned so that it is easy to chill the patient's skin with the topical refrigerants. Several minutes before surgery, the patient should be given reusable gel cold packs wrapped in towels to hold in place over the operating sites. This prechilling prepares the skin for topical refrigerant anesthesia.

Modern wirebrush dermabrasion is performed using a motorized hand engine fitted with a circular wirebrush. The hand engine has largely replaced the original cable-driven dental unit employed in the past. The most commonly used hand engine is produced by Bell International, Burlingame, CA. This hand held device is light and maneuverable and is attached to a small console by a coiled electric cord. A newer engine, the AEV-12, is produced by Ellis International, Madison, NJ. The AEV-12 engine provides up to 30,000 rpm and more torque than on the Bell engine (maximum 18,000 rpm). This is more important for diamond fraise dermabrasion since the shaft of wirebrush may bend or rupture above 20,000 rpm. Wire brushes are currently available in 3 and 6 mm widths and 17 mm diameter (Fig. 10.6). They are available in 3 calibers of wire: fine, medium, and coarse in the 3 mm width. Only the medium caliber wire is available for the 6 mm brushes.

Only a simple surgical tray is required which holds the hand engine with the appropriate size wire brush locked in place. The surgeon must ensure that the assistant has properly secured the brush to the engine to prevent the possibility of a flying missile. Also on the tray are sterile cotton towels. These can be autoclaved and reused. Red towels are less likely to show stains. Gauze pads are not used as they may become entangled in the wire brush. Several cans of Fluor Ethyl should be on the tray as well. The surgeon and the assistants should be capped, masked, and gloved. In addition face shields should be used to prevent blood splatter. Low penetration surgical masks and goggles can provide further protection.

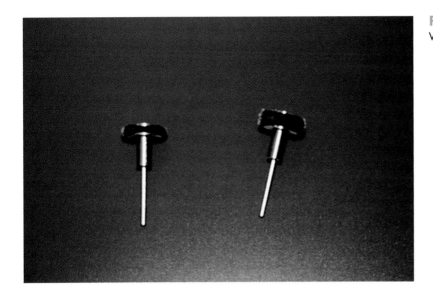

FIGURE 10.6
Wire brushes for dermabrasion.

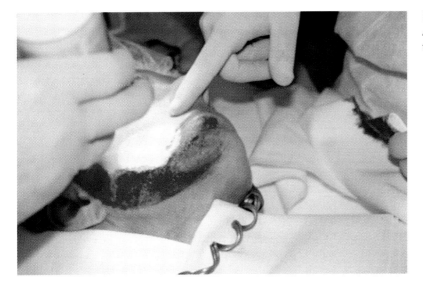

FIGURE 10.7
An area is frozen that the surgeon can abrade before the skin thaws.

WIRE BRUSH TECHNIQUE

It is more efficient for the right-handed surgeon to perform dermabrasion from the right side of the operating room table. The hand engine should be adjusted so that the wire brush rotates in a clockwise direction. Left-handed surgeons usually feel more comfortable abrading from the left side with the wire brush rotating counter clockwise. The surgeon or assistant should spray the refrigerant on a portion of the face to be dermabraded, holding the can 5 to 7 cm from the face to prevent dripping. The frozen area should be one that the surgeon can easily abrade before the skin thaws (Fig. 10.7). This is normally about 6 or 7 cm in diameter. The area should be frozen for about 10 seconds. Over freezing the skin results in longer thaw times and cryogenic injury and may lead to hypopigmentation or scarring. The surgeon must develop a system of rapidly freezing and then putting down the can on a nearby

table so that abrading can begin without delay. This can be facilitated by the assistant handing the spray can to and taking it from the surgeon. If an assistant does the spraying, there must be good communication between the surgeon and assistant to avoid over freezing. Special handles are available to attach to the commercial spray can nozzles to facilitate an even discharge of the cryogen on the face.

After the skin is frozen sufficiently, the surgeon should immediately begin dermabrading. The skin should be held taut. A convenient approach is for the assistant to pull in two directions and the surgeon pulling in a third direction using the nondominant hand. The sterile towels facilitate holding onto the slippery surface of previously abraded skin. A sterile white cotton glove may also be used by the surgeon or assistant to improve the grip. If the skin is loose, the instrument may skip and gouge the face.

FIGURE 10.8
Proper dermabrasion technique with the hand in firm control making strokes horizontal to the skin surface.

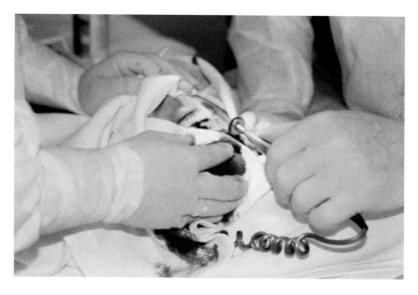

It is extremely important that the surgeon maintain a firm grip on the handle of the hand engine. Grasping the handle with the palm and fingers with the thumb placed over the neck helps to maintain control. The surgeon should make careful strokes across the skin in a horizontal direction (Fig. 10.8). The stroke should be unidirectional, perpendicular to the plane of rotation of the brush, and light and rapid allowing the brush to do most of the work. A feeling of pressure or friction indicates too deep of a stroke. Abrading in a back and forth manner will only gouge the skin. As the brush enters the papillary or superficial reticular dermis, white parallel lines appear indicating bundles of collagen. Proceeding further into the mid or lower reticular dermis causes intermittent fraying of these bundles. Deeper abrasion would penetrate through the dermis leading to scar formation.

The typical wire brush dermabrasion proceeds segmentally. Each surgeon should develop a planned sequence of moving from one part of the face to the other. If dependent areas of the face are abraded first, bleeding will not obscure adjacent unabraded skin. Thus, the outer cheek may be approached first, leading to the medial cheek followed by the chin, the upper lip, and the nose. Next, the other cheek is approached from lateral to medial and the forehead abraded last. Many surgeons prefer to abrade the forehead last because freezing is more painful in this area probably due to minimal subcutaneous tissue.

Around the nose, the refrigerant spray should be aimed away from the nostrils to avoid patient inhalation. Dermabrasion near the vermillion border should be performed with strokes directed perpendicular to the mouth. The abrasion should be continued up to the vermillion border, carefully eliminating any minor rhytides which are often found here. Patients should be instructed to pull their lips over the teeth to facilitate a

firm site upon which to abrade. Some surgeons alternatively prefer to grasp the lip in their nondominant hand to immobilize it.

Dermabrasion can be performed on the lower eyelids, but the skin is quite thin here and the procedure is technically more difficult. Eyelids are abraded more safely with a diamond fraise. The tissue must be frozen solid while held tautly to avoid any wrinkling. Often the entire eyelid is not abraded, but the procedure should at least extend over the orbital rims. Superficial abrasion can be used to feather this area to avoid a line of demarcation. Some surgeons prefer to use chemical peeling or laser resurfacing of the lower lids instead of abrading the eyelids. Chemical peeling of the brow also helps to blend in this area. Peeling or laser resurfacing may also be used on the upper eyelid but dermabrasion is rarely employed here.

The most common line of demarcation after dermabrasion is found at the mandibular margins. The surgeon should ensure that abrasion is continued over the mandible and slightly down onto the neck. Dermabrasion of the neck is unpredictable as this tissue heals in an erratic manner and may scar easily. However, dermabrading 1 cm below the mandibular margin is safe. Superficial abrasion should be used to feather into this zone to minimize contrast between the abraded and nonabraded skin. Additionally, light chemical peeling may be performed on the neck to improve actinic damage or dyschromia and minimize contrast between the abraded and nonabraded skin.

At the end of the dermabrasion, the surgeon should carefully examine the entire face to ensure that no areas were skipped. If a skipped area is found, it can be lightly frozen and abraded. When the surgeon is satisfied that the dermabrasion is complete, the assistant applies gauze squares soaked in lidocaine without epinephrine. This provides additional anesthesia and hemostasis.

POSTOPERATIVE CARE

In the past, open techniques for wound care after dermabrasion were preferred. However, with the development of biologic dressings closed care for at least the first 24 to 48 hours is now standard (16). Although there are a variety of biologic dressings available Vigilon (CR Bard, Inc., Murray Hill, NJ), is ideally suited to the abraded wound.

When the patient is ready for dressing application, a layer of petrolatum, Aquaphor (Beiersdorf, Inc., S. Norwalk, CT) ointment, or an antibiotic ointment is applied. Over this, sections of Vigilon are placed and secured together with waterproof tape. Next gauze squares are applied and likewise secured. These dressings are then further supported by wrapping Kling gauze (Johnson & Johnson Inc., Arlington, TX) over and around the entire face leaving gaps for the eyes, nose, and mouth. Alternatively, an absorbent mask or elastic mesh can be used to secure the dressings.

The patient is discharged with detailed home instructions. Because they have usually been sedated, patients should be accompanied by a responsible adult and escorted directly to their bed. The head should be kept upright on several pillows to minimize edema. Some serosanguineous drainage should be expected. The patient should remain in bed except to go to the bathroom until the following morning.

Ice packs are useful in helping to minimize swelling. Commercial gel packs are efficient. Alternatively, ice packs may be prepared by placing miniature ice cubes or frozen vegetables in plastic food bags which are then wrapped in towels. The aim is to chill, but not over chill the abraded skin. The ice packs should be applied intermittently 10 minutes on and 10 minutes off for the rest of the day after surgery. This should be continued until the patient is ready to go to bed for the night.

Some patients may have trouble sleeping the first few nights after surgery. Elevation on several pillows, drainage, and slight discomfort all combine to make sleep difficult. Sleeping pills dispensed by the physician are often appreciated. The attendant or spouse should be informed that the patient may be groggy after surgery or after taking sleeping pills and they should be accompanied even to the bathroom.

We prefer to see our patients as often as possible after dermabrasion to ensure they are healing properly. We normally see our patients the day after the abrasion and remove the surgical dressing. If the patient is uncomfortable with complete facial occlusion, open care can be instituted at this point. Other patients prefer to have the face covered and a new Vigilon dressing can be reapplied for an additional 24 hours. Open care consists of frequently cleansing the abraded sites with tap water followed by the application of a bland ointment such as petrolatum, Aquaphor or a non sensitizing antibiotic ointment. This cleansing should be performed as often as possible, but at least 6 times daily. Patients often find that water applications makes them more comfortable especially when the abraded sites begin to dry out. Showering and shampooing as necessary is encouraged.

Soap use can usually begin on the third postoperative day; any earlier and the soap may cause some burning. A mild superfatted soap is appropriate. The patient should wash using only their fingers and not a wash cloth. Gentle rubbing of the skin will debride the thin crusts that have formed without causing bleeding. Soap and water followed by application of a bland ointment 4 times a day usually continues until the skin has re-epithelialized (postoperative day 7 to 10).

Once re-epithelialization has occurred, the heavy ointments are replaced by soothing moisturizers such as Eucerin cream (Beiersdorf, Inc., S. Norwalk, CT). This can be replaced subsequently by Eucerin lotion or Cetaphil lotion (Owen/Galderma Laboratories, Inc., Ft. Worth, TX) which are thin enough to allow cosmetics to be applied over them. Once the patient can apply cosmetics, they often feel more comfortable about their appearance and are ready for work or social situations. Many men are uncomfortable with cover ups and may require a longer period of hiding from the public. However, all patients should be informed preoperatively that they will feel well enough to perform some work at home usually after the first postoperative day.

Once the patient has returned to public life, they should be careful to avoid the sun. Sunscreens usually irritate the newly abraded skin and cannot be applied for 1 to 2 weeks postoperatively. Once the sunscreens can be used, the patient should still do his/her best to avoid prolonged periods of sunlight as this will lead to burns and potentially dyspigmentation. Generally the patient should avoid significant sun exposure for 3 months postoperatively.

Patients with Fitzpatrick type III skin type and higher are prone to postoperative hyperpigmentation. This result should be expected, and the patient should be informed of it before the dermabrasion. There is a clinical impression that the use of tretinoin and hydroquinones preoperatively may reduce the severity of this postoperatively, but this has not been scientifically validated. It is however, advantageous to use hydroquinones preoperatively to be sure the patients are not sensitive to them. Four percent hydroquinone cream can generally be tolerated approximately 2 to 3 weeks postoperatively. Hydroquinone use should be instituted with all darker skin patients and at the earliest sign of hyperpigmentation in lighter skin patients. As soon as the skin tolerates it, tretinoin can also be applied to facilitate the effect of the hydroquinone. These bleaching agents should be used for several months after the hyperpigmentation has resolved.

Because of the use of occlusive ointments after dermabrasion, many patients are prone to acne or milia. In the early postoperative period, topical antiacne medications are not tolerated. Appropriate acne antibiotics should be employed (tetracycline, minocycline, erythromycin). Once the skin is healed sufficiently, benzoyl peroxides, azelaic acid, tretinoin, and topical antibiotics can be employed as required. Many dermabrasion patients have an intrinsic tendency for acne (which has often caused their scarring) and they must be carefully treated to prevent cystic lesions that could lead to new scarring.

Milia occur frequently after dermabrasion. In some patients this problem can be quite severe. Milia do not require treatment as they gradually dissolve spontaneously. If desired by the patient, milia can be treated by manual unroofing or light electrodesiccation. Alternatively, 70% glycolic acid peels can be employed weekly to loosen these small cysts. Aggressive acne surgery should not be employed as this may cause scarring. Tretinoin is somewhat useful in dissolving milia but is quite slow in action. Many patients cannot tolerate tretinoin during the first month postoperatively, but it should be reintroduced when feasible. Low concentration cream formations are used early and then the patient can be switched over to stronger creams or gels as the skin tolerates.

Erythema is quite common after re-epithelialization has occurred. However, this erythema should gradually fade, 50% or more by the end of the first month postoperatively. Persistent erythema, particularly in a focal area may be evidence of an incipient scar. Focal persistent erythema should be treated initially with topical steroids. If this does not help, intralesional steroids may be required. Intralesional steroids should be used in low concentrations at first (2 to 3 mg/ml of triamcinolone). The concentration may be adjusted as required. Silicone sheeting may also be helpful in preventing early hypertrophic scars. If the erythema begins to thicken into a true scar, aggressive intralesional therapy and topical steroid-impregnated tape are often helpful. If this aggressive therapy fails, treatment with a flashlamp pulsed-dye laser can be pursued. With early intervention, permanent scarring rarely occurs after dermabrasion.

LONG TERM CARE

Many patients are initially excited about the results of dermabrasion because wrinkles or scars appear to be ablated which have really been improved by edema. After the swelling subsides, these scars or wrinkles may appear. Patients should be forewarned that it is very rare for dermabrasion to remove all scars or wrinkles and that some will not be eliminated even when the best techniques are employed. However, a measure of disappointment is expected when the final results become apparent 3 to 4 months postoperatively. At this time, the patient should be reminded that perfect results were not expected and that they have had significant improvement in most areas.

If additional dermabrasion is required to further improve the pathology treated, it should probably be deferred for about 1 year. This allows complete dermal recovery before another abrasion and allows the patient to adjust to the facial improvement and to make an informed decision as to whether they are interested in undergoing additional resurfacing. If subsequent dermabrasion is required, it can often be done in a "spot" manner without the need for a full face abrasion. These spot abrasions heal nicely without a line of demarcation when performed on previously abraded skin. Severe scars may require several spot abrasions at 1 year intervals until they finally reach a satisfactory result. After 2 or 3 abrasions however, there are usually diminishing returns and the patient must weigh the prolonged recovery from dermabrasion against the minimal additional gains they might achieve.

Permanent hypopigmentation occurs in a small percentage of all patients who undergo resurfacing. This complication is most likely after phenol peeling. However, it does occur after dermabrasion and usually in a focal manner. Hypopigmentation can be traced back to problems that occurred immediately after the abrasion such as infection. Often however, there appears to be no reason why one part of the face heals with loss of pigment and other areas heal satisfactorily. There is no satisfactory treatment for hypopigmentation. However, this problem can be disguised by superficial abrasion or medium chemical peeling around the hypopigmented segments. These additional resurfacing approaches are used to blend areas of hypopigmentation; however, they are never 100% effective. All patients must be informed before hand that hypopigmentation is a possibility after dermabrasion and that there is no-good treatment for it.

OTHER COMPLICATIONS

Bacterial infection is quite rare after dermabrasion when modern wound care techniques are employed. However, it does occur in a small percentage of individuals. Preoperative prophylaxis with oral antibiotics is not recommended as this may induce resistant species of bacteria, although topical antibiotics intranasally and in the ear canals can be useful. If infection does occur, appropriate broad spectrum oral antibiotics should be employed after cultures are taken. The physician should not wait for the results of the culture before instituting therapy. In contrast to laser resurfacing, monilial infections are quite rare after dermabrasion.

Herpes simplex infections can be devastating after dermabrasion. The newly abraded skin can allow proliferation of the infection throughout the face which may result in scarring. All patients who have a history of herpes simplex should be treated with prophylactic doses of acyclovir. If infection does occur, the physician can switch the patient over to valcyclovir or famcyclovir. These new generation antivirals provide high blood levels of acyclovir and are useful in resistant cases.

COMPARING DERMABRASION TO OTHER RESURFACING TECHNIQUES

A surgeon who is highly skilled in the use of resurfacing lasers and chemical peeling cannot provide patients with all of the potential benefits unless he or she also performs dermabrasion. Dermabrasion requires manual dexterity and good judgement; however, it is no more difficult to learn than any other surgical procedure. There is a natural learning curve during which the neophyte abrader should proceed cautiously as is the case with other resurfacing techniques.

Dermabrasion probably gives better results for facial scars than does laser resurfacing or chemical peeling. This is particularly true of surgical and traumatic scars. Deep acne scars also appear to obtain better results after dermabrasion than with other resurfacing approaches. Dermabrasion has also been shown to achieve long term prophylaxis against actinic keratoses. Postoperatively, patients with multiple precancerous lesions often remain free of these for a minimum of 4 years (16), which is twice as long as the prophylaxis provided by chemical peeling (17). The effect of laser resurfacing on precancerous lesions is currently unknown since the technology is so new. Dermabrasion has also been shown to be effective for a variety of benign dermal and epidermal growths (See Table 10.1). Chemical peeling is generally not effective in removing these lesions. Laser resurfacing may or may not be useful for removing many tumors. This will become clear with longer experience with this technology.

Abrasive wounds are cleaner than chemical or thermal burns. After dermabrasion, wound healing begins immediately without the need for macrophage scavenging of devitalized tissue as is the case with chemical peeling or laser resurfacing. Bacterial, viral, and monilial infections appear to be less common with dermabrasion than with deep chemical peeling and laser resurfacing. Although the wound looks worse to the patient in the first postoperative week, usually dermabraded skin is far less erythematous at 30 days than skin treated by deep chemical peeling or laser resurfacing.

Dermabrasion has been practiced by physicians for thousands of years. It remains an important part of the surgical armamentarium of those who practice skin resurfacing. The best trained surgeon should be able to perform all types of skin resurfacing to offer patients the widest array of modalities for improving their skin.

REFERENCE

1. Kurtin A. Corrective surgical planning of the skin. Arch Dermatol Syph 1953;68:389.
2. Kromayer E. Rotationsinstrumente: ein neues techisches Verfahren in der dermatologischen Kleinchirurgic. Dermatol Z 1905;12:26.
3. Kromayer E. Cosmetic Treatment of Skin Complaints. New York: Oxford University Press, 1930 (English translation of the second German edition, 1929).
4. Iverson PC. Surgical removal of traumatic tattoos of the face. Plast Reconstr Surg 1947;2:427.
5. Lowenthal L. Punch biopsy with autograft. Arch Dermatol Syph 1953;67:629-631.
6. Wilson J, Ayres S, Luikart R. Mixtures of fluorinated hydrocarbons as refrigerated anesthetic. Arch Dermatol 1956;74:310-311.
7. Burks J. Wirebrush Surgery. Springfield, IL: Charles C. Thomas, 1955.
8. Yarborough JM. Ablation of facial scars by programmed dermabrasion. J Dermatol Surg Oncol 1988;12:292-294.
9. Rubenstein R, Roenigk HH, Stegman SJ, et al. Atypical keloids after dermabrasion of patients taking isotretinoin. J Am Acad Dermatol 1986;15:280-285.
10. Alt TH, Goodman GJ, Coleman WP III, et al. Dermabrasion. In: Coleman WP III, et al., eds. Cosmetic Surgery of the Skin (2nd ed). St. Louis: Mosby, 1997:112-151.
11. Wentzell JM, Robinson JK, Wentzell JM Jr., et al: Physical properties of aerosols produced by dermabrasion. Arch Dermatol 1989;125:1637-43.
12. Coleman WP III, Guice W. Office surgery and the law. Adv Dermatol 1987;2:207-227.
13. Hanke CW, O'Brian JJ, Salow EB. Laboratory evaluation of skin refrigerants in dermabrasion. J Dermatol Surg Oncol 1985;11:45-49.
14. Coleman WP, Klein JA. Use of the tumescent technique for scalp surgery, dermabrasion, and soft tissue augmentation. J Dermatol Surg Oncol 1992;18:130-135.
15. Goodman G. Dermabrasion using tumescent anesthesia. J Dermatol Surg Oncol 1994;20:802-807.
16. Coleman WP III, Yarborough JM, Mandy SH. Dermabrasion for prophylaxis and treatment of actinic keratois. J Dermatol Surg 1996;22:17-21.
17. Lawrence N, Brody H, Alt T. Chemical peeling. In: Coleman WP III, et al. eds. Cosmetic Surgery of the Skin. St. Louis: Mosby, 1997:85-111.

CHAPTER 11

Diamond Fraise Dermabrasion

■ William P. Coleman III
Naomi Lawrence

In 1957 the diamond fraise was introduced as an alternative to the wire brush for dermabrasion (1). These rough wheels were shown to abrade the skin less aggressively than the wire brush. They were easier to control and less likely to gouge the skin. At the time, some dermatologists preferred the newer instrument over the old; the debate over which is superior continues today (2-4). Both instruments can be used effectively to abrade human skin and achieve similar results. Because the techniques are different, most surgeons prefer to use one or the other consistently rather than switch back and forth between these two different approaches.

Because the diamond fraise is inherently less efficient in abrading skin, more powerful hand engines have been developed which rotate the fraise at high revolutions per minute (rpm). Although the wire brush cannot be used efficiently over 20,000 rpm because the shaft may bend, diamond fraises may be used at speeds up to 60,000 rpm. The high speed Derma 3 Dermabrader (A. Schumann, Düsseldorf, Germany) provides a variable speed of 15,000 to 60,000 rpm. This machine requires special high speed diamond fraises with a thicker shaft to withstand the high rpm. The combination results in a more aggressive, powerful instrument than the lower rpm motors.

Another available engine, the AEV-12 hand engine (Ellis International, Madison, NJ) can operate at speeds from 1,000 to 30,000 rpm. The widely used Bell hand engine (Bell International, Burlingame, CA) is available in models that operate up to 20,000 rpm (Fig. 11.1). Standard diamond fraises can be used in either of these medium rpm machines. The diamond fraise is an effective instrument for achieving deep dermabrasion even at speeds below 20,000 rpm.

Diamond fraises are available in a wider variety of designs than the wire brush. Standard fraises are found in diameters ranging from 10 to 17 mm and widths from 2.5 to 10.5 mm. They are also produced in three different grits: standard, coarse, and extra-coarse. The greater the width of the fraise, the more efficient it is and the less tendency it has to gouge the skin. The coarser the fraise is, the more easily it will penetrate the skin (Fig. 11.2).

Fraises are also available in "pear" and "bullet" shapes (Fig. 11.1). The smaller fraises are primarily used by surgeons to feather the margins of deep scars. They are also useful for abrading around concave areas, such as the supraralar region of the nose and the philtrum of the lip.

PREPARING FOR DIAMOND FRAISE DERMABRASION

The indications, consultation, and preoperative preparations for diamond fraise dermabrasion are the same as for wire brush dermabrasion (see Chapter 10). Although some surgeons prefer one instrument over the other, similar clinical results can be achieved using either instrument. Because of the aggressive nature of the wire brush and its potential to "run" or gouge tissue, even those experienced with its use may often employ the diamond fraise for delicate areas. Some surgeons are uncomfortable using the wire brush on the upper lip or lower eyelids, for example, and the standard grit diamond fraise is very forgiving in these more difficult to abrade locations. Also, since the wire brush cannot be manufactured into unusual shapes, such as the pear or bullet, many wire brush surgeons use the smaller diamond fraises to feather scars or abrade concave anatomical locations.

FIGURE 11.1
The popular Bell hand engine fitted with a bullet shaped diamond fraise.

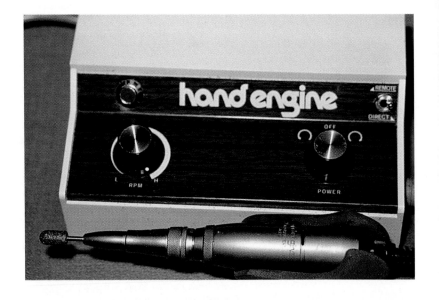

FIGURE 11.2
Extra coarse diamond fraises.

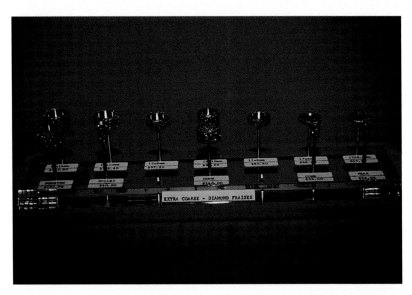

ANESTHESIA

Classic cryoanesthesia is commonly used for diamond fraise dermabrasion as with wire brush surgery. However, local anesthesia can be employed as an alternative and is more feasible with the fraise than with the wire brush, which requires an absolutely firm surface. The upper lip can be easily abraded using only local infiltration of 2% Xylocaine with 1:100,000 epinephrine using the diamond fraise. Regional dermabrasion of the nose can be accomplished in the same manner (Fig. 11.3). Full face diamond fraise dermabrasion, however, is not feasible using stock solutions of 2% lidocaine with 1:100,000 epinephrine due to the potential for lidocaine toxicity. In full face dermabrasion the 2% full strength solution is used for regional nerve blocks of the supra-

orbital, infraorbital, and mental nerves. The rest of the face can be efficiently anesthetized using tumescent anesthesia with 0.1% lidocaine and 1:500,000 epinephrine. Enough anesthesia must be infiltrated to render the skin firm and blanched (Fig. 11.4). Even when several hundred ml of the anesthesia solution are employed, it is still well within the bounds of the maximum recommended dose for lidocaine (7 mg/kg) (5).

Although tumescent anesthesia has been shown to be safe in doses of up to 55 mg/kg for body liposuction, higher doses have not been tested for safety on the face. High doses of lidocaine are not required because only 250 to 300 ml of 0.1% lidocaine is necessary to achieve the proper tumescence. The use of EMLA cream (Astra USA, Inc., Westboro, MA) 1 hour before dermabrasion further enhances the effect of tumescent anesthesia (6).

The tumescent solution is injected systematically beginning radially from the preauricular area using a spinal needle until the skin is firm and blanched. This indicates adequate infiltration and good vasoconstriction. Manual infiltration with 10 ml syringes allows the surgeon to draw back on the plunger and avoid accidental intravascular injections. As the surgeon empties a syringe, the assistant exchanges it for a full one. Tumescing an entire face may take 20 to 30 minutes. Another option is to use a peristaltic pump set on a slow infiltration rate. This avoids the syringe exchange maneuver but does not allow drawing back on the plunger to avoid intravascular injection. The tumescent anesthetic approach is more compatible with diamond fraise than wire brush dermabrasion since the skin is not rendered as firm as after freezing with fluorinated hydrocarbons.

Tumescent anesthesia significantly decreases bleeding during dermabrasion and reduces blood splatter and risk of blood born pathogens to operating room personnel (Fig. 11.5). It also provides another advantage not feasible during cryoanesthesia. Some scars extend deeper than are apparent preoperatively. During dermabrasion, it may become clear that a scar extends down through the reticular dermis. Rather than attempting to dermabrade too deeply and risk further scarring, these defects can be excised during dermabrasion and repaired (Fig. 11.6). Due to the massive re-epithelialization that occurs after dermabrasion, these excisional wounds heal quite rapidly. Often the sutures need to be removed

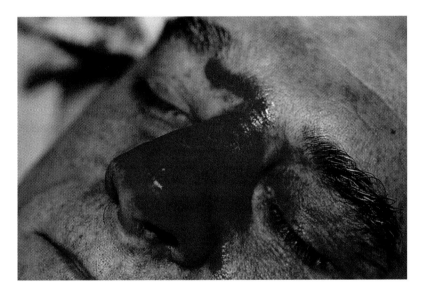

FIGURE 11.3
Regional dermabrasion of the nose and brow scar performed using local anesthesia.

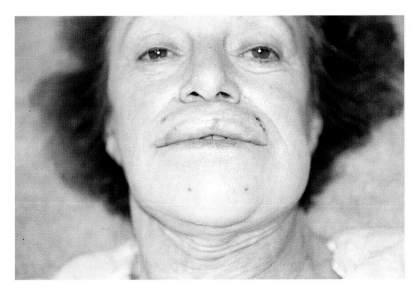

FIGURE 11.4
A blanch in the overlying skin indicates sufficient tumescence.

FIGURE. 11.5
Tumescent anesthesia was used on the chin with standard cryoanesthesia on the cheek. Notice the diminished bleeding in the tumesced skin.

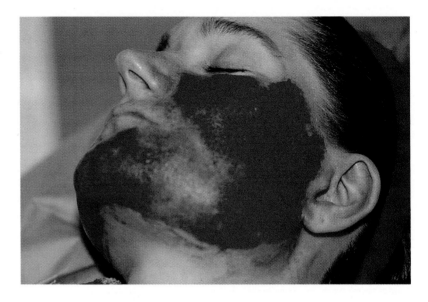

FIGURE 11.6
A, A deep scar is unmasked during dermabrasion.
B, The scar is excised and repaired simultaneously.

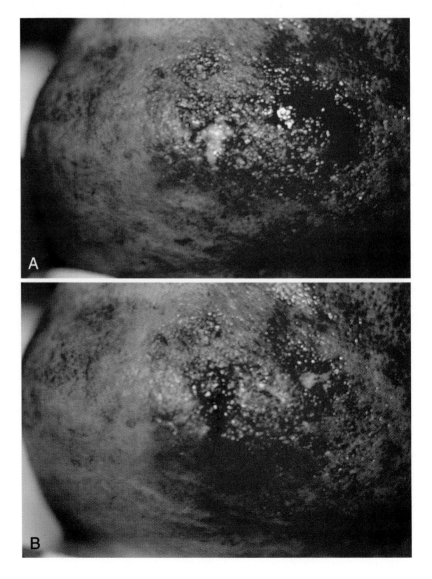

within 3 days postoperatively or they may become buried in the healing skin.

This technique provides a good alternative to preoperative *punch grafting* or *punch elevation,* which are two stage procedures. Punch grafting or punch elevation are usually employed 6 to 8 weeks *prior* to the dermabrasion. Thus, the patient has to endure two periods of facial healing. Punch grafting and punch elevation may be indicated when the surgeon decides that certain scars are too deep to be sufficiently improved by dermabrasion alone (3, 7, 8). Punch elevation is used when the lining of the scar is still intact skin. Using a dermal punch, this depressed segment can be elevated to surface level after detaching its fibrous connections.

Punch grafting is employed when the base of the depression is scar tissue. The scar is punched out and replaced with a small dermal graft taken from the postauricular area. These grafts can be secured with small sutures or steri strips. The advantage of punch grafting is that healthy unscarred skin is used to replace the original defect. However, there is a possibility that the donor skin will not be an exact match for its new facial location and even after dermabrasion differences in color and texture may be apparent. Also, a small circular scar can sometimes remain. When direct excision and repair of the scar is feasible, preferably during dermabrasion, these problems are avoided. However, even the most carefully repaired scar at times has a tendency to become depressed postoperatively and only partially improve the defect. In these cases, punch grafting would often provide a better result (Fig. 11.7).

DIAMOND FRAISE TECHNIQUE

The patient is prepared and sedated similarly to wire brush dermabrasion. Whether local or cryoanesthesia is used, many of the same techniques are employed. Prechilling of the skin with ice packs is favored by some experts, but not necessary. If cryoanesthesia is used, the surgeon should freeze the skin sufficiently to obtain a firm surface upon which to operate. However over freezing the skin creates an injury additional to the abrasion and may result in increased potential for scarring and hypopigmentation. Furthermore, the skin does not need to be as "rock hard" to perform diamond fraise dermabrasion as with the wire brush. The assistant and surgeon employ a three-point traction maneuver as with wire brush surgery to secure the skin.

Some surgeons prefer to use gentian violet or other dyes to indicate the bottom of deeper scars, others prefer to abrade the deeper scars first and then feather the rest of the face with a shallower abrasion. Still others systematically abrade the entire face and proceed deeper over scarred segments.

One advantage of diamond fraise dermabrasion is that fraises of varying coarseness can be employed to modulate the aggressiveness of the abrasion. It is possible to deeply abrade the facial skin using 18,000 rpm and a standard diamond fraise. However, the surgeon will have to exert a great deal of manual pressure to achieve this. Also, the hand engine will gradually heat up indicating motor fatigue. These problems can be resolved by using a higher rpm level (or a more powerful hand engine) or a coarser fraise. A 17 mm, 6 mm wide, extra coarse diamond fraise at 20,000 rpm is nearly as aggressive as the same size wire brush. The surgeon must apply slightly more manual pressure with the fraise than with the brush but can easily abrade deeply into the dermis.

The white parallel lines of collagen bundles are less apparent in the abraded dermis when the diamond fraise is used than when the wire brush is used. With diamond fraise dermabrading the surgeon uses signs such as the capillary loops found in the papillary dermis and the sebaceous glands in the upper reticular dermis to determine the depth of the sanding. The capillary loops are seen as short, red, linear structures that bleed as the skin thaws. Transected sebaceous glands are small, yellow globules. These are difficult to see in the face of brisk bleeding. When tumescent anesthesia is employed, there is far less bleeding and anatomic structures such as transected sebaceous glands can be more easily identified. However, fine bleeding points in the papillary dermis and coarser reticular bleeding are less apparent (Fig. 11.5).

POSTOPERATIVE COURSE

Patients heal after diamond fraise dermabrasion identically to those who are treated with the wire brush given that the level of the abrasion is the same. Therefore, the same techniques are used to heal the skin and help to minimize complications. Long term results are also similar. Although some wire brush advocates occasionally claim that they achieve better results by "lacerating" collagen fibers, it is likely that given equal depths of dermal injury, the two techniques produce identical results (9).

Diamond fraise dermabrasion is more user friendly than wire brush dermabrasion. The neophyte will feel comfortable with this instrument more rapidly than the wire brush. Practice on oranges or other skin simulators allows the surgeon to practice technique. Using the diamond fraise, excellent results can be achieved with acne scars (Fig. 11.8), actinic keratoses (Fig. 11.9), seborrheic keratoses (Fig. 11.10), rhinophyma (Fig. 11.11), traumatic scars (Fig. 11.12), wrinkles (Fig. 11.13) and many of the other abnormalities also treatable by wire brush dermabrasion.

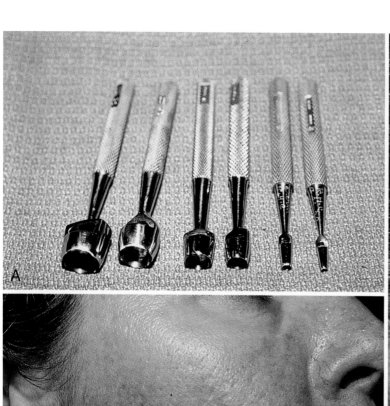

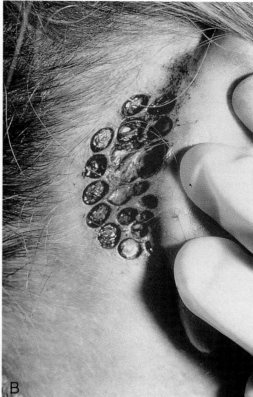

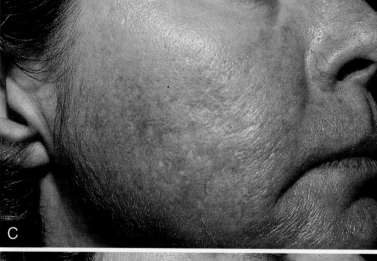

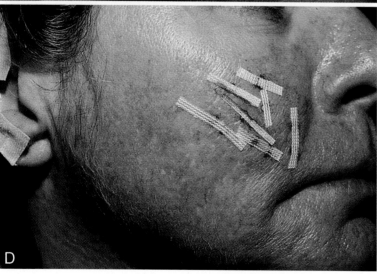

FIGURE 11.7

Punch grafting prior to dermabrasion. A, Surgical punches in various sizes can be utilized to excise scars and harvest full-thickness skin grafts. B, The post-auricular area is a useful donor site for punch grafts. C, A 50 year old woman has a variety of acne scars on the cheek. D, Ten pit-type scars have been punched out and have been replaced with postauricular grafts. The grafts are secured with narrow paper strips for 48 hours. (Reprinted with permission from C. William Hanke, MD.)

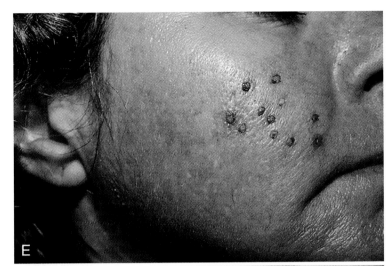

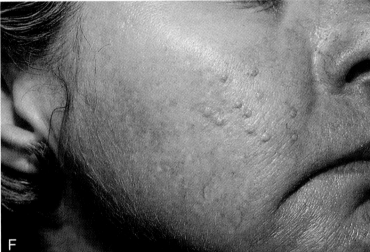

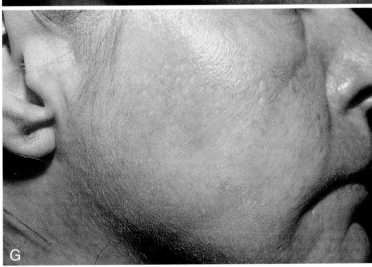

FIGURE 11.7 *(continued)*
E, The grafts are crusted at seven days. F, The majority of the grafts are elevated above the skin surface eight weeks after punch grafting. The patient is ready for dermabrasion of the cheeks. G, The patient's skin is relatively smooth 6 months following dermabrasion. The punch replacement grafts are barely detectable. (Reprinted with permission from C. William Hanke, MD.)

FIGURE 11.8
A, Acne scars before diamond fraise dermabrasion. B, Acne scars six months after diamond fraise dermabrasion.

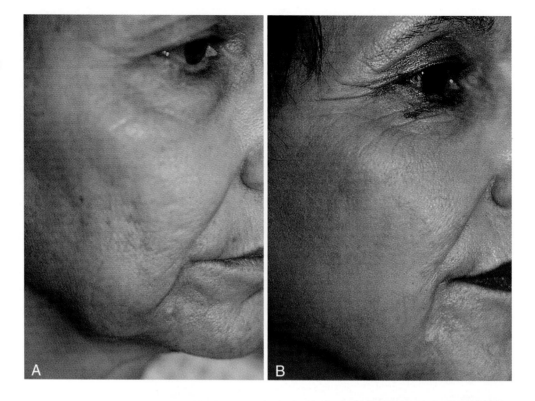

FIGURE 11.9
A. Multiple actinic keratoses of the forehead prior to diamond fraise dermabrasion. B. Nine years after diamond fraise dermabrasion there is no recurrence of actinic keratoses in the abraded areas.

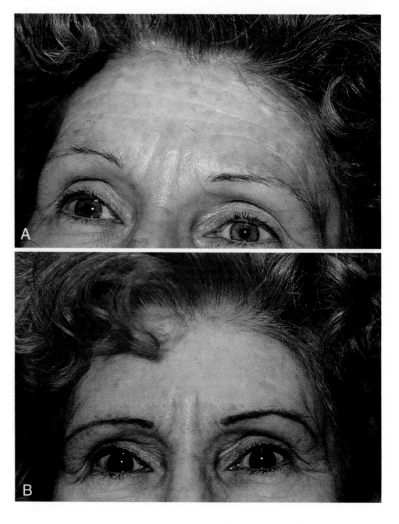

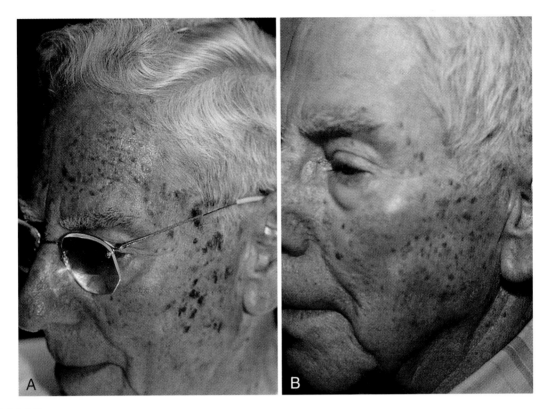

FIGURE 11.10

A, Multiple seborrheic keratoses before dermabrasion. B, Four years after dermabrasion of the forehead there has been no recurrence of the seborrheic keratoses. Note the continued presence of seborrheic keratoses in the non-abraded areas.

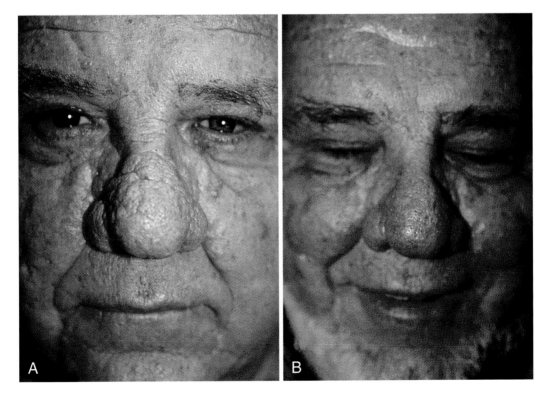

FIGURE 11.11

A, Rhinophyma prior to diamond fraise dermabrasion using the tumescent technique. B, One year postoperatively the contours are significantly improved.

FIGURE 11.12
A, Traumatic scars of the cheek and upper lip 6 weeks after an automobile accident. B, Four months after diamond fraise dermabrasion these scars are satisfactorily diminished.

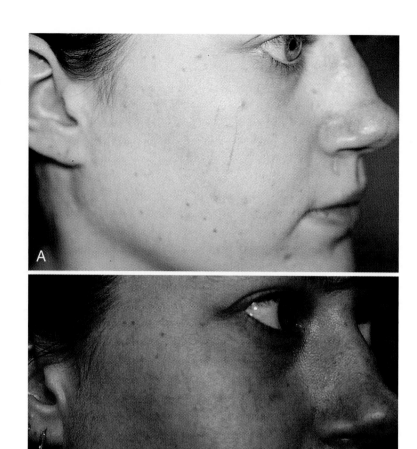

FIGURE 11.13
A, Multiple rhytides of the face.
B, Six months after dermabrasion.

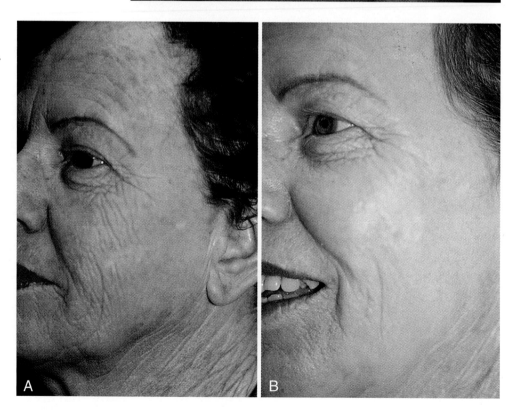

REFERENCES

1. Luikart R, Ayres S, Wilson J. Surgical skin planing. NY State J Med 1957;59:3413-3447.
2. Alt TH. Technical aids for dermabrasion. J Dermatol Surg Oncol 1987;13:638-648.
3. Alt TH, Goodman GJ, Coleman WP III, et al. Dermabrasion. In: Coleman WP III, et al. eds. Cosmetic Surgery of the Skin. 2nd ed. St. Louis: Mosby, 1997:112-151.
4. Yarborough J. Dermabrasive surgery. Clin Dermatol 1987;5: 57-80.
5. Coleman WP III, Klein JA. Use of the tumescent technique for scalp surgery, dermabrasion, and soft tissue reconstruction. J Dermatol Surg Oncol 1992;18:130-135.
6. Goodman G. Dermabrasion using tumescent anesthesia. J Dermatol Surg Oncol 1994;20:802-807.
7. Lowenthal L. Punch biopsy with autograft. Arch Dermatol Syph 1953;67:629-631.
8. Johnson W. Treatment of pitted scars: Punch transplant technique. J Dermatol Surg Oncol 1986;12:260-265.
9. American Academy of Dermatology Committee on Guidelines of Care: Guidelines of care for dermabrasion. J Am Acad Dermatol 1994;31:654-657.

CHAPTER 12

Manual Dermasanding

■ David R. Harris

Resurfacing, initially performed with primitive abrasive tools, has been a part of mankind's effort to beautify for as long people have been adorning themselves with cosmetics and tattoos. In modern times the use of motor-driven dermabrasion was reported by Kromayer in 1905 (1). After the second world war, Kurtin introduced wire brush dermabrasion, creating a renaissance of interest in resurfacing techniques, primarily to improve acne scarring (2). However, the use of dermabrasion to improve abnormalities in texture suffered a decline in popularity in the 1960s (3). In the early 1970s, research into the mechanism of superficial wound healing encouraged interest in motor-driven dermabrasion using the diamond fraise (4, 5). Traditional motor-driven techniques, either with the diamond fraise or with wire brush, often resulted in sharp lines of demarcation, especially in the periorbital and mandibular areas. Most patient dissatisfaction was not so much with the less than complete improvement in scar revision, than with these sharp lines between abraded and unabraded skin. In the mid 1980s, a communication by Maliner described the use of various grades of silicone carbide sandpaper that he used manually to improve acne scars (6). Modern reports of manual resurfacing go back at least as far as Iverson, who, in 1947, used hand sandpaper to remove traumatic tattoos (1). Also, abrasive material, such as "dragon-skin," was used for scar revision before the second world war (7).

Experiments with various grades of silicone carbide sandpaper and wallscreen (silicone-coated carbide granules on a wire mesh) in combination with low strength trichloroacetic acid (TCA) were carried out with the goal of improving both acne scars and actinically injured skin, the results of which were published in 1994 (8). Manual dermasanding was again revisited with some

new "wrinkles" by Chiarello in 1996 (9). The following discussion explores the author's approach to manual dermasanding, patient selection and education, and variations on the technique including combined laser resurfacing, and a discussion of dermasanding as part of a process of care including the use of topical modalities.

ADVANTAGES AND DISADVANTAGES OF MANUAL DERMASANDING

Advantages

There are several advantages over both motor driven and laser resurfacing. First, the manual technique is simple to master and safe to use. For those who are used to motor driven abrasion, the use of manually held papers is much more controlled, especially when abrading the difficult periorbital areas, even to the tarsal margin and the commissures of the lips. Moreover, manual dermasanding allows for a very smooth, soft feathering at the edges of the abraded areas which are easily carried into the hairline and over the mandibular margin onto the neck. This feathering is possible because of the many random scratch marks at the edge of the abraded area that are reflected in soft blending between abraded and unabraded zones.

More important, the technique has parity with the results achieved by both motor-driven and laser resurfacing, especially for acne scarring and the full measure of rhytides seen in photoaged skin. Healing time, usually between 5 and 8 days, as with other forms of resurfacing, is no different from the rest. The erythema associated with this resurfacing fades quickly over the same time period as seen with motor-driven techniques. Moreover, manual dermabrasion does not cause as much erythema as an average resurfacing with the laser, while postinflammatory hyperpigmentation is no different with this procedure than with motor-driven equipment. However, experience to date suggests that the problem of pigment loss, which can be permanent, is not seen as frequently with the manual technique as it is with the motor drive procedure.

The great advantage to manual resurfacing is that it is technically safe and inexpensive to use; a piece of motor driven equipment operating at 22,000 revolutions per minute can cause a great deal of damage if a mistake is made and too many passes with a laser can lead to unpredictable results. With manual resurfacing, uniform bleeding points (a common end point in resurfacing) appear slowly over time with many opportunities to reassess as one proceeds. Large errors are less apt to happen. Moreover, unlike carbon dioxide (CO_2) lasers, which are expensive, require set up and appropriate use, and due to technology advancement can make the unit obsolete, sandpaper does not change.

Finally, manual resurfacing allows small or even larger "touch-up" procedures with ease. Many patients may need a second or third, either full or partial procedure to further improve residual rhytides or scars. With the manual dermasanding technique and local anesthesia, many of these "touch-up" procedures can be done rapidly, in an extended office visit, at low cost with little time necessary for set up.

Disadvantages

Use of 25% TCA *following* manual abrasion, can produce a great deal of burning even with appropriate analgesia and local anesthesia. Subsequently, application of TCA *before* dermasanding was as effective with minimal burning. Moreover, the frost from TCA application finds the base of folds, rhytides and scars, creating a white "marker" to be abraded.

The CO_2 laser offers one important advantage over dermasanding in its ability to achieve the same uniformity of epidermal wounding on the upper and lower eyelids. Other than this one caveat, I do not believe that either motor driven dermabrasion or laser resurfacing is superior to what can be achieved with the manual dermasanding technique alone.

PATIENT SELECTION AND EDUCATION

Before undertaking any resurfacing procedure the physician should appreciate that mastering the art of appropriate patient selection and education is as important as a thorough grasp of the technique itself.

Patient Selection

A technically appropriate patient for resurfacing has either the sequelae of photoaging or facial scarring. Actinic injury includes a dull, muddy tone with dyschromia, keratoses and/or the presence of rhytides. The acne scarred or traumatically scarred patient who most benefits from dermabrasion has relatively shallow saucer-shaped depressions, fine pitting or depressed or raised linear scars of various types. Those with deep valley scarring with decided tissue deficits are less likely to be helped after epidermal resurfacing alone.

However, appropriate scars and wrinkle lines that can be revised with resurfacing constitute only one facet of an appropriate candidate. The candidate also should have a mature and realistic attitude, a reasonably good self-image, and a positive outlook on life. Conversely, patients who have chosen multiple cosmetic procedures to improve life or find happiness are constantly disappointed when these procedures do not make their life better; they are difficult to satisfy regardless of the outcome. In like manner, patients who are in a depressed emotional state are less rewarding candidates in spite of appropriate scars and rhytides to resurface. An individual who has the unrealistic expectations that a cosmetic procedure will change the nature of their existence will indeed be a disappointed and angry patient.

Patient Education

The primary reason to choose an appropriate candidate with a good psychological outlook and a mature attitude is because the resurfacing procedure is often not perfect! The prospective patient must learn, by both in depth discussion and written materials, that the resurfacing procedure is part of a process of improvement and restoration that takes time and may need to be repeated for adequate satisfaction. The patient must understand that while initial improvement may be excellent and that 60% to 80% of the unwanted wrinkles may be erased, there will be a measure of disappointment. This is because not every rhytid or scar can be removed in a single procedure and that uniform skin tone may take months to return. At the end of the procedure, patients often only see what is left, and only a preoperative photograph will serve as a reminder of what was there before. Part of this educational process includes a discussion of what can be done about the disappointment. This discussion includes a review of "touch-up" or repeated procedures and how they work and what the cost would be. As part of the educational process, a pretreatment program should be undertaken so there is time for reassessment and prepare the patient for the procedure.

PATIENT PREPARATION

Test Site

Most patients undergoing a deeper peel or resurfacing procedure are subject to possible depigmentation as a postoperative sequela. While most pigment loss occurs after delayed healing, there is a subset of patients who lose pigment with any local trauma. These include patients who are genetically predisposed to vitiligo. Some of these patients can be identified by peeling or resurfacing a test spot in a post auricular area. The post auricular test site is important for two reasons. First, there is a need to wait a minimum of 6 weeks to 2 months to identify the predisposed individual, providing a reasonable period for reflection for both the physician and patient. Second, this is a valuable medical/legal strategy. While it is true that a substantial number of patients who lose pigment during delayed healing cannot be identified by a test site, the physician has done all that he or she can to eliminate a patient who is prone to early pigment loss with trauma. The patient can honestly be told that to the best of the physician's knowledge, the test site does not indicate that the patient is apt to lose pigment. Most test sites in the post auricular fold are accompanied by a prolonged rosy or pink hue. This is usually evident at the end of the second month of observation. Some patients are quite concerned with this pinkness, which can last longer than postoperative rosiness or pinkness on the face, but they can be reassured that the postoperative skin can easily be camouflaged with make-up.

Patients who are prone to hyperpigmentation (those of Mediterranean, African, Latino or Asian descent) may or may not pigment at the test site. However, one must assume that all darker skin types will hyperpigment with resurfacing and part of the patient preparation should be topical care to ameliorate such an event.

Preoperative Skin Care

All patients who are appropriate candidates for manual dermasanding should be placed on a preoperative skin care program. At the minimum, this program should include application of sunscreen and an alpha hydroxy acid or retinoid. For the acne prone patient, it is important to provide at least topical prophylactic therapy before the resurfacing procedure because the greasy postoperative topical preparations commonly cause an acne flare.

A case could be made for placing all nonacne prone patients on a preoperative lightening program. This is because even some of the lightest skinned individual hyperpigment after resurfacing, especially those of Nordic descent. Patients with a history of hyperpigmentation, either postinflammatory or melasma, or a subtle discoloration of the lip or malar eminence, should begin pretreatment lightening. A typical lightening program includes equal parts of a SPF 30 sunscreen and a 5% to 10% hydroquinone preparation. 8% to 10% hydroquinone in equal parts of 20% azelaic acid is also an excellent pretreatment for evening application. Any of these preoperative regimens should be started at least 1 month prior to resurfacing. I do not feel the initiation of such a program *after* the procedure is wise because patients have become irritated or sensitive to a lightening agent that was not started before the procedure and end up with dramatic hyperpigmentation. Remember, in the predisposed individual, relief of hyperpigmentation may take many months of emotional support, topical care and peeling. Hypopigmentation or depigmentation following resurfacing may be permanent, and resistant to attempts to restore normal skin tone.

Preoperative Instruction

Preoperative consultation with the patient 1 or 2 days before the procedure is helpful. The physician should be present at part or all of the discussion. Frequently, the patient has questions that the physician might need to review. The physician, nurse, or staff member can "walk through" the procedure with the patient again, explaining what will happen before, during and following the manual dermasanding. All of the written materials including informed consent forms and a separate "touch-up" consent form (Fig. 12.1), are once again reviewed

---

OUR SKIN BUFFING AND PEELING PROCEDURE
WHAT OUR PATIENTS SHOULD KNOW FIRST

Why do we do this procedure? We introduced our skin buffing and peeling procedure to counteract the major effects of sunlight and aging on facial skin. Some of these problems include a loss of luster, with a flat, opaque-appearing skin, irregular pigmentation (brown spots), and the onset of superficial as well as deep wrinkle lines. This procedure can also be used in an attempt to lessen scars from acne, chickenpox, or other causes. In addition to looking better, the skin actually becomes healthier with less precancerous, sun damaged cells.

What is this procedure? Sterile buffing material and/or a power driven abrasive wheel is utilized to remove a superficial layer of facial skin in those areas which require attention. A peeling solution is then applied to the entire surface. The procedure is usually accomplished in a quiet office setting under light sedation and local anesthetic. Most patients perceive some discomfort during the buffing procedure and some degree of a transient burning sensation during the application of the peeling solution; iced compresses are then applied to soothe the skin. Alternatively, the procedure may be done in a surgery center with sedation/anesthesia administered by an anesthesiologist at additional cost. If this is done, any additional risks will be discussed with you by the anesthesiologist prior to the procedure. The whole procedure usually takes about one-half to one hour, after which the patient rests a while before returning home. The patient must obtain a ride to and from the office for the procedure. Because of the medications used prior to and during the procedure, the patient cannot drive him/herself.

FIGURE 12.1

Written materials should include both a tailored informed consent form and a separate "touch-up" consent form so there are no surprises when further resurfacing is required for satisfaction. *(continued)*

What happens after this procedure?   Most patients experience a period of warmth for the first hour or two. Over the first 3–5 days there is a degree of swelling over the entire face and especially the eyelids. A thin, flexible brown crust forms which feels somewhat tight. Some patients experience some itching, but few complain of burning and severe discomfort. During the following 5–7 days the swelling quickly disappears and the thin crust peels off, much like the peeling after a severe sunburn. Complete separation occurs in about 7–14 days, allowing the patient to return to normal activity.

Infection during healing is possible but unlikely if postoperative care instructions are followed and follow up visits are kept. If healing is delayed, pus drains from the skin or you have a history of cold cores, you must notify your doctor since these signs may indicate a potential infection problem. Although unlikely, an allergic reaction is always possible to the topical and oral medications used in connection with this procedure.

Patient's initials_____

What can patients expect over a longer period?   After the swelling disappears and the crust separates, most patients note areas of pinkness or redness, much like one would expect after any scab falls off. For the most part this color difference is appreciated in the areas that have received the buffing. While the pink discoloration is easily covered with most foundation and makeup programs, some patients note persistence of color change for several months. On occasion, some people gain a degree of brown or excessive pigmentation of the skin. This varies from individual to individual and is most commonly seen in darker skin types. We have found that brown excessive pigmentation can be treated with lightening preparations and generally improves in a matter of months. A few people are prone to loss of pigmentation, which can be permanent in a few cases. Because of this, we first buff and peel a hidden test site to check for these pigmentary problems. However, these tests may not be totally predictive of what will occur when the entire face is treated. Although unlikely, scarring may occur especially if there is a problem with healing (such as an infection).

Can we guarantee satisfaction?   No cosmetic surgeon can guarantee to make a patient happy but can only promise to do the best work possible. We offer this procedure because the majority of our patients are pleased with the outcome. Satisfaction is based on a realistic expectation. No one should expect our efforts will remove every abnormal pigment spot, every wrinkle or smooth skin perfectly. Moreover, deeper folds are not affected by this procedure. If there are problems with healing, preexisting scars may be made worse or new ones created.

Patients should understand that friends and family generally appreciate beneficial changes less than they do. This is because we are much more critical of our own appearance than we are of other people. Moreover, some people seek this kind of procedure expecting it to make them happier; not only happier about personal appearance but about life in general. If one feels that a satisfactory result will change his or her life, meet someone new or get a better job, disappointment is bound to occur. A realistic attitude is absolutely necessary for satisfaction.

What can we do to make our patients satisfied?   We do everything within our power to maximize patient satisfaction. We consider this procedure part of an overall continuing skin rejuvenation program which may include topical care, collagen augmentation, further procedures or "touch ups".

I have read the above and discussed this information with my doctor. I feel I have a clear understanding of the procedure and the possible side effects. I have been informed that this procedure will not be covered by insurance and that payment is my responsibility before the procedure is done.

_____
Patient

_____
Witness

_____
Date

OUR IMAGE ENHANCING "TOUCH-UP" PROGRAM
A Special Service for Dermasanding and Peel Patients

Improving wrinkled skin lines, abnormal pigmentation, or scarring, involves a skilled type of texturing of the skin. We are proud of the results of our dermasanding and peeling procedures, the success of which is a product of over 20 years of experience.

However, no single texturing procedure can guarantee 100 percent satisfaction. We tell our patients they will generally appreciate anywhere from 30 up to 80% improvement in scars, pigmentation or wrinkle lines. This is to say that in some spots there may be a complete eradication, but in other areas there may be less satisfactory improvement.

This means that for some people there may be a measure of *dissatisfaction* with any one procedure.

Because of this fact and our desire to continue working with each patient to find the greatest level of satisfaction possible, we offer our "Touch-up" program. Simply stated, we will continue to work for one year on those areas where scars and wrinkles remain for $_____ per "touch-up" session. We encourage our patients to participate in a quest for continued improvement by keeping "touch-ups" affordable. This entire program is an investment in one's own sense of self image. To have an unwanted spot here and there is a continuing disappointment. With our "Touch-up" program, the physician and patient work with one another to enhance satisfaction with a modest investment of time and money.

I have read the above, discussed and understand the "Touch-up" program.

_____
Date

_____
Patient

_____
Witness

FIGURE 12.1 *(continued)*

TIPS FOR BUFF-PEEL PATIENTS DURING THE HEALING STAGE

1. Immediately after your buff-peel you will be partially sedated when you return home. During this first day you will need to take several different kinds of pills.

   It is important that your eat and drink a normal amount of food and water during the course of the first day. We recommend an eight ounce glass of fluid each hour, even if a family member must wake you.

2. Sometimes patients are concerned about swelling around the face and eyes. This is a part of the healing process and perfectly normal. At times the eyes may swell completely shut for a few hours or even a day. We have given you special medication to decrease the swelling and ice compresses also help. This usually decreases significantly by day 4 or 5. Scabs usually separate by day 7 to 10.

3. Occasionally some patients find a mild degree of nausea over the first two or three days. We have given you a prescription for Tigan suppositories for the nausea if necessary. Note the list of drug stores in the Santa Clara Valley that are open overnight to fill any prescription.

FACIAL CARE INSTRUCTIONS

1. Cleanse face three to four times daily with our soap-free cleansing lotion, using a soft wash cloth moistened with water. Rinse your face several times with tepid water after cleansing and gently pat dry. You may shower and shampoo as usual. Many patients find the shower a convenient way to cleanse the skin.

2. After patting dry, apply a thin film of Silvadene cream and Elta melting moisturizer mixed together in equal amounts. Continue to apply mixture three to four times daily, until all scabbed areas have fallen off. If you experience burning or stinging for more than a minute or two—call. You may be sensitive to the Silvadene.

3. A few patients become sensitive to the cream which you have been given. If you become sensitive you will note an increase in stinging and irritation rather than a cool relief when the medicine is applied. If this occurs, please call and we will make an adequate adjustment.

ALL NIGHT PHARMACIES

(Physicians can provide a list for patients)

FIGURE 12.2
Postoperative instructions should be written out and easy to understand.

and signed. All of the written pre- and postoperative instructions are also discussed. Preoperative instructions should include the need for the patient to be off any psychotropic drugs at least 24 hours, eating a normal meal, and the taking of preoperative medication at least 1½ hours before presentation. The patient should not drive to or from the procedure. Postoperative instructions include a detailed description of skin care and medications (Fig. 12.2). Another very useful written statement concerns what the patient should expect including all the sequelae that may or may not occur (Fig. 12.3).

During this preoperative consultation the patient can be given a tote bag that contains a number of postoperative topical preparations including a cleanser and the ointment for the abraded skin. The tote bag can also contain prescriptions for any preoperative and/or postoperative medications (Fig. 12.4). It is prudent to reinforce what will most likely be accomplished and what areas might not be improved satisfactorily with the procedure. This is a powerful second or third repetition and should be done at the end of the preoperative consultation just before the patient leaves. The same message should be repeated when the patient arrives for the procedure.

THE PROCEDURE

Materials

The manual dermasanding technique involves applying 25% or 35% TCA to defatted skin. After uniform frosting, the surface of the skin is abraded or "buffed" with various strengths of sterilized silicone carbide sandpaper. I use Wetordry (3M Company, St. Paul, Minnesota) sandpaper, which can be obtained in three grades (fine grade #400, medium grade #220-320, and coarse grade #180). The fine grade is used primarily on the thin rhytides around the eyes and the medium and coarse grades over the rest of the face. The coarse grade is the most useful (Table 12.1). Cut the sandpaper into 1½-inch squares or 2 × 3-inch pieces, and autoclave several pieces together in a bulls-eye bag (Fig. 12.5). For an average case of scars or actinically injured skin, 3 to 6 pieces of sandpaper may be used, primarily coarse and medium grades.

The treatment stand should have several pieces of each grade of silicone carbide paper, a cup containing water for moistening the paper, 2 × 2 gauze pads that are used as rolls to hold the paper, an appropriate number of 4 × 4 gauze sponges, and TCA (Fig. 12.6). A

WHAT TO EXPECT AFTER YOUR SKIN RESURFACING

When sun damaged or acne scarred skin is treated with our special resurfacing procedures, our patients are given complete instructions concerning postoperative care. Here is a reminder of the important changes that may occur during the healing phase.

1. OOZING.   When the old skin is removed, and before the new fresh, smooth surface is restored, there is a measure of oozing and draining for the first two to four days. Most of the fluid is either clear or slightly yellow-tinged over a surface which is moist and light pink. Because we apply ointments to keep the skin moist, this drainage is entirely appropriate.

2. SWELLING.   Swelling occurs and is most intense between day two and five. For some, the swelling occurs most intensely around the eyes and upper cheeks. At times, for a day or so, the eyes may be swollen almost shut. This is an entirely natural phenomenon and is in no way detrimental to healing or harmful to you, the patient.

3. A ROSY HUE.   When the skin has finished growing, usually by day six to ten, the skin takes on a rosy or pink color. This pinkness is the new fresh skin before it assumes its natural color tones. The pinkness fades a lot over the first several weeks, but some people will note a measure of pinkness for some months. The rosy or pink tones can be easily camouflaged with appropriate foundation or make-up and will not be a problem with daily activities.

4. ITCHINESS AND DISCOMFORT.   Some patients note a degree of itchiness during the healing phase, totally normal, for skin which is regrowing or healing. However, increased *PAIN* AFTER the first **48** hours is a important sign that there may be a problem. While rare, increasing pain after **48** hours should be reported immediately to the physician or nurse in charge of your case.

5. RESIDUAL LINES OR SCARS.   Your physician has discussed the fact that not every scar or wrinkle line will be removed by our resurfacing procedure. This is because each scar and wrinkle is a separate problem and some are far more resistant to our treatment than others. While we enjoy a high degree of patient satisfaction, some measure of disappointment may occur when the patient recognizes that not every line or scar has been removed. As we discussed, we then can further improve those residual wrinkle lines and scars by a "touch-up" procedure at a later time.

6. CHANGE IN PIGMENTATION.   In spite of appropriate preparation, some darker skinned patients will recognize a measure of deeper pigmentation after the resurfacing procedure. This darkening, which may occur at any of the resurfaced areas, will be treated and will fade over time.

   An occasional patient, in spite of our efforts to test beforehand, may note over some months the occurrence of a lighter than normal spot in the resurfaced skin. This occurs in a few because of unusual response to the healing process. While this is rare, it can occur and remain permanently. These areas can be covered with make-up and at times can be blended satisfactorily to the surrounding skin.

FIGURE 12.3
A statement reviewing all that could be expected after dermasanding.

FIGURE 12.4
During a preoperative visit, patients receive a "tote bag" containing instructions, medications and prescriptions.

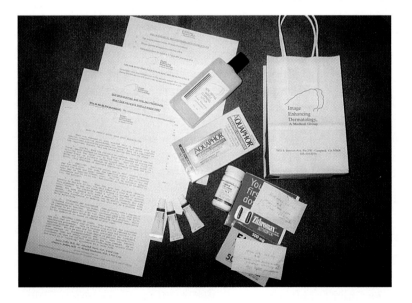

separate area should contain those medications necessary for analgesia and sedation. I use 4 10 ml syringes, two of which contain equal parts of 2% Xylocaine and 0.25% Marcaine with epinephrine. The other two syringes contain equal parts of 1% Xylocaine and Marcaine. In addition, unless intolerant or allergic, I administer 75 to 100 mg of Demerol (Sanofi Winthrop Inc., New York, NY) and 25 mg of Phenergan (Wyeth-Ayerst

Laboratories, Philadelphia, PA) on arrival. Iced compresses should be available to apply after the application of TCA, although burning is minimal with adequate local anesthesia (Fig. 12.7).

TABLE 12.1

SILICONE CARBIDE SANDPAPER

Grade	Purpose
400-Fine	Fine rhytides, especially eyelids
220-320 Medium	Eyelids and fine rhytides around vermilion. Use after one or two passes with a laser with debris removed.
180-Coarse	Generally used for most scars and rhytides with the exception of eyelids.

Preoperative Patient Care

One to two hours before presentation, patients can take 20 mg of Valium (Hoffman LaRoche, Nutley, NJ) by mouth. A light meal should be eaten by the patient and the routine of the day followed up to the time of the operation. If the patient is using other psychotropic drugs, they must be stopped the night before and day of the procedure. Asking specifically about psychotropic medications is important because some patients are reluctant to indicate that they are on antidepressants or another medication that may have a synergistic effect with Valium and Demerol. If the patient has taken the Valium preoperatively, he or she can arrive at the office in a relaxed, mildly groggy or slightly somnolent condition. If the 20 mg of Valium does not have any noticeable effect on the patient, it may require more than the normal amount of medication to secure adequate analgesia. Preoperative photographs can be taken at this time and

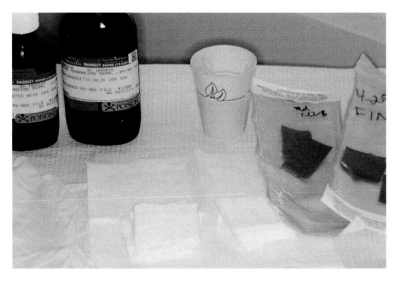

FIGURE 12.5
Several pieces of 1.5 × 2-inch silicone-carbide sandpaper is autoclaved in bulls-eye bags.

FIGURE 12.6
The treatment stand holding sandpaper, a cup of water for moistening, 2 × 2 gauze pads for use as rolls to hold the paper, sponge and TCA for the preabrasion peel.

FIGURE 12.7
Flexible iced compresses are prepared by placing several individual pieces of wet 4 × 8 gauze pads between plastic wrap and freezing the package.

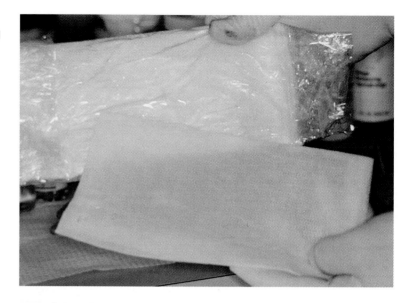

FIGURE 12.8
Regional blocks are effective for anesthetizing both the mid portion of the face and the forehead.

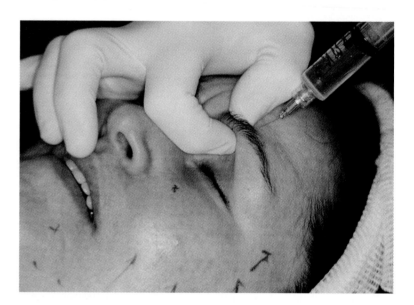

the patient can receive an intramuscular injection of 75 to 100 mg of Demerol and 25 mg of Phenergan, a combination, which I believe, supplies adequate, smooth and safe analgesia.

After waiting 10 to 15 minutes, the buccal mucosa at the first and second incisors is anesthetized with viscous Xylocaine and 2 ml of equal parts of 2% Xylocaine and 0.25% Marcaine, both with epinephrine, is injected into each of the infraorbital foramina. In like manner 1 ml of this anesthetic is injected into the mental foramen as is 1 ml into both the supraorbital foramina. With these injections, adequate anesthesia is achieved for most patients over the entire forehead, in the mid portion of the face including the nose (Fig. 12.8).

The next set of injections, using the 2% Xylocaine mix, anesthetizes a field beginning at the deep preauricular area and follows a line around the angle of the

mandible to the tip of the mentum on each side (Fig. 12.9). Then 1% Xylocaine mix is injected by fan technique from lateral to medial and medial to lateral over the malar surfaces and the temple (Fig. 12.10). Injecting the band of 1% mix in the inferior and superior orbital rims to anesthetize the eyelids is useful. Generally two 10 ml syringes of 2% Xylocaine/Marcaine mix and one 10 ml syringe of the 1% Xylocaine/ Marcaine mix is sufficient for regional and field blocks. With practice, all anesthetizing of the face should take 10 minutes or less. Warn the patient to expect a measure of rapid heart beat or "pounding" pulse for several minutes following the anesthesia injections.

Application of TCA

The skin is aggressively cleansed and defatted with one of two mixtures. Many prefer acetone and alcohol, scrubbing vigorously with 2 × 2 gauze pads and re-peating the combination of acetone and alcohol, two or three times. A convenient end point is about 5 minutes of vigorous defatting. Some like to scrub the face with a detergent or antibacterial soap first, but this is not necessary with vigorous defatting. Remember, these efforts are aided by a preoperative instruction to carefully remove any make-up before presentation. I use a 10% or 15% glycolic acid astringent in an isopropyl alcohol/propylene glycol base. Patients seem to tolerate glycolic acid more easily than acetone and the same uniform frost is obtained with 25% or 35% TCA peel. Any scars or rhytides that are to be marked should be done so before proceeding. Remember, patients often reveal these specific areas for attack more effectively if he or she sits and has light shadow from the back or side.

Both 25% and 35% TCA peels produce similar results before manual dermasanding. If one is resurfac-ing severely actinically injured sebaceous skin with a large measure of dyschromia, a 35% TCA application is favored. TCA is applied vigorously with 2 × 2 gauze pads (Fig. 12.11). The face is divided into sections with the forehead completed first, followed by each side of the face. The end point for applying TCA is the beginning of a uniform frost and stinging. Remember that the patient is anesthetized, so the perception of pain is greatly blunted in untraumatized skin. Nonetheless, most patients feel some mild degree of stinging or burning, and ice compresses are applied for 5 to 10 minutes (Fig. 12.12).

The Dermasanding

Many physicians choose to resurface patients in one or more cosmetic units. For example, patients who have a significant problem with tone but only a few rhytides in the periorbital or oral areas, may receive dermasanding

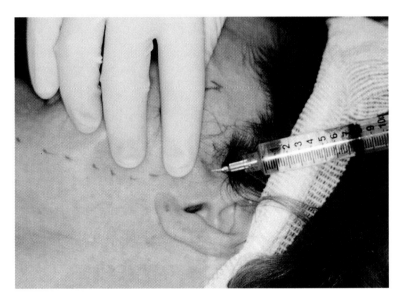

FIGURE 12.9
The periphery of the face is anesthetized by an injection beginning preauricular and proceeding down and around the angle of the mandible of the chin.

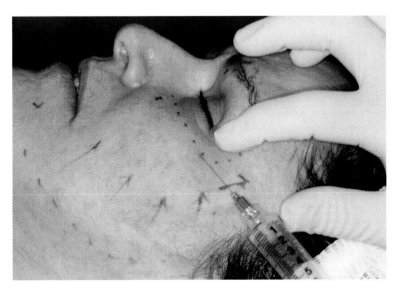

FIGURE 12.10
The lateral face is blocked by "fanning" anesthesia from the mandible and preauricular areas medially (note *arrows*).

only in these areas. In like manner, those with acne scars over a portion of the malar surface may be derma-sanded only in these areas. Nonetheless, in all cases the entire face is peeled. However, it is preferred to resurface the entire facial skin because, from time to time, those who have only specific cosmetic units resurfaced will notice a permanent tone or texture difference between the unresurfaced and the resurfaced skin. Sometimes matching this difference exactly in follow-up procedures is difficult. I now lightly dermasand only the finest of rhytides over the upper lip and periorbital areas if the entire facial skin is not being abraded.

For patients who are receiving a full face resurfacing, treatment begins on the forehead. Two 2 × 2 gauze pads are rolled tightly to resemble a dental roll and a piece of medium or coarse paper is wrapped around the roll (Fig. 12.13). Before "buffing" the skin, the entire roll is dipped into water because wet silicone carbide paper is a more efficient abrasive. Actual dental rolls do not retain water as effectively as the gauze pads. While rubbing the sandpaper back and forth or in circular strokes does not require great skill, with time, one does gain a "feel" for this technique. Light abrasion, without much pressure, done repeatedly over the same area gives the smoothest results. More pressure can and should be used in problem areas such as deep rhytides and scars, but start with a light hand. The end point of the abrasion is a uniform bleeding surface with the evidence of smooth collagen (Fig. 12.14). If the collagen fibers begin to get a ragged or frayed appearance, the abrasion has

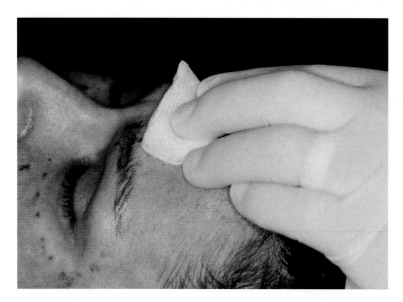

FIGURE 12.11
25% to 35% TCA is massaged vigorously into the skin with coarse 2 × 2 gauze pads.

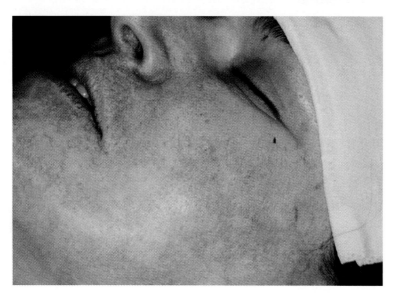

FIGURE 12.12
After each zone is peeled (forehead, followed by each side of the face), iced compresses are applied for about 10 minutes.

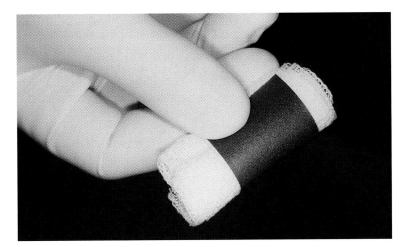

FIGURE 12.13
Sandpaper is wrapped around two 2 × 2 gauze pads rolled tightly to resemble a dental roll.

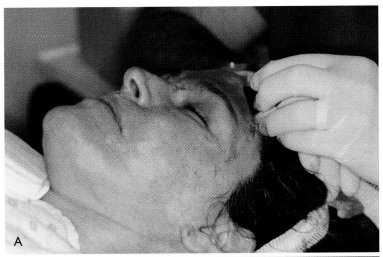

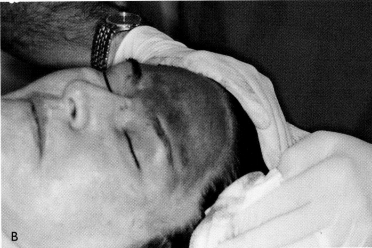

FIGURE 12.14
A, Dermasanding is best accomplished with a light hand, slowly going over the same areas until uniform bleeding points are achieved. B, The end point is a smooth, uniformly bleeding surface, without ragged collagen.

gone too far into the skin. In this manner, with little experience, a safe end point can be achieved.

After the forehead is completed, a new piece of sandpaper wrapped around 2 or 3 fresh rolled 2 × 2 pads should be used for the temple, malar surface, upper lip and chin on one side. Care is required to use light pressure over the malar eminence and mandible, because the presence of a superficial bony surface can easily allow unnecessarily deep abrasion, delayed healing and hypopigmentation. Both back-and-forth motions and a circular motion with a light hand should be used to go over the same area to achieve uniform bleeding points over time. Dermasanding each side of the face takes about 10 minutes (Fig. 12.15).

Difficult areas at the vermilion and commissure are treated by simply lifting and stretching the inside of the lip to meet the paper (Fig. 12.16). A special focus should be placed on perioral furrows as they merge into the vermilion and onto the lip as they are resistant to superficial resurfacing. One must abrade onto the lip surface from the vermilion to achieve eradication of these lip line furrows (Fig. 12.17).

When sanding the periorbital areas, use one tightly rolled premoistened gauze pad to create a uniform, firm surface to wrap medium or fine paper. This allows an easier approach to dermasanding the lower lid, almost to the tarsal margin and the lateral one-half of the upper lid (Fig. 12.18). While manual derma-sanding cannot reach quite the uniformity of the laser, satisfactory results can be achieved with the majority of patients (Fig. 12.19).

The nose should also be sanded. Even if there is virtually no visible defect, the entire facial skin should be resurfaced and manual dermasanding of the nose is done with ease. Frequently, patients note one or another small defect and complain if the nose is not resurfaced.

When dermasanding is complete, moist gauze is applied until bleeding has ceased and the smooth coagulated surface is carefully examined under magnification for remaining unabraded or inadequately abraded areas, scars, or rhytides needing further work. An advantage of manual resurfacing is the ease in identifying areas that need further sanding, which can then be approached with confidence and control. These areas can be lightly "burnished," buffed or brushed with the paper to achieve the desired end point.

POSTOPERATIVE CARE
Systemic Medication

For patients with any history of herpes simplex virus, a short course of appropriate systemic drugs, such as acy-

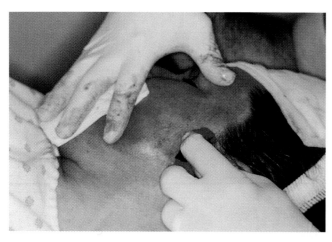

FIGURE 12.15
Each side of the face is dermasanded to uniform bleeding points, a task which takes about 10 minutes a side.

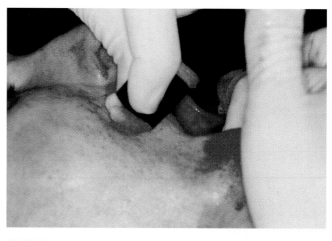

FIGURE 12.17
Sanding of the vermilion to eradicate lip line furrows.

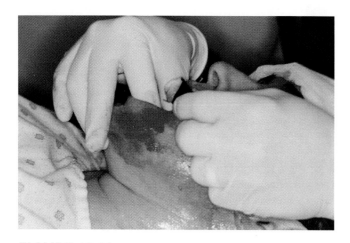

FIGURE 12.16
The vermilion, commissures and the entire lips are abraded in a uniform manner by stretching the tissue with your fingers.

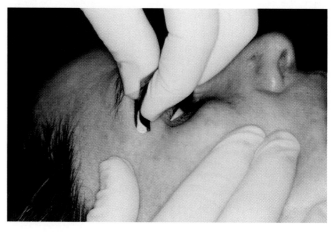

FIGURE 12.18
Wrap fine or medium paper around one tightly rolled 2 × 2 gauze pad when approaching abrasion of the eyelids.

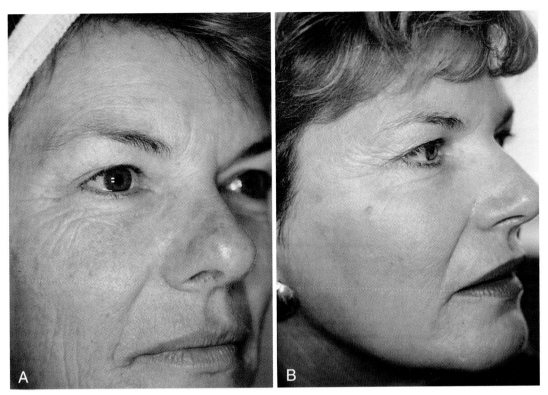

FIGURE 12.19
A, Appearance pre-dermasanding. B, Appearance post-dermasanding. Note the improvement in the periorbital rhytides.

clovir, is indicated. Such patients should begin a 5-day prophylactic course at the time of the procedure. Occasionally, a patient will experience an outbreak of herpes simplex after completion of this prophylactic course and the disease may even be apparent as long as 1 week after healing. Susceptible patients should have a supply of appropriate drugs on hand for this possibility. In addition, patients should receive a 5-day course of antibiotics, usually a cephalosporin, again beginning at the time of the procedure. Finally, an appropriate amount of postoperative pain medication should be prescribed. Most patients favor Vicodin (Knoll Pharmaceuticals, Inc., Mount Olive, NJ), which does not require a triplicate prescription. Sleeping pills should not be prescribed or used with Vicodin.

Topical Medication

Patients should apply a semiocclusive ointment frequently to ensure a moist healing environment. Many studies have shown that split thickness wounds, such as seen with resurfacing procedures, heal about twice as fast with far less discomfort when kept moist. This is because new epidermis regenerates from transected appendages, primarily sweat glands and hair follicles, and migrates across the denuded surface. When this denuded collagenous surface is free of a dry crust, which represents both dried serous transudate and dry dead dermis, the epidermis migrates unimpeded. A combination of equal parts Silver-sulfadiazine cream in Aquaphor (Beiersdorf, Inc., S. Norwalk, CT), or an ointment alone, such as Aquaphor or petrolatum should be used on the face. Frequent cleansing with a soap-free cleanser, such as Cetaphil (Owen/Galderma Laboratories, Ft. Worth, TX) or Aquanil (Person & Covey, Inc., Glendale, CA) is recommended followed by reapplication of the ointment 6 or 7 times daily. Use of the shower for debridement is often superior to a washcloth or gauze.

Serous oozing and edema occur during the first 3 to 4 days postoperatively. The edema may be severe enough to impair vision between the second and fourth day. Ice compresses and postoperative 40 mg triamcinolone diacetate given intramuscularly can help ameliorate the edema. Epithelization over the moist surface should be largely complete within 5 to 7 days. The presence of *increasing* pain during the postoperative period, burning or tenderness to a greater extent than the first 48 hours, or delayed healing after 10 days demands attention. The most common complication is infection that is resistant to the postoperative antibiotics. Cultures and aggressive therapy and daily visits should be initiated.

Postoperative Visits

In the uncomplicated case, the patient can be seen 24 or 48 hours postoperatively and again at 3 to 5 days. As a physician becomes confident enough in the procedure, the patient without complications may be seen as late as 1 week postoperatively. However, follow up phone calls with the patient to determine postoperative healing at the end of the procedure day and every other day up to the postoperative visit are recommended. These calls, usually placed by an experienced nurse, are extremely helpful in monitoring patients and cementing an excellent patient relationship.

FOLLOW-UP CARE

When healing is complete, at about 1 week, patients may have a rosy or pink hue, some remaining edema and a measure of dissatisfaction. Patients should be reassured that things are going very well and a subsequent visit should be scheduled between 2 weeks and 1 month. As the patient recovers and erythema fades, the areas of residual scarring or rhytides that were unresponsive to manual dermasanding will become evident (Fig. 12.20). Many patients will be reasonably satisfied with the results, but an equal number will at some time in the future desire further treatment. Two to four months should elapse between procedures to allow the erythema to fade toward normal. For some patients, repeated procedures may not satisfactorily eliminate all

rhytides or scars. Some unresponsive or residual rhytides are due to excessively active muscles of expression in the periorbital, glabellar or forehead area. Other approaches may need to be explored, such as filling agents, excision and undermining of scars as well as BOTOX (Allergan Inc., Irvine, CA) injections for dynamic muscles of expression (Fig. 12.21).

Continuing Care

Patients who were on preoperative topical programs should resume this care as soon as tolerated. This is especially true of patients who are prone to hyperpigmentation. Patients can be cautiously reintroduced to the topical lightening program as soon as healing is completed, usually at 7 days postoperatively. Some patients may find the topical ointments irritating at this early phase of healing. It is important to use pretreatment lightening agents if possible, or switch to another to avoid hyperpigmentation. Hyperpigmentation is difficult to manage because patients with this problem are usually dissatisfied with the results of the resurfacing until the pigmentation is adequately eliminated. While the use of sunscreens are important, especially if patients are going to have prolonged or intense sun exposure, most resurfacing patients are not more sun sensitive or sunburn prone than those who have not been

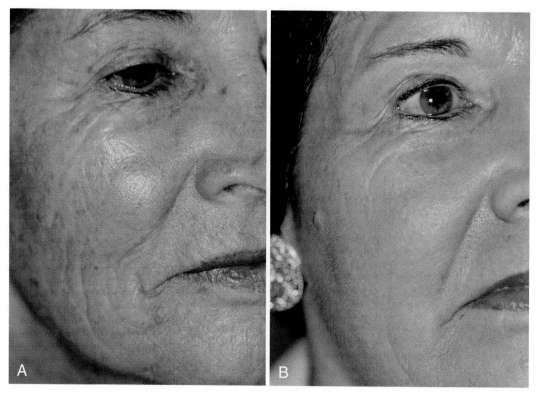

FIGURE 12.20

A, Pre-dermasanding patient with extensive rhytides. B, Appearance post-dermasanding. While decided improvement is appreciated, residual rhytides are present which may give a measure of disappointment.

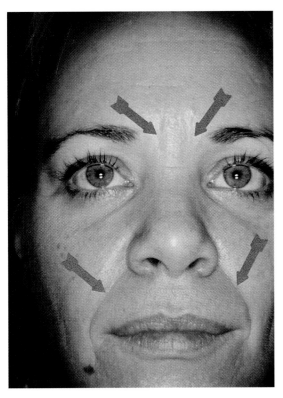

FIGURE 12.21
Some patients require other therapeutic measures to eliminate residual rhytides and folds, such as BOTOX (glabella *arrows*), or space filling substances (nasolabial furrow *arrows*).

resurfaced. For some, pinkness is a problem and may remain for several months. Established relationships with aestheticians skilled in cosmetic camouflage are useful for referring patients with residual pinkness or hyperpigmentation. It is less than ideal to simply suggest your patients seek counsel "some place" when it comes to postoperative make-up care.

VARIATIONS ON THE THEME

Tumescent Dermasanding With Cryospray

Recently, Chiarello introduced his variation of the manual dermasanding procedure. He reported the use of combined tumescent anesthesia, especially in the perioral areas, stereoscopic magnification, and meticulous dermasanding using silicone carbide sandpaper (9). Probably any name brand silicone carbide sandpaper will work equally well. In addition, other hand held abrasive instruments are used, such as the sandpaper cylinder from the Dremel (Emerson Electronic Inc., Racine, WI) sanding tool, dermabrasion fraises and diathermy head cleaner sanding paper. These smaller tools are helpful for sanding the shoulders of saucer-shaped depressions such as individual varicella scars. A light liquid nitrogen spray with a thaw time of 7 sec-

onds or less is used right after dermasanding which allows a finer feathering of edges and the option of more destructive therapy in areas that may need more treatment. Spraying the vermilion border is also helpful.

Combined Dermasanding and Laser Resurfacing

The combined use of a CO_2 ultrapulsed laser with manual dermasanding is effective for treating patients with resistant rhytides or redundant folds and deeper rhytides in periorbital areas. Using 250 mJ, 60 Watts with a density of 5, the CO_2 laser is used to cover the entire upper and lower lids to tarsal margins. The necrotic debris is removed with moistened applicator sticks. A second pass is accomplished without removal of debris. The remainder of the skin is treated with one or two passes using the ultrapulse laser at 300 mJ, 60 Watts with a density of 7. Then, all of the dry debris in the periorbital areas and elsewhere is manually dermasanded, usually with medium grade paper, until adequate bleeding points are reached in a uniform pattern. This technique combines the advantages of the laser in the periorbital areas with the safety, efficacy and ease of manual dermasanding feathering in the remaining areas (Fig. 12.22). Peeling is not advocated as an adjunct to this procedure at this time because no apparent additional advantages are known.

Undermining or Subcision

Recently, Orientrich reported his experience using subcision to soften and raise facial scars (10). A similar technique, called "undermining," tears or lyses scar tissue at the base of depressed valley scars using two types of needles (a 16-Gauge, 1½-inch needle and a No-kor 1½-inch needle with a "spear-like" head [Becton Dickinson, Rutherford, NJ]) (Fig. 12.23). The needles are inserted beneath carefully marked valley scars after tumescent anesthesia. The scar is lysed using a back and forth motion to create tears or tunnels in the collagen. A fibrin clot, migration of fibroblasts and new collagen deposition frequently results in satisfactory improvement of the depressed scars. Patients are reevaluated 2 to 4 weeks postoperatively to determine if further undermining is necessary before resurfacing.

SUMMARY

For any resurfacing procedure for actinic injury or scarring to be successful, the procedure must be part of a process of care beginning with patient selection and education, appropriate pre- and postoperative topical care, and one or more "touch-up" procedures that are frequently necessary for adequate patient satisfaction. All too often the inexperienced cosmetic surgeon looks at *doing* the procedure as an end point instead of a

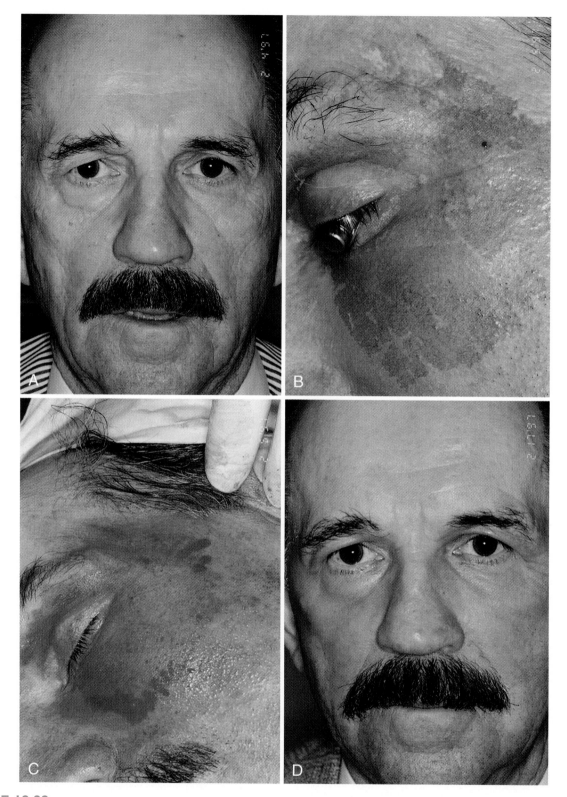

FIGURE 12.22

A, Combined laser and manual dermasanding to treat periorbital rhytides. B, Two passes using the CO_2 laser CPG are completed over the upper and lower lids. C, The lased surface and surrounding skin then is lightly dermasanded using medium grade paper to uniform bleeding points. D, Appearance 14 days after the laser and dermasanding procedure. Note soft margins of treated skin and minimal erythema.

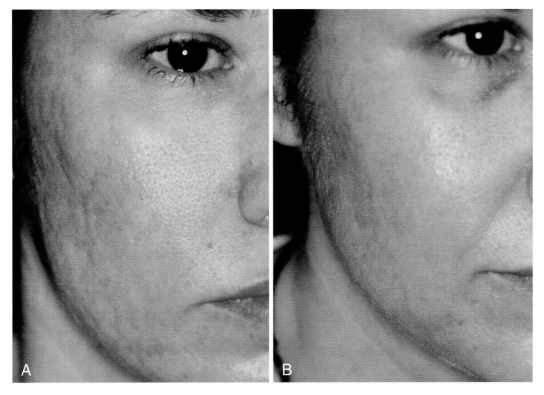

FIGURE 12.23

A, Pre-treatment appearance of irregular depressed valley scars. B, Post undermining (subcision) and manual dermasanding. Appreciable improvement is noted both in skin lifting and the texturing of the scars.

process of *continuing care* for patient satisfaction. For those who have chosen to add peeling and resurfacing to an armamentarium of cutaneous care, skill is demanded, not only in the execution of the procedure itself, but in understanding and nurturing the psychological desires and the cutaneous needs of the patient.

REFERENCES

1. Epstein E. Dermabrasion. In: Skin surgery. 5th ed. Springfield, IL: Charles C. Thomas Publisher, 1982:593-610.
2. Burks JW. Wire Brush Surgery. Springfield, IL: Charles C. Thomas Publisher, 1956.
3. Yarborough JM. Wherefore dermabrasion. Dermatol Surg 1995;21:381-382.
4. Harris DR. Healing of the surgical wound: basic considerations. J Am Acad Derm 1979;1:197-207.
5. Harris DR. Healing of the surgical wound: factors influencing repair and regeneration. J Am Acad Derm 1979;1:208-215.
6. Malner JS. Regional hand dermabrasion. In: Plastic and Reconstructive Surgery of the Head and Neck, the Third International Symposium, Vol I: Aesthetic Surgery. New York: Grune and Stratton, 1981;1:191-194.
7. Personal Communication, Dr. Paul Jacobs, 1989.
8. Harris DR, Noodleman FR. Combining manual dermasanding with low strength trichloroacetic acid to improve actinically injured skin. J Dermatol Surg Oncol 1994;20:436-442.
9. Chiarello SE. Tumescent dermasanding with cryospraying: a new wrinkle on the treatment of rhytids. Dermatol Surg 1996;22:601-610.
10. Orientreich DS, Orientreich N. Subcutaneous incisionless (subcision) surgery for the correction of depressed scars and wrinkles. Dermatol Surg 1995;21:543-549.

IV

Laser
Resurfacing

CHAPTER 13

Skin Response to Laser Resurfacing

■ Sue Ellen Cox

Clay J. Cockerell

Patients have long desired a procedure that can safely and effectively help to reverse the cutaneous signs of aging. Public demand is great for such a procedure as is reflected in the number of cosmetic procedures for this performed each year. In 1992, the American Society for Plastic and Reconstructive Surgery conducted a survey that documented the performance of 104,000 dermabrasions at a cost of $468 million and 141,000 facial peels at $21 million. The pressure to develop such techniques has been steadily increasing as a consequence of several factors, the most important of which is our society's equation of youth as beauty, a myth perpetuated by industry and the media. Although both medical and surgical approaches to this challenge are available, these have traditionally suffered from either lack of efficacy or unpleasant side effects. Recently, a novel application of the carbon dioxide (CO_2) laser was developed that has transformed the approach to dealing with cutaneous photoaging.

The CO_2 laser was first developed in 1964 by Bell Laboratories (Murray Hill, NJ). It emits light in the far infrared portion of the electromagnetic spectrum at 10,600 nm, a wavelength that is highly absorbed by water, which is the primary component of most human tissues. Because of its ability to cut and vaporize tissue and to photocoagulate blood vessels, surgical applications were developed using the CO_2 laser in ophthalmology for photocoagulation of diabetic retinopathy. The CO_2 laser was also used in surgery with the promise of "bloodless" excisions due to its ability to cut tissue while simultaneously coagulating small blood vessels. The CO_2 laser could also vaporize tissue when used in a defocused mode, and applications in dermatology were developed for the removal of superficial lesions, such as verrucae and actinic cheilitis. In the late 1980s, David and Lask were the first to conceive of the idea of CO_2 laser skin resurfacing for photodamaged skin (1). They used a standard CO_2 laser with a 3 to 8 mm spot size at a target distance of 4 to 12 cm. While effective at vaporizing superficial layers of the skin only, the laser had a very narrow therapeutic range that led to variable results with a significant risk for scarring. In 1990, Coherent Laser Corp. (Palo Alto, CA) introduced a high energy output, ultra short pulse laser system that could be used safely and effectively. Shortly thereafter, Sharplan Laser, Inc. (Allendale, NJ) developed an alternative method for achieving safe facial resurfacing that used a continuous wave CO_2 laser with an attached microprocessor-controlled scanner. This device rapidly scans a defocused laser beam on the tissue causing superficial vaporization (2, 3). Because the beam does not remain on any point of tissue for more than 1 msec, it effectively acts within the thermal relaxation time of tissue thereby limiting the thermal damage to surrounding normal skin markedly lessening the risk of scarring and other complications (4).

CLINICAL AND HISTOLOGIC CHANGES OF THE AGING FACE

Aging of the skin can be divided into two types: intrinsic and extrinsic. Intrinsic aging refers to changes that develop as a consequence of the passage of time alone. In the skin, these are relatively minor and consist primarily of slight epidermal thinning, loss of elasticity and some loss of substance. Extrinsic aging essentially refers to photoaging, which is a consequence of the long-term effects of sun damage to the skin. Other forms of extrinsic aging of the skin are a consequence of exposure to other forms of cutaneous injury such as x-rays and infrared irradiation. Photoaging is manifested as wrinkling particularly around the mouth and eyes, as a yellowish, sallow discoloration, as telangiectasia, hyperpigmented and hypopigmented macules and as keratoses, both solar and seborrheic keratoses. Because of its depth of penetration into the papillary dermis, the technique of laser resurfacing is ideally suited for treatment of photoaging. While not primarily indicated for significant laxity of the skin, a tightening effect does occur with CO_2 laser use that is not seen with the other methods of resurfacing.

Histologically, intrinsic aging is characterized by alteration of the epithelium and its adnexa and the dermal connective tissue. Flattening of the dermal-epidermal junction also occurs as does effacement of the rete ridge pattern (5). Eccrine and apocrine glands are decreased in size and their activity lessens. In contrast, sebaceous glands increase in size on the face, although the degree of secretion may vary among individuals and may be either increased or decreased.

Fibroblasts play an important role in maintaining dermal architecture. In addition to producing collagen and elastin, they participate in the inflammatory process producing collagenase and other proteolytic enzymes when the skin is wounded. Fibroblasts are also targets for growth factors that can either stimulate fibroblast proliferation and procollagen production or inhibit their production of collagenase. In aged skin, there is a decrease in the number of fibroblasts in the dermis that is associated with a decrease in collagen and elastin content as a consequence of underproduction of procollagen and over expression of collagenase. The dermal connective tissue matrix is normally composed of 70% collagen, which provides tensile strength, and 2% to 4% elastic tissue that provides elasticity and resilience. The rate of collagen loss is approximately 1% per year of adult life. Quantitation of elastin loss is less precise, but it decreases markedly after age 30. Morphologically, individual collagen bundles become thinned and may be either tangled or straight fibers that are loosely woven. The net result is an inability to maintain structural integrity of the dermis (6). There is also a decrease in the number of macrophages, mast cells and dendritic cells in the dermis.

Photoaging induces a number of histological changes that are often superimposed on those of intrinsic aging. In addition to effacement of epidermal rete ridges, there is often slight atypia of keratinocytes with hyperpigmentation. Skin that is chronically exposed to sun has almost twice the number of melanocytes as nonexposed skin. The melanocytes are larger and tend to cluster and, in some cases, lead to the development of lentigenes. Ultraviolet irradiation induces a decrease in both the number and function of Langerhans cells (5, 7). Solar elastosis develops within the papillary dermis as a consequence of degeneration of elastin and is manifested by a bluish-gray discoloration of collagen bundles primarily in the papillary dermis but with extension into the reticular dermis (8, 9). The ground substance of the dermal matrix, which consists primarily of dermatan sulfate and hyaluronic acid, is also decreased. There is also a modest reduction in vascularity (10). Elastic fibers at the dermoepidermal junction appear cylindrical in shape and arranged vertically when examined by scanning electron microscopy. In the reticular dermis, elastic fibers appear more branched and larger; in the deep reticular dermis, elastic fibers often appear as large, thin, broad sheets (11). Transmission electron microscopy demonstrates diminished electron density of collagen fibrils, decreased contrast in cross striations and fragmentation of individual fibrils into filaments in photoaged skin (12).

MEDICAL TREATMENT

Several medical therapies have been demonstrated to be efficacious in improving photoaged skin. Significant improvement in photoaged skin can be achieved when patient education is combined with sun avoidance and photoprotection. Current topical therapies include retinoids, alpha hydroxy acids (AHAs) and antioxidants. Medical therapy is slow, however, and patients must be committed to long-term therapy and to a lifestyle change. Furthermore, the tolerance levels of individual patients to these agents varies greatly as the agents can induce significant irritation.

Retinoic acid (tretinoin) is the most carefully studied of the topical agents used for the treatment of photoaging and is generally regarded as the most effective agent that can be applied by the patient. It has several different effects on the skin at the levels of both the epidermis and the dermis. Griffiths et al showed that topical application of tretinoin directly induces collagen synthesis. In a study comparing the effects of application of topical tretinoin and a vehicle, tretinoin induced an 80% increase in the formation of type I collagen compared to only a 14% increase when the vehicle was applied alone (13).

Application of tretinoin has also been shown to reduce excess epidermal melanin, decrease keratinocytic atypia and diminish angiogenesis (14, 15). Recent research suggests that tretinoin may exert some of its effect by inhibiting proteins that degrade collagen and elastin as a result of sun overexposure (16).

Topical therapy with AHAs has gained popularity in the last few years as an alternative to tretinoin. These agents have not been studied as extensively as retinoids, although they have been shown to increase stratum corneum thickness and reduce corneocyte cohesion (17). These agents offer the advantage of being less irritating to the skin than tretinoin but are generally not as effective.

SURGICAL TREATMENT

For more than 30 years, chemical peeling with phenol, trichloroacetic acid (TCA), other acids and dermabrasion have been the mainstays of surgical rejuvenation of the aging face. Descriptions of these techniques are found in other chapters, and can also be found in a number of excellent reference works. Since laser resurfacing is becoming more popular, and in many areas is replacing these time-honored techniques, it is important to assess how the laser compares in efficacy and safety. Fitzpatrick et al recently conducted an animal study comparing the effects of pulsed CO_2 laser skin resurfacing with 35% TCA chemical peel, Bakers-Gordon 50% phenol peel and dermabrasion (18). They evaluated the histologic effects of skin damage induced by different pulse energies and differing numbers of passes and compared the depth of vaporization and thermal damage to the depth of tissue removal achieved by other resurfacing modalities. A 4 μm punch biopsy was taken immediately after treatment and at 7, 21 and 42 days. They found that application of 35% TCA resulted in tissue necrosis to a depth of 75 μm in the dermis, dermabrasion resulted in tissue removal to 350 μm and 50% Baker's phenol resulted in necrosis in the reticular dermis to 1000 μm. The depth of thermal necrosis with a single pass of the laser at the various energies was <40 μm. A second and third pass with the various energy levels resulted in thermal damage from 53 to 106 μm. Both the depth of vaporization and residual thermal damage were directly related to pulse energy and varied from 60 to 150 μm but was usually less than 100 μm. By varying the pulse energy and the number of passes, the depth of necrosis could be finely controlled to 400 μm in the dermis.

Re-epithelialization of all sites was complete by 7 days with the exception of the phenol treated skin, which required approximately 3 weeks. Healing of the TCA treated skin was similar to that of the laser treated skin at lower energy levels with one or two passes.

Healing of the dermabraded skin was similar to laser-treated skin at the higher (250 to 450 mJ per pulse) energies and with two or three passes. Although laser-tissue interaction resulted in heat-induced collagen contraction, the degree of thermal damage did not interfere with wound healing. No scarring resulted from any of the treatments.

Superficial chemical peels with AHA improve dyspigmentation of the skin but are only minimally effective at reducing fine wrinkles. Medium depth combination chemical peels with Jessner's solution and TCA are more effective at removing pigmentary abnormalities and, because of greater depth of penetration, also remove solar keratoses and solar lentigines and can diminish fine wrinkling. Deeper wrinkling around the mouth and eyes are not greatly improved, however. Phenol peeling does achieve removal of the deeper rhytides but sometimes at the expense of permanent hypopigmentation and an unnatural appearance to the skin. Laser resurfacing improves both fine as well as deep wrinkles. Furthermore, laser resurfacing normalizes dyschromia and has an added benefit of skin tightening. Hypopigmentation is only a rare complication with laser resurfacing and if it does develop, it is usually minimal in extent.

Laser resurfacing affords a number of other advantages over other techniques. It avoids variables inherent in chemical peeling that are operator dependent and cannot be fully controlled, such as penetration of the acid, defatting, application of pressure and number of coats of acid applied by the operator. Phenol peeling produces such deep injury to the reticular dermis that there is a risk of scarring. In contrast, laser resurfacing is never carried out to the depth of a deep chemical peel, yet the combined effects of tissue removal, collagen contraction and collagen remodeling produce comparable degrees of improvement with less risk of scarring. Furthermore, phenol peeling is associated with the potential for cardiotoxicity so that all patients who are treated with this agent must undergo cardiac monitoring. Finally, laser resurfacing avoids many of the risks of dermabrasion including exposure to blood-borne pathogens and inadvertent tissue trauma (4). Laser resurfacing is "forgiving" in that an inadvertent pass over an already treated area does not produce significant additional damage. In contrast, dermabrasion requires more manual dexterity.

Thus laser resurfacing has significant promise for treating photoaged facial skin (Fig. 13.1). Most studies of laser resurfacing reveal a greater than 50% clinical improvement. This technique is currently the subject of intense study and the reader is referred to additional review articles (4, 19-25).

FIGURE 13.1
A, Photodamage with lentigenes and rhytides before treatment and B, 6 weeks after full face laser resurfacing.

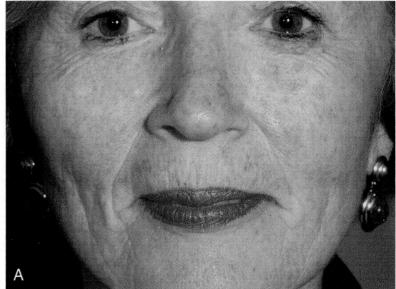

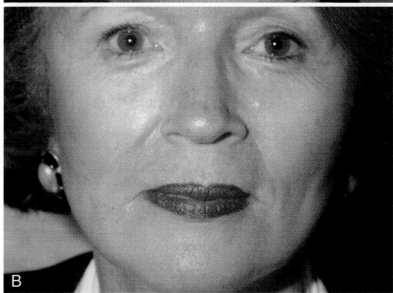

COMPARATIVE HISTOLOGY OF CUTANEOUS EFFECTS OF RESURFACING LASERS

Cotton et al were among the first to evaluate the histologic effects of a high-energy, short-pulse CO_2 laser system (Surgica XJ-150 direct current laser, [Sharplan Laser, Inc.]) on human skin and compare it to the effects of various chemical peels (26). The Surgica XJ-150 laser is a superpulse system and was used to treat 2×2 cm areas with a 3 mm collimated laser beam and a 3 mm spot size without overlapping. Energies of 250 mJ, 300 mJ and 400 mJ, all at 10 W with a 0.33 second interval, were used and both single and double passes were made on the skin. Surface debris was not removed before the second pass was made. Skin biopsy specimens were obtained at 1, 3, and 90 days following laser resurfacing at

two different locations (preauricular and postauricular skin).

Although they evaluated only 4 patients, Cotton et al made a number of important observations. One finding was that, at 90 days, a papillary dermal "repair zone" comprised of compact collagen bundles in parallel with the epidermal surface was present. The degree of fibrosis was noted to increase as the laser energy increased. A similar dermal repair zone has been previously documented with both medium and deep chemical peels (27, 28). It is thought that fibrosis seen histologically probably accounts for the clinical benefits of laser resurfacing as photodamaged collagen and elastin are replaced with newly formed collagen. Cotton et al also found that the depth of injury increased both with increasing pulse energy and with additional passes. The depth of dermal coagulative necrosis was 0.07 mm with a single pass at 250 mJ and 0.25 mm with a double pass at 400 mJ.

Kauvar et al looked at depth of thermal injury produced by three different laser systems: the UltraPulse 5000 laser (Coherent Laser Corp.), the superpulsed Surgica XJ-150 system and the scanned SilkTouch system (Sharplan Laser Inc.). A continuous wave laser was used as a control. In their study, it was not possible to test the same laser parameters due to the different technologies; however, the parameters chosen are considered standard for each laser system. Their results are depicted in Figure 13.2 (29).

We recently evaluated biopsy specimens taken from 4 patients in 5 different locations on the face (periocular, forehead, mandible, corner of the mouth and cheek) fol-

lowing laser resurfacing. We used the Surgica XJ-150 and the SilkTouch laser. In addition, two of these patients had a medium depth chemical peel (Jessner's solution followed by 35% TCA) on non-laser treated facial skin (30). Biopsies were taken 1 day following laser resurfacing and chemical peeling in all patients, and 60 days following full face laser resurfacing in 1 patient who underwent the procedure for acne scarring. In this patient and one other, a split face design was used in which the right side of the face was treated with the SilkTouch laser and the left side was treated with the Surgica XJ-150. The pulse parameters chosen were those considered to give optimal clinical results. The Surgica XJ-150 was used in the periocular location at 300 mJ with a 3 mm collimated handpiece at 10 W. In the other areas of facial skin the power was increased to 400 mJ with all other parameters remaining the same.

The SilkTouch laser settings used were 7 W with 0.2 second exposure times with a scanned 3 mm diameter. When two passes were made, proteinaceous debris was removed between passes. Histologic evaluation revealed that the Surgica XJ-150 laser ablated with 1 pass the entire epidermis with minimal inflammation in the periocular area (Fig. 13.3). In the same patient, the medium depth peel necrosed three-fourths of the epidermis with vacuolar alteration of the basement membrane, smudging the papillary dermis and producing minimal inflammation (Fig. 13.4).

Biopsies taken from the cheek, forehead and mandible of the two patients in which the facial split paradigm was performed were evaluated. One pass with the SilkTouch laser was approximately equal to the Surgica XJ-150 laser with both leading to ablation of the epidermis. The SilkTouch laser ablated slightly deeper but the difference was insignificant. Two passes with these laser systems revealed deeper thermal coagulation with the Surgica XJ-150 than the SilkTouch system.

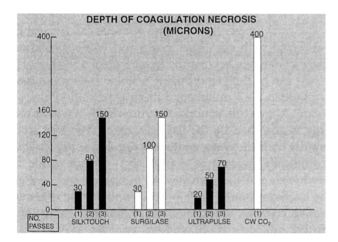

FIGURE 13.2

Depth of coagulation necrosis produced with one, two or three passes with each of the lasers. (Used with permission from Kauvar ANB, Waldorf HA, Geronemus RG. A histopathological comparison of "char-free" carbon dioxide lasers. Dermatol Surg 1996;22:343-347.)

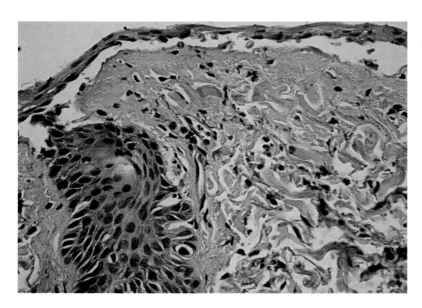

FIGURE 13.3

Skin biopsy taken from periocular skin following 1 pass with the Surgica XJ-150 resurfacing laser. The epidermis is necrotic and has separated from the dermis. There is slight coagulation of the upper papillary dermis and minimal inflammation. (Hematoxylin and eosin, original magnification ×400.)

There was necrosis to the upper reticular dermis with a greater inflammatory infiltrate present with the Surgica XJ-150 (Fig. 13.5). One observation noted on histologic examination was that there was not a marked difference in depth between one and two passes with the Silk-Touch system (Fig. 13.6). However, the depth of destruction increased more with the Surgica XJ-150 between pass one and two. This suggests that the SilkTouch laser may be more "forgiving" while the Surgica XJ-150 might be more destructive and that the two might be able to be used in different, perhaps complementary, settings.

Biopsies taken at 60 days following treatment demonstrated fibrosis of the papillary dermis in a pattern similar to that reported in other studies with lamellar, compact horizontally oriented collagen bundles with a

normal appearing epidermis overlying. No difference in the thicknesses of the dermal repair zone between the right and left sides were appreciated and no significant variability was seen in biopsies taken from different areas of facial skin were noted. As this was a pilot study and biopsy specimens of pretreated skin were not obtained, no exact measurements of the thicknesses of injury were made and no studies to evaluate the precise collagen subtypes were performed.

Thus, the studies performed by Cotten et al, Kauvar et al and by us support that two passes with the Surgica XJ-150 extends slightly deeper than 2 passes with both the UltraPulse 5000 and SilkTouch lasers (26, 29). The Surgica XJ-150 superpulse system in which the energy is delivered in a pulsed pair may deliver the laser energy over a longer period than the 1 msec thermal relaxation

FIGURE 13.4

Skin biopsy taken from periocular skin following medium depth chemical peel (Jessner solution followed by 35% TCA). There is complete coagulation necrosis of the epidermis with re-epithelialization beneath the necrotic epidermis. There is minimal degeneration of the papillary dermis with minimal inflammation. (Hematoxylin and eosin, original magnification ×400.)

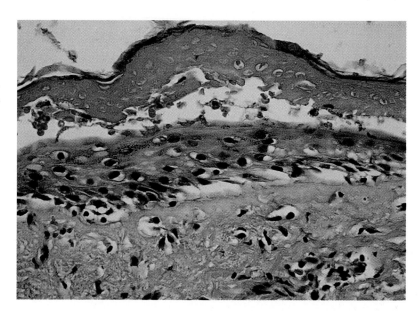

FIGURE 13.5

Skin biopsy taken from left mandibular skin following two passes with the Surgica XJ-150 resurfacing laser. The epidermis is absent and there is coagulation of the papillary dermis and upper reticular dermis. There is a moderate degree of inflammation with lymphocytes and neutrophils. (Hematoxylin and eosin, original magnification ×400.)

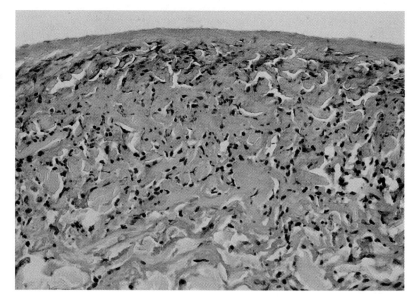

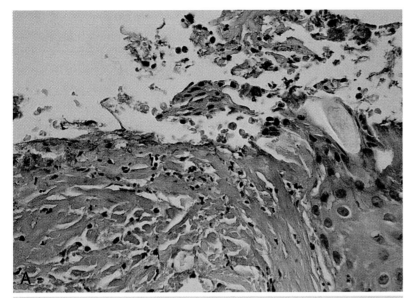

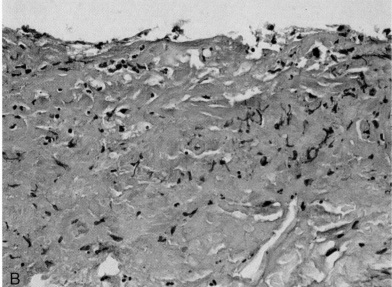

FIGURE 13.6

A, Skin biopsy taken from right mandibular skin following two passes with the SilkTouch resurfacing laser. There is complete absence of the epidermis and the papillary dermis has been ablated. There is a sparse inflammatory infiltrate of lymphocytes and scattered neutrophils in the upper reticular dermis. There is overlying crust. Note that, even though there have been 2 passes, the reticular dermis is intact. Similar findings were noted with 1 pass of this laser suggesting that it is more "forgiving" (Hematoxylin and eosin, original magnification ×400). B, Skin biopsy taken from the forehead of the same patient following 1 pass with the SilkTouch resurfacing laser. Note the lesser degree of inflammation and the less extensive degeneration of the dermal collagen. (Hematoxylin and eosin, original magnification ×400.)

time of tissue, allowing for heat diffusion away from the target. In addition in the study by Cotton et al, the failure to wipe away vaporized tissue may act as a "heat sink" to absorb additional laser energy without vaporization producing diffusion away from the target (4).

In a pilot study performed with the assistance of Robert Briggaman, MD, electron microscopy was performed on tissue immediately following resurfacing and thereafter at intervals of 4 and 10 months. A biopsy of preauricular skin taken after treatment with the Silk-Touch laser (1 pass at 7 W with a 6 mm spot, 0.2 seconds on skin, 0.4 seconds off skin, and removal of vaporized skin) revealed complete absence of the epidermis with the surface of the specimen consisting of lamina densa. There was thermal necrosis of the entire papillary dermis with spread to the upper reticular dermis. The necrosis extended to a depth of 6 to 7 μm from the lam-

ina densa to the upper reticular dermis. Figure 13.7 clearly shows necrosis of the more superficial portion of a single dermal fibroblast while the deeper portion appears uninjured. Results of electron microscopic evaluation of specimens taken at 4 and 10 months following treatment are currently in the process of evaluation.

THERMAL EFFECTS OF LASER RESURFACING

The birth of the cosmetic resurfacing laser was developed out of the need to minimize thermal damage and heat diffusion to normal skin structures. Ideally, the effects of the laser would be confined to the site of treatment. As heat is potentially damaging to normal skin, minimizing its effects is of prime importance. Different tissues have different sensitivity to the effects of heat.

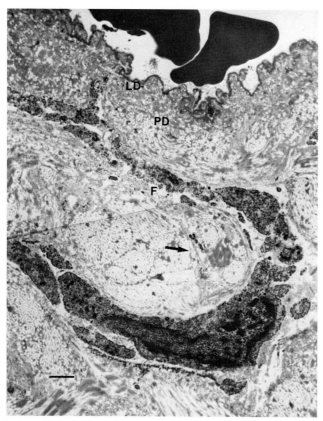

FIGURE 13.7

Preauricular skin treated with Silk Touch Laser (1 pass at 7 W with 6 mm spot) followed by wiping away the damaged epidermis. Post-treatment electron micrograph shows lamina densa (*LD*) portion of the basement membrane zone with several red blood cells at the surface. Thermal injury involves necrosis of the entire papillary dermis (*PD*) and extends into the upper reticular dermis to the level of the arrow. The more superficial portion of a dermal fibroblast (*F*) is necrotic while the deeper portion appears uninjured. Depth of thermal injury from the lamina densa to the arrow is approximately 6 to 7 μm (Bar = 1 μm).

For example, skin and cornea are more sensitive to thermal damage than the aorta and myocardium. This sensitivity is likely a consequence of the content of the individual tissue as the major extracellular matrix protein of corneal stroma and dermis is collagen while that of aorta and myocardium is muscle (31). When used in the cutting mode, continuous wave CO_2 lasers generate temperatures greater than 300°C at the immediate zone of impact leading to almost instantaneous carbonization of tissue. Adjacent to the immediate zone of impact, the depth of injury produces zones of vacuolization (100 to 200 μm) and edema (100 to 200 μm) (32). Furthermore, collagen shrinks as a consequence of heat, a finding that was first noted with surgical corneal reshaping in 1898 (33).

Three zones of collagen alteration have been identified following treatment of skin with an electrically pulsed continuous wave CO_2 laser (31). The innermost zone, occurring at a pulse duration of 2 msec, is referred to as "char" and is several microns deep. The next zone, 5-15 μm wide, is manifest as a bluish staining of collagen with hematoxylin and loss of its fibrillar appearance. Shorter pulse durations showed more hematoxylin staining of collagen than normal, but less than the inner zone. In a study of rat skin, heat induced collagen shrinkage occurred in three phases: denaturization of the triple helix, unwinding of the helix, and hydrolysis of collagen cross-links. This was associated with dermal relaxation which increased as the temperature increased (34). Fitzpatrick further elaborated on the three distinct zones of thermal damage of the skin induced by CO_2 lasers. The "zone of direct interaction" refers to the changes induced by direct action of laser on the tissue itself and results in vaporization of intracellular water and tissue ablation. Underlying this is the "zone of irreversible thermal damage and denaturation" which consists of frank tissue necrosis. Beneath this is the "zone of reversible thermal damage." In this zone, there is collagen shrinkage with minimal necrosis. As the skin undergoes repair, there is fibroblast proliferation and new collagen synthesis. The skin tightens as myofibroblasts contract leading to lessened laxity clinically (20).

The thermal effect on the skin differentiates laser resurfacing from other skin resurfacing modalities. In a recent presentation, Fitzpatrick described various effects of heat on collagen. He noted that isolated collagen fibers shrink up to one-third of their length. This contraction occurs at temperatures between 55° and 60°C with degeneration occurring at 70°C. He also noted that new collagen formation develops for the first 6 months after laser resurfacing and increases up to 4-fold. Thus, many of the desired effects of skin resurfacing such as tightening of lax skin, smoothing of rhytides, and improvement of cutaneous texture over time occur as a consequence of thermal effects on the skin.

Therefore, it is obvious that the optimal thermal spread for resurfacing lasers be determined as it has important implications for the therapeutic effects of the laser. For example, the SilkTouch system has greater thermal spread than the UltraPulse 5000 (35). This may be a consequence of increased change in tissue temperature but it may increase the risk of scarring. The clinical observation of immediate "tightening" of tissue after laser treatment is most likely secondary to dehydration of the skin by the laser; however, long-term tightening is most likely a consequence of collagen synthesis. Fitzpatrick has noted that it is not known whether thermally altered collagen persists indefinitely in its new form or acts as a matrix for new collagen formation that recapitulates its shortened overall structure (20).

Immediate physical changes of laser resurfaced skin have recently been described by Gardner et al. They evaluated 305 excised skin samples which were then treated with either the UltraPulse 5000 or the SilkTouch laser. Parameters assessed included lateral skin shrinkage, transient temperature change, isometric tension development, elasticity change and histologic features. Gardener et al found that tissue shrinkage was linearly correlated to the number of passes with no statistical difference between the two laser systems. Tissue temperature increase was statistically greater with the SilkTouch system (19.5°C) than with the UltraPulse 5000 laser (15.4°C). The magnitude of temperature increase was independent of the number of passes. Tissue tension plateau was attained after the second pass with the SilkTouch and after the third pass with the UltraPulse 5000 laser. The elasticity of laser-treated specimens decreased as the number of laser passes increased. The histologic findings were similar to those seen in other studies with the exception that Gardener et al did not report an increase in depth of coagulative necrosis with increasing number of passes (35). This is contrary to the findings of both Kauvar et al and Cotton et al in which the zone of residual thermal damage increased with subsequent passes (26, 29). The study by Gardner et al is important in defining the skin's physical changes that develop immediately following laser resurfacing; how-

ever, the study is limited as only in vitro skin samples were studied.

THE CLINICAL RESPONSE OF SKIN TO LASER RESURFACING

When teaching laser resurfacing to the novice, specific changes in the skin are often described as indicators of tissue response to both laser penetration and the depth of penetration. Deciphering the skin indicators has been described as an "art" that consists of learning to recognize tissue color changes and tissue reactions. These changes provide a rough estimate of tissue penetration that may vary by measurements of tens to hundreds of microns (36). It is generally said that with the first pass of the laser, a whitish bubbled appearance of the skin surface is observed. This change represents intracellular water vaporization and residual desiccated protein debris (Fig. 13.8). When this debris is removed with saline, intact, smooth pink tissue representing the papillary dermis is revealed (Fig. 13.9). With the next laser pass, there is obvious visual contraction of the skin and its color assumes a yellowish hue. These fea-

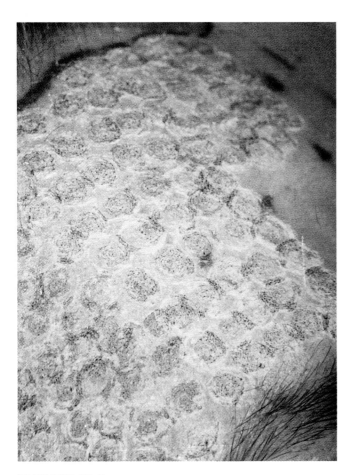

FIGURE 13.8
Initial pass with the SilkTouch laser showing desiccated protein debris.

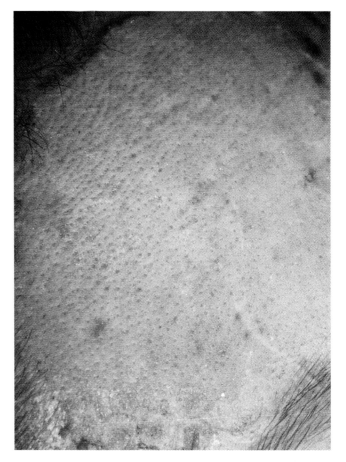

FIGURE 13.9
Skin appearance immediately after removing the debris reveals a pink papillary dermis.

tures are more obvious in areas of thicker skin such as that around the mouth. Thin skin, such as that of the upper eyelid, has marked contraction with less obvious tissue yellowing. When three or more passes are performed, dehydrated yellow-brown proteinaceous material, which represents degenerated collagen of the reticular dermis, is seen. Involvement of the reticular dermis is an end-point, beyond which charring and thermal diffusion may occur resulting in unwanted tissue necrosis.

For the practitioner of laser surgery, a working knowledge of both laser systems is important to understand the concept of beam uniformity. The UltraPulse 5000 laser system functions with a gaussian distribution of energy within each pulse. The energy at the periphery of the pulse is lower than that at the center. Therefore, by overlapping slightly (approximately 10%), a more uniform tissue response is achieved. In contrast all the tissue within the scanned area is vaporized to a uniform depth with the SilkTouch system. The scanned focused beam moves within a spiral so that the center and edges of the treated tissue are exposed to the same power density. Therefore, the clinician should not overlap individual pulses when using the SilkTouch system. Furthermore, when using the SilkTouch for full face laser resurfacing, the use of the 6 mm spot size allows for more uniform heat distribution without dissipation. Clinically, greater contraction of the skin is noted.

CONCLUSION

The advent of the CO_2 resurfacing laser for treatment of photoaged skin is one of the most promising developments in cosmetic dermatology in many years. Wound healing studies which address extracellular matrix repair are ongoing and should better define the science behind contraction of the skin. As the effects of lasers on the skin become better understood, it is anticipated that the current lasers will be used more effectively, that new applications will be discovered and that new generations of lasers will be developed that take advantage of information about the skin's response to them.

Acknowledgment. The authors acknowledge and appreciate the expertise of Dr. Robert Briggaman in preparing and evaluating the electron microscopy for this chapter.

REFERENCES

1. David LM, Lask GP, Glassberg E, et al. CO_2 laser cosmetic and therapeutic treatment of facial actinic damage. Cutis 1989;85:247.
2. Chernoff WG, Schoenrock LD, Crammer H, et al. Cutaneous laser resurfacing. Int J Aesth Reconstr Surg 1995;3:154-158.
3. Chernoff WG, Slatkine M, Zair E, et al. SilkTouch: a new technology for skin resurfacing in aesthetic surgery. J Clin Laser Med Surg 1995;13:97-100.
4. Hruza G, Dover J. Laser skin resurfacing. Arch Dermatol 1996;132:451-455.
5. Kurban RS, Bhawan J. Histologic changes in skin associated with aging. J Derm Surg Oncol 1990;16:908-914.
6. Fitzpatrick RE. Facial resurfacing with the pulsed carbon dioxide laser. Fac Plast Surg Clin N Am 1996;4:231-240.
7. Gilchrest BA, Murphy GF, Soter NA. Effect of chronologic aging and ultraviolet irradiation on Langerhans cell populations. J Invest Dermatol 1982;78:85-88.
8. Braverman IM, Fonferko E. Studies in Cutaneous aging: The elastic fiber network. J Invest Dermatol 1982;78:434-443.
9. Mitchell RE. Chronic solar dermatosis: A light and electron microscopic study of the dermis. J Invest Dermatol 1967;43:203-220.
10. Gilchrest BA, Stoff JS, Soter NA. Chronologic aging alters the response to ultraviolet-induced inflammation in human skin. J Invest Dermatol 1982;79:11-15.
11. Lavker RM, Zheng P, Dong G. Aged skin: A study by light, transmission electron, and scanning electron microscopy. J Invest Dermatol 1987;88:44s-51s.
12. Braun-Falco O. Die Morphogenese der senil-aktinischen Elastose. Arch Klin Exp Dermatol 1969;235:138-160.
13. Griffiths CEM, Russman AN, Majmudar G, et al. Restoration of collagen formation in photodamaged human skin by tretinoin (retinoic acid). N Engl J Med 1993;329:530-535.
14. Yamamoto O, Bhawan J, Hara M, et al. Keratinocyte degeneration in human facial skin: documentation off new ultrastructural markers for photodamage and improvement during topical tretinoin therapy. Exp Derm 1995;4:9-19.
15. Griffiths CEM, Voorhees JJ. The tretinoin story. Fitzpatrick's J Clin Dermatol 1995;3:14-25.
16. Fischer GJ, Datta SC, Talaur HS, et al. Molecular basis of sun-induced premature skin aging and retinoid antagonism. Nature 1996;379:335-339.
17. Stiller MJ, Bartolone J, Stern R, et al. Topical 8% glycolic acid and 8% I-Lactic acid creams for the treatment of photodamaged skin. Arch Dermatol 1996;132:631-636.
18. Fitzpatrick RE, Tope WD, Goldman MP, Satur NM. Pulsed carbon dioxide laser, trichloroacetic acid, Baker-Gordon phenol, and dermabrasion: A comparative clinical and Histologic study of Cutaneous resurfacing in a porcine model. Arch Dermatol 1996;132:469-471.
19. Chernoff WG, Schoenrock LD, Crammer H, Wand J. Cutaneous laser resurfacing. Int J Aesth Reconstr Surg 1995;3:154-158.
20. Fitzpatrick RE, Goldman MP, Satur NM, Tope WD. Pulsed carbon dioxide laser resurfacing of photoaged facial skin. Arch Dermatol 1996;132:395-402.
21. Lowe NJ, Lask G, Griffin ME, Maxwell A, Lowe P, Quilada F. Skin resurfacing with the UltraPulse carbon dioxide laser: observation on 100 patients. Dermatol Surg 1995;21:1017-1019.
22. Waldorf HA, Kauvar ANB, Geronemus RG. Skin resurfacing of fine to deep rhytides using a char-free carbon dioxide laser in 47 patients. Dermatol Surg 1995;21:940-946.
23. Lask G, Keller G, Lowe N, Gormley D. Laser resurfacing with the SilkTouch flashscanner for facial rhytides. Dermatol Surg 1995;21:1021-1024.

24. Ho C, Nguyen Q, Lowe NJ, Griffin ME, Lask G. Laser resurfacing in pigmented skin. Dermatol Surg 1995;21:1035-1037.
25. Alster TS, West TB. Resurfacing of atrophic facial acne scars with a high-energy, pulsed carbon dioxide laser. Dermatol Surg 1996;22:151-155.
26. Cotton J, Hood AF, Gonin R, et al. Histologic evaluation of preauricular and postauricular human skin after high-energy, short pulse carbon dioxide laser. Arch Dermatol 1996;132:425-428.
27. Baker TJ, Gordon HL, Mosienko P, et al. Long-term histological study of skin after chemical face peeling. Plast Reconstr Surg 1974;53:522-525.
28. Brody HJ. Histology and classification and wound healing. In: Brody HJ, ed. Chemical Peeling. St. Louis: Mosby Year Book, 1992:7-22.
29. Kauvar ANB, Waldorf HA, Geronemus RG. A histopathological comparison of "char-free" carbon dioxide lasers. Dermatol Surg 1996;22:343-347.
30. Monheit G. The Jessner's + TCA peel: A medium-depth chemical peel. Dermatol Surg Oncol 1989;15:9:945-950.
31. Walsh JT, Flotte TJ, Anderson RR et al. Pulsed CO_2 Laser Tissue Ablation: Effect of tissue type and Pulse Duration on Thermal Damage. Lasers Surg Med 1988;8:108-118.
32. Nelson JS, Berns MW. Laser-tissue interactions. In: Goldman L (ed): Laser Non-Surgical Medicine. Lancaster, PA: Technomic Publishing Co., 1991:23-54.
33. Tans LJ. Experimentelle Untersuchungen uber Entstehung von astigmatismus durch nicht-perforirende Corneawunden. Graefes Arch Opthalmol 1898; 45:117-152.
34. Allain JC, Lous LE, Cohen-Solal L, et al. Isometric tensions developed during hydrothermal swelling of rat skin. Connective Tissue Res 1980;7:127-133.
35. Gardner ES, Reinisch L, Stricklin GP, et al. In vitro changes in non-facial human skin following CO_2 laser resurfacing: a comparison study. Lasers Surg Med 1996;19:379-387.
36. Fitzpatrick RE. Understanding Lasers. J Derm Surg 1995 Nov;(Suppl):7-8.

CHAPTER 14

Physics of Resurfacing Lasers

■ Elizabeth I. McBurney

The pulsed carbon dioxide (CO_2) laser is one of the latest surgical instruments available in the high technology revolution of medicine. The underlying concept of lasers was formulated by Albert Einstein in 1917. In 1959, Theodore Maiman designed the first prototype laser by stimulating a ruby crystal to produce red laser light. Dr. Leon Goldman published the first account of using a laser system on skin in 1963 (1). In 1965 the continuous wave CO_2 laser was developed. In the three and one half decades, there has been mercurial rise in the types of lasers used in medicine (2).

HISTORY

Einstein's original concept of lasers is based on the simple physics that when a molecule is in a high energy state it is unstable and quickly reverts to its resting state, and in doing so releases a photon of light. He proposed that an excited state is more likely to produce a photon when in the presence of a photon of like energy. What Einstein theorized, and what subsequent scientists proved, is that if a volume of the same element is affected by controlled stimulus, it will generate stimulated emission of monochromatic, coherent and collimated light. The word *LASER* is an acronym for *Light Amplification by Stimulated Emission of Radiation* and describes the physical process by which laser light is produced.

Since the development of the first ruby laser, there has been the continuous development of new lasers. To date, there have been hundreds of different lasers developed throughout the electromagnetic spectrum (Table 14.1, Fig. 14.1). Many different substances can be stimulated to emit laser light: solids such as ruby crystal, liquid dyes, gas mixtures containing CO_2, and others. Regardless of the type of laser, four components

make up all lasers: (1) A medium composed of the element or compound, (2) A source of excitation energy to stimulate the medium, (3) Highly reflective mirrors at either end of laser tube, and (4) A delivery system such as fiberoptic wand or articulated arm. To generate a laser beam, the laser medium must be stimulated by a source of energy such as high intensity light, radio frequency emission, or high voltage electricity. This external energy source stimulates all the atoms or molecules within the laser medium. If more than half the atoms within the laser medium are excited, the condition called population inversion occurs and there is an excess energy of photons. As one atom releases a photon of energy it collides with other excited atoms, resulting in the generation of two photons. The photons are in perfect alignment with the same amount of energy wavelengths and the resultant laser beam is coherent, collimated, and monochromatic.

LASER-TISSUE INTERACTION

Lasers react with tissue through chemical, thermal and photoacoustic reactions. Lasers within the visible spectrum (approximately 400 to 700 nm) and above in the infrared red range react with tissue on a thermal or photoacoustic basis. When laser light comes in contact with the surface of the skin, it can be reflected, absorbed, transmitted, or scattered (Table 14.2, Fig 14.2). The primary medical uses for lasers involve affecting tissue by absorption or scattering.

The three primary organic chromophores of tissue are water, hemoglobin, and melanin. Tissue chromophores are essential for absorption of laser energy. In the use of the resurfacing CO_2 laser, the water is the dominant tissue target. Besides these primary chromophores,

TABLE 14.1

ELECTROMAGNETIC SPECTRUM SITE OF LASERS AND SKIN ABSORPTION TARGET

Laser	Spectrum Position	Wavelength (nm)	Skin Chromophore	Laser	Spectrum Position	Wavelength (nm)	Skin Chromophore
Excimer lasers	Ultraviolet		Protein	Copper Vapor	Green	511	Melanin, blood
ArF		193			Yellow	578	Melanin, blood
KrCl		222		Dye Laser	Yellow	585	Melanin, blood
KrF		248		Ruby	Red	694.7	Melanin
XeCl		308		Alexandrite	Infrared-A	755	Melanin
XeF		351		Nd:YAG	Infrared-A	1,064	Melanin, blood
Argon	Blue-Green	488-514.5	Melanin, blood	Holmium:YAG	Infrared-A	2,100	Water
KTP	Green	532	Melanin, blood	Erbium:YAG	Infrared-A	2,940	Water
Krypton	Multi-Color	531.7-647.1	Melanin, blood	Carbon Dioxide	Infrared-B	10,600	Water

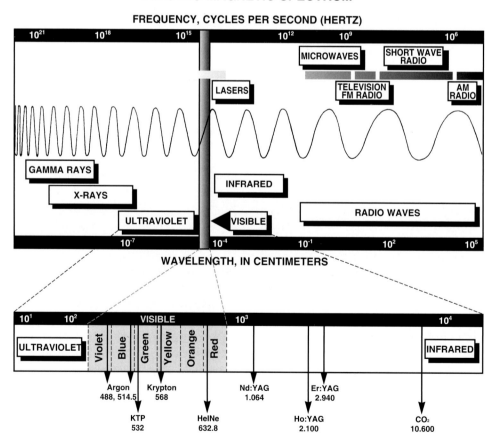

FIGURE 14.1

Electromagnetic spectrum.

TABLE 14.2

TISSUE EFFECTS FROM THERMAL ENERGY

Temperature	Visual Change	Biological Change
37–60°C	No Change	Warming, welding
60–65°C	Blanching	Coagulation
65–90°C	White/Gray	Protein denaturization, necrosis
90–100°	Puckering	Drying
100–150°C	Plume	Vaporization
150–210°C	Carbonization	Potential scar

INTERACTION OF LASER LIGHT AND TISSUE

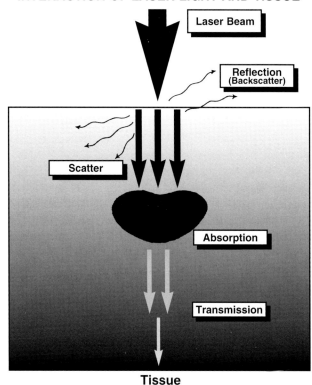

FIGURE 14.2
Interaction of laser light and tissue.

some lasers will determine their effect by tissue color, vascularity, or foreign pigment, such as tattoos. The laser effect on the tissue is primarily a thermal one, and the resultant tissue effects occur within distinct thermal ranges from 37°C to 210+°C (Table 14.2).

The absorption of light in tissue is described by Beer's law, which states that for a given distance of absorbing material that light passes through, a fixed fraction of the light that entered that length of absorbing medium is absorbed. It is customary to describe the absorption strength of a given material at a given wavelength by the depth at which the light penetrates before being absorbed to the point when only 10% of the light that entered remains. This depth is called the extinction length. Most of the laser energy is absorbed in the first extinction length, but some (10%) penetrates deeper. After two extinction lengths, about 1% continues to propagate. A closely related and more commonly used measure of absorption is the absorption length. This is the depth to which light must penetrate to be 63% absorbed. There are approximately 2.3 absorption lengths in each extinction length. The absorption length of clinical lasers in water varies over a wide range, depending on the wavelength of the laser. As can be seen in Figure 14.3, the absorption length of the blue/green argon laser in water is extremely high. In contrast, the CO_2 laser has an absorption length of 20 μm (3).

The summation of the laser tissue effects is controlled through three parameters: the laser power, the spot size, and the length of time the light dwells on the tissue. When the laser beam exits the laser tube, it is passed through a series of mirrors within an articulating arm to a hand piece or through fiber where it is focused behind a lens. This focusing of the laser beam controls the rate of tissue ablation.

The intensity, or strength of the laser beam, is referred to as the power density and is measured in power per unit of tissue area (watts/cm²). Power density varies inversely with the square of the diameter of the beam. As the diameter of the laser beam, or spot size, is made smaller, the power is increased four fold. Thus, for the highest cutting power, the smallest, most focused spot size is used. Power density is a static measurement and does not take into account the length of time that the laser beam is applied. The total amount of laser energy delivered to the tissue is measured by multiplying the power, or watts (W), by the delivery time and is measured in Joules. The dosage is derived by dividing the energy delivered by the cross-sectional area of the beam and is described in Joules/cm² (J/cm²). This is known as the fluence. For a given spot size, the only two variables are power (watts) and time.

One watt per 100 seconds delivers the same amount of Joules as does 10 W for 10 seconds, but common sense dictates that the tissue effect between these two levels is dramatically different. It is not only important to establish the power and the spot size for the procedure, but also to control the exposure time on the tissue for the desired results. The longer the tissue is exposed to the laser, the greater the spread of thermal energy to collateral tissues. To limit exposure time and still achieve the desired tissue effect, the laser power must be increased to compensate.

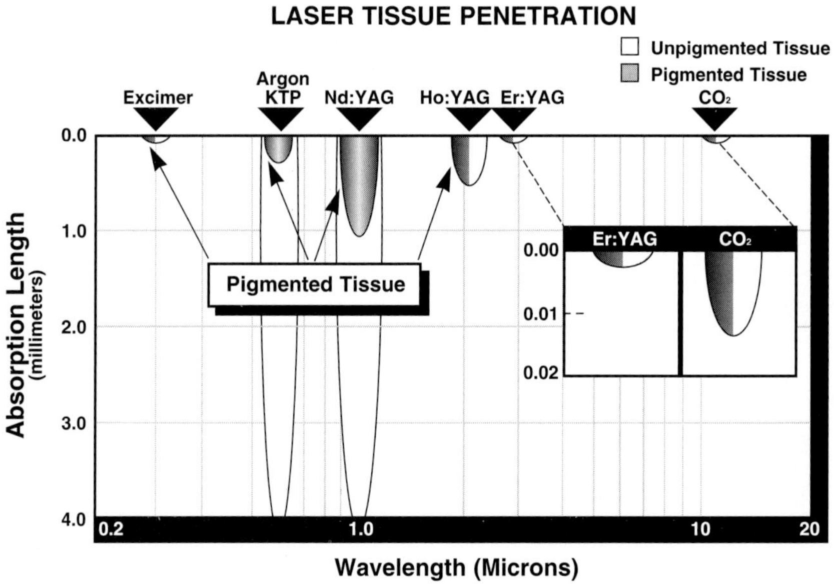

FIGURE 14.3

Laser tissue penetration. (Modified from Smith MFW. Neurological surgery of the ear. Hamilton, Ontario: BC Decker, 1992:146.)

LASER TISSUE PENETRATION

When the lasers are used effectively in surgery, histologic studies show that the minimum depth of tissue damage tends to be between one absorption length and one extinction length (Fig. 14.3). The difference in absorption plays a critical role in the use of selection and application of clinical lasers. Once laser light is absorbed by tissue, it immediately converted into heat. Upon completion of heating the absorbent tissue, the heat begins to diffuse to adjacent tissue by conduction. The process by which heat diffuses within the tissue by conduction is called thermal relaxation. The thermal relaxation time of a given tissue is the time required for the heated tissue to lose 50% of its heat through diffusion. Significant thermal damage, for example heat conduction, will not occur if the duration of the laser pulse is shorter than the time it takes the heated layer to cool. The time it takes heat to penetrate a given distance is proportional to the square of the distance; thus, if after one second, the tissue 1 mm below the surface has reached a temperature of 70°C, the time required for tissue 2 mm below the surface to reach 70°C will be four times as long, or 4 seconds.

When heat energy impacts the surface of the tissue, it directly heats the tissue within an absorbing length. Heat is also conducted into surrounding tissue by thermal relaxation. The heat that is not conducted into adjacent tissue may vaporize or ablate the tissue near the surface. There is, therefore, a competition between the ablation of tissue that absorbs the laser energy and a coagulation of deeper tissue. The rate of ablation is determined by the rate of deposition of the laser energy into the tissue. The higher the power of the laser, the faster the water is evaporated and the faster the ablation. **The key to clean ablation with minimal thermal damage is to ablate tissue faster than heat is conducted into surrounding underlying tissue** (3). This guarantees that

coagulation is limited to the absorption length of the laser.

Because the rate of ablation depends on the power density for each type of laser, there is a critical power density for minimal thermal damage. Whenever the power density is above this value, thermal damage is least possible for that type of laser. When ablation is attempted at less than critical power density, charring may result. Charring is avoided by doing ablation only at power densities greater than the critical value. It is something of a paradox, but critically important, that minimal thermal damage occurs at high power densities. The concept of working at low power in the interest of safety and position may produce exactly the opposite result. Precise tissue removal with minimal thermal damage to the surrounding structures can only be accomplished by using the laser at high power densities for a short time rather than a low power density for a longer time. In the CO_2 laser, the absorption length (minimum damage) shown is 0.02 mm. The thermal diffusion time is 0.002 seconds. The critical power density is 50 W/mm^2, and the critical pulse energy, therefore, is 0.040 J/mm^2 (3).

The theory of selective photothermolysis proposed by Anderson and Parish in the early 1980s refined the methods of using CO_2 laser light (4). By selecting the correct laser wavelength and delivering it in the appropriate time and energy, a particular target can be destroyed with little or no damage to the surrounding skin. This principle of selective thermolysis states that selective heating can be achieved by preferential laser light absorption and heat production in the target chromophore with heat being localized to the target by a pulse duration shorter than or equal to the thermal relaxation time (time for the target to cool by 63%) of the chromophore. The thermal relaxation time for 20 to

30 μm thickness of water-containing tissue that absorbs CO_2 laser light is less than 1 msec (5). Other wavelengths in addition to the CO_2 laser are capable of ablating skin, but have disadvantages. The erbium:yttrium aluminum garnet (Er:YAG) laser produces an infrared light of 2,940 nm, which is well absorbed by water and ensures superficial absorption. The Q-switched Er:YAG laser, with its extremely short nanosecond pulse durations, ablates approximately 5 to 10 μm of tissue, leaving behind only a few microns of thermal damage that cannot even seal small blood vessels. Once bleeding starts, the Q-switched Er:YAG laser loses its ability to ablate further, as all the energy is absorbed by the blood. In its normal mode, with a pulse duration of 250 msec, the Er:YAG laser ablates more tissue per pass, leaving a zone of thermal necrosis of approximately 50 μm. The longer pulse duration allows for more thermal conduction and, consequently, is sufficient to be hemostatic (5).

Applying the theory of selective photothermolysis to the CO_2 laser allows very precise cutaneous ablation by laser-tissue interaction, which is not achievable with dermabrasion, chemicals or cold steel. The first step is the selection of the correct wavelength, which is based on absorption of laser light by the target and the tissue. The CO_2 laser emits energy at 10,600 nm, a wavelength that is strongly absorbed by water (Fig. 14.4). This laser light is absorbed within a 20 μm radius of tissue (5).

The second concept is to choose a laser that produces sufficient energy to destroy the target, and at the same time, can deliver the energy in high enough bursts to destroy the target but not allow disbursement of thermal energy resulting in scars. With modifications of newer CO_2 lasers, this certainly is possible. The depth of penetration is very small due to the fact that the water in the epidermis immediately absorbs the laser energy. It has been recognized to achieve tissue ablation with no conduction of heat to adjacent tissue, at least 5 J/cm² are required (5). The latest generation of CO_2 lasers are able to achieve precise control of tissue vaporization, hemostasis, and minimal residual thermal changes.

When the CO_2 laser interacts with tissue, there are three different and distinct zones of thermal tissue alteration. The zone of direct interaction of the laser on target tissue results in vaporization of intracellular water and tissue ablation. Beneath this layer is a zone of irreversible thermal damage and denaturization resulting in thermal necrosis. Under this layer is a zone of reversible thermal damage. Fitzpatrick et al hypothesize that repair of this layer of reversible thermal damage during healing accounts for the tightening of the sagging skin and improvement of the wrinkles (6). When the new CO_2 lasers impinge upon the surface of the skin, there is immediate ablation of the tissue. This is followed by some desiccation and collagen shrinkage and then biological factors or cytokines are released. Ninety percent of the CO_2 laser pulse is absorbed in upper 20 to 30 μm of skin. The depth of penetration per pulse is generally 35 μm. So in theory, it will take 7 to 8 passes to remove a 300 μm wrinkle, when in actuality it is only 2 to 3 passes (7).

The CO_2 laser can be operated in a continuous wave mode, in singular repeat pulses of a continuous wave mechanically blocked by a shutter, varying from 0.05 second to 1 second, or in a Q-switched super pulse beam that exposes the tissue to extremely high powers

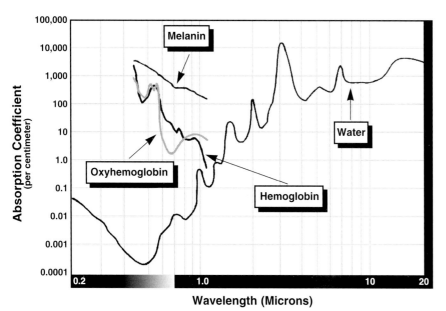

ABSORPTION OF TISSUE CHROMOPHORES

FIGURE 14.4

Absorption of tissue chromophores. (Reprinted with permission from Smith MFW. Neurological surgery of the ear. Hamilton, Ontario: BC Decker, 1992:146.)

for thousandths to millionths of a second. It has been proven that the superpulse beam works best on tissue and allows thermal relaxation in surrounding tissue to release any energy. Also, there is a transmission from a thermal effect to a photoacoustic effect. While heat of the laser creates tissue effect by warming the tissue above 100°C, the superpulse beam avoids carbonization. Carbonization removes the user's ability to selectively warm tissue because it heats to over 945°C when exposed to a laser beam, and, therefore, carbon becomes its own heat source. By applying a superpulse beam to tissue, there is an acoustic shock created by the sudden and intense beam that bounces carbon from the surface and away from the laser contact. This aerosol carbon and debris form the tissue plume that can be removed by a smoke evacuator. Applications that require warming tissue enough to achieve anastomosis, hemostasis, or shriveling of tissue are best accomplished through a continuous wave used at lower power.

To confine the thermal energy of a CO_2 laser, a pulse duration of approximately ≥ 1 msec is necessary and enough energy has to be delivered to completely vaporize the water in the tissue target. This requires 5 J/cm² to be delivered in 1 msec or less (5).

Recent studies by Ross et al have shown that, although pulse duration is an important determinant in ablation and thermal damage, irradiation is more critical as an independent parameter in predicting the effects of the CO_2 laser (7). Ross et al found that to achieve ablation with minimal thermal damage, pulse duration should be less than or equal to 1 msec per radiant energies exposures between 7.5 and 14 J/cm² (7). The results achieved by CO_2 laser resurfacing are the effects of several mechanisms. The epidermis and superficial dermis of the photodamaged skin are physically ablated by the laser. Below this top layer, the laser injury departs a zone of thermal heating, changing the dermal characteristics. Type I collagen has been shown to contract up to 60% when heated to 55 to 60°C. Cutaneous collagen contraction has been reported in rat and pig models. Finally, a delayed wound remodeling may explain the continued improvement that is seen postoperatively (5).

Cutaneous laser resurfacing was initially performed using the old continuous wave CO_2 laser in a defocused mode for simple tissue vaporization (8). Despite excellent results of these procedures, application of the recontouring techniques was limited by the skill of the laser operator and by the excessive heat conduction to the surrounding normal skin.

Recent improvements in CO_2 laser technology have eliminated the problems of nonspecific heat conduction. Two different types of CO_2 lasers have been developed to obtain selective char-free tissue ablation that is necessary for cutaneous resurfacing. The first type is a high-peaked power pulsed CO_2 laser that produces up to 500 mJ of energy per 600 μsec to 1 msec pulse (9, 10). A variation on this is another laser that produces energy up to 400 mJ by closely pairing two mJ pulses. The second type of CO_2 laser is the conventional continuous wave laser that is attached to a microprocessor-controlled scanner which rapidly scans the focused laser beam across the surface. The dwell time of the laser beam on any given area is less than 1 msec. The effect on tissue is similar to being lased with the consecutive 1 msec pulses (2).

The high energy pulsed or scanned CO_2 laser systems are being used in a number of cosmetic applications including cutaneous resurfacing of rhytides and benign tumors, scar modification, and hair transplantation (11). These new generation CO_2 lasers allow ablation of epidermis and dermis down to a variable depth with a bloodless and char-free environment. This improved, controlled tissue destruction combined with enhanced visualization maximizes outcomes and minimizes complications and risks.

REFERENCES

1. Goldman L, Blaney DJ, Kindel DJ, et al. Effect of the laser beam on the skin: preliminary report. J Invest Dermatol 1963;40:121.
2. Grossman MC. What is new in cutaneous laser surgery? Dermatol Clin 1997;15:1-8.
3. Trost D, Zacherl A, Smith MFW. Surgical laser properties and their tissue interaction. In: Smith MFW, ed. Neurological surgery of the ear. Hamilton, Ontario: BC Decker, 1992:131-162.
4. Anderson RR, Parrish JA. Selective photothermolysis: precise microsurgery by selective absorption of pulse radiation. Science 1983;220:524-527.
5. Hruza GJ. Laser skin resurfacing. Arch Dermatol 1996: 451-455.
6. Fitzpatrick RE, Goldman MP, Satur M, et al. Pulsed carbon dioxide laser resurfacing of photoaged facial skin. Arch Dermatol 1996;132:395-402.
7. Ross EV, Domankevitz Y, Skrobal M, et al. Effects of CO_2 laser pulse duration in ablation and residual thermal damage: implications for skin resurfacing. Lasers Surg Med 1996;19:123-129.
8. David LM, Lask GP, Glassbert E, et al. Laser abrasion for cosmetic and medical treatment of facial actinic damage. Cutis 1989;43:583-587.
9. Cotton J, Hood AF, Gonin R, et al. Histologic evaluation of preauricular and postauricular human skin after high-energy short-pulse carbon dioxide laser. Arch Dermatol 1996;132:425-428.
10. Alster TS. Comparison of two high-energy, pulsed carbon dioxide lasers in the treatment of periorbital rhytides. Dermatol Surg 1996;22:541-545.
11. Alster TS, Lewis AB. Dermatologic laser surgery: a review. J Dermatol Surg 1996;22:797-805.

CHAPTER 15

A Comparison of Lasers Currently in Use for Skin Resurfacing

■ Arielle N.B. Kauver
Roy G. Geronemus

Skin resurfacing with high energy, short-pulsed or scanned carbon dioxide (CO_2) lasers has recently emerged as a widely accepted modality for aesthetic skin rejuvenation. The resurfacing CO_2 lasers predictably vaporize thin layers of tissue and produce narrow zones of thermal damage. The desired degree of skin resurfacing is achieved by means of applying one or more laser passes in order to remove the epidermis and a variable thickness of the dermis. This technique offers potential advantages of improved control and reproducibility compared with the traditional methods of chemical peeling and dermabrasion. Superb clinical results have been obtained with these lasers in treating facial rhytides, surgical scars, acne scars, and photodamaged skin with a minimal risk of long term side effects (1-5).

With the development of various new technologies for resurfacing lasers, including CO_2 lasers, Erbium: YAG (Er:YAG) lasers and other mid-infrared wavelengths, histologic studies are employed to assess the ability of these lasers to produce thin-layer tissue ablation with minimal thermal damage to the adjacent skin. Based on these studies, guidelines are developed for the appropriate number of passes required to achieve the desired depth of resurfacing with each system. Histologic studies comparing laser resurfacing lasers with chemical peeling and dermabrasion provide useful information regarding the relative depths of tissue destruction and wound healing that occurs with each of these techniques. Microscopic analysis of tissue speci-

mens taken following laser resurfacing procedures provides insight into the mechanisms of re-epithelialization, new collagen production and collagen remodeling following these procedures.

LASER TISSUE INTERACTION IN SKIN RESURFACING

CO_2 lasers have been used for approximately three decades, but it was not until the last few years that these lasers have been modified to remove thin tissue layers with minimal heat damage to the surrounding skin. CO_2 lasers were quickly adopted as surgical tools because of their ability to both vaporize tissue in the defocused mode and rapidly incise tissue in the focused mode. Small nerve endings, blood vessels and lymphatics are coagulated as tissue is incised with the CO_2 laser, creating a bloodless surgical field and minimizing postoperative edema. With the original continuous wave models, the laser light is strongly absorbed by tissue, but continued application of the laser beam results in thermal diffusion and damage to zones of tissue approximately 0.5 to 1.0 mm in diameter. As a result, the use of the continuous wave CO_2 lasers for the vaporization and incision of skin lesions resulted in an unacceptable rate of scarring and pigmentary change (6-9).

Theoretical thermal models suggested that suitably short pulses of CO_2 radiation could ablate tissue while minimizing the production of thermal damage in the surrounding tissue (10-17). The earliest modification of the continuous wave lasers involved electronic shuttering of the beam to produce individual "pulses" of radiation ranging from 0.1 to 1.0 second in duration. There were no clinical advantages demonstrated with these models compared to the conventional continuous wave CO_2 lasers.

The next advance in CO_2 laser technology was the development of the "superpulsed" systems that could obtain peak powers 2 to 10 times higher with pulse durations 10 to 100 times shorter than conventional models. These laser systems are incapable of producing high peak power pulses; they deliver a train of 20 to 100 pulses per second to attain average powers comparable to continuous wave CO_2 lasers. Although the superpulsed lasers produced narrower zones of thermal damage in some animal studies, clinical outcomes in humans were no better than those seen with continuous wave lasers (18-21).

The ideal pulse parameters necessary to achieve thin layer vaporization of tissue with minimal residual thermal damage using CO_2 lasers were established based on the concepts of selective photothermolysis (22). This theory states that selective heating of a target chromophore in tissue can be achieved by preferential laser light absorption and heat production in the target chromophore by using a pulse duration shorter than or equal to the thermal relaxation time. The thermal relaxation time is the time it takes the target to cool by 63%.

For infrared lasers, the main chromophore in skin is water, which comprises approximately 90% of the tissue content. The 10,600 nm wavelength of the CO_2 laser has a high water absorption coefficient, which means this wavelength is absorbed strongly by tissue. As a result, 90% of the incident CO_2 laser light energy is absorbed in a 20 to 30 μm layers of tissue with only minimal light scattering, if the light is deposited faster than the thermal relaxation time (i.e., the cooling time) of skin (23-25). The thermal relaxation time for the 20 to 30 μm thickness of tissue absorbing CO_2 laser light is less than 1 msec.

In addition to the pulse duration requirements, resurfacing CO_2 lasers must be capable of delivering sufficient energy to achieve tissue vaporization during the laser pulse or scan. The energy density necessary to vaporize tissue with the CO_2 laser is approximately 5 J/cm^2 (23-25). Lower power CO_2 lasers that are incapable of reaching this fluence will coagulate and desiccate tissue, causing tissue temperatures to exceed 600°C. Extensive zones (1 to 5 mm) of thermal damage are produced in the surrounding tissue, comparable to those seen with electrocautery. In summary, tissue ablation of 20 to 30 μm layers of tissue will occur with minimal residual thermal damage if the laser delivers light at a fluence greater than 5 J/cm^2 within a radiation impact time under 1 msec (26).

Er:YAG lasers have recently been introduced for laser skin resurfacing. The 2,940 nm emission wavelength of this laser matches the main peak of water absorption, and its water absorption coefficient is ten times that of the CO_2 laser. Pulsed Er:YAG lasers therefore, ablate even thinner layers of tissue than CO_2 lasers, and leave behind inconsequential amounts of residual thermal damage. The thermally-coagulated layer of tissue produced beyond the point of vaporization is sufficiently small that pinpoint bleeding may occur with dermal ablation.

LASER SYSTEMS

Appropriate tissue ablation parameters for CO_2 lasers were first achieved with two varying types of technology, a high energy, short-pulsed system and a rapidly scanned technology. The UltraPulse 5000 laser (Coherent Laser Corp., Palo Alto, CA) is a high power laser that is capable of producing single pulses for peak energies up to 500 mJ, delivered within pulse durations of 600 sec to 1 msec. When used with the 3 mm collimated spot size, energy fluences of 5 to 7 J/cm^2 can be achieved. A computerized pattern generator (CPG) can be used in conjunction with this laser system to produce larger scanning sizes up to 19 mm in diameter, and several different geometric patterns. These patterns are comprised of individual 2.25 mm collimated beams, which can be overlapped by 10% to 60% to vary the total energy delivered to the tissue and achieve varying depths of ablation.

The other type of CO_2 skin resurfacing laser technology uses a conventional continuous wave CO_2 laser with an attached microprocessor-controlled scanner that rapidly scans a focused laser beam across the tissue. The SilkTouch laser (Sharplan Lasers Inc., Allendale, NJ) is the prototype for this technology. In order to achieve high energy densities, the CO_2 laser beam is focused to a spot size of 125 to 200 μm, depending on the handpiece in use, and the scanner moves the beam around a geometric pattern with consistent velocity to ensure that the radiation dwell time on any given point of tissue is under 1 msec. This system can deliver energy fluences of 5 to 15 J/cm^2 or more, depending upon the power of the continuous wave laser. Scan sizes with this system can be varied from 3 mm to 16 mm in diameter and take on several geometric shapes.

Several other skin resurfacing CO_2 lasers are now available (Table 15.1). The SurgiPulse XJ-150 (Sharplan Lasers Inc., Allendale, NJ) laser produces 600 μsec pulses that are delivered in pairs, and the two paired high energy peaks combine to a maximum of 400 mJ of energy per pulse. The TruPulse CO_2 laser (Tissue Technologies, Albuquerque, NM) has a pulse duration ranging from 60 to 100 μsec and produces narrower zones of thermal damage while abating thinner layers of tissue with each pass compared to the other resurfacing CO_2 lasers. Several other superpulsed CO_2 laser

* Axiom → 5 J/cm² @ 1 msec. ↗ necessary for CO_2 laser

TABLE 15.1

TABLE 15.1

CO₂ RESURFACING LASERS

Model	Pulse/Scan Duration (μsec)	Pulse Energy (mJ)	Scanner Available
Coherent UltraPulse	900	500	Yes
Surgilase SurgiPulse	600	400	Yes
Sharplan SilkTouch/ FeatherTouch	<890	1400	N/A
Palomar TruPulse	100	500	Yes
Luxar Nova Pulse	superpulsed	500	Yes

TABLE 15.2

ERBIUM:YAG RESURFACING LASERS

Model	Average Power (W)	Pulse Energy (J)	Rep Rate	Scanner Available
Candela	15	1	15	Yes
Con-Bio	10	1	10	Yes
SEO	5	1	10	Yes
ESC	20	1	10	Yes

systems, such as the Nova Pulse (Luxar Laser Corp., Bothell, WA) have been developed for skin resurfacing. This laser focuses the CO₂ beam to a small diameter of 0.8 mm in order to reach the ablation threshold of tissue, and when used with scanning devices that shorten the effective pulse duration, the laser can produce consistent clinical results. A variety of pulsed Er:YAG lasers have now received FDA clearance. Many of the manufacturers are now developing higher power systems that can produce pulse energies up to 2 J (Table 15.2).

HISTOLOGY OF RESURFACING LASERS: IMMEDIATE EFFECTS

Histologic evaluation of human skin after treatment with resurfacing lasers provides an understanding of the effects of these lasers on tissue. These studies provide the framework for selecting the right parameters to use with each resurfacing laser system, depending on the clinical indication and skin type being treated. To reliably predict the depths of tissue ablation and the amount of residual thermal damage produced with single or multiple laser passes, Kauver et al developed a model for in vivo treatment of human skin (27). In these

studies, one or more laser passes were performed on human skin, using clinically appropriate parameters for each laser system tested. Wet applicators were used to remove the coagulated debris after each laser pass, and the skin was blotted dry immediately before the next laser pass. Both high energy short-pulsed and scanned CO₂ laser technologies were tested. The UltraPulse laser was evaluated using a 3.0 mm collimated handpiece with a pulse energy of 450 mJ, at a power of 4 W. The SurgiPulse XJ-150 was tested with a 3.0 mm beam, operating at 10 W. Tests were also performed with the Silk-Touch laser using a 6.0 mm spot size, exposure times of 0.2 seconds and a power setting of 18 W. Control sites were applied using a Surgicenter 40 laser (Sharplan Laser Inc., Allendale, NJ) with a power setting of 10 W and 0.2 sec exposure times.

Using these parameters, one pass with either the SilkTouch or SurgiPulse lasers ablate entirely through the epidermis, producing a measurable zone of coagulation necrosis in the superficial papillary dermis. In contrast, one pass with the UltraPulse laser left behind foci of intact epidermis. A second pass was needed to ablate entirely through the dermal-epidermal junction with this laser. The depth of ablation with the SilkTouch and SurgiPulse lasers measured 30 to 50 μm, and 20 to 30 μm with the UltraPulse system. Each laser system produced increasing zones of thermal damage with the first three successive laser passes, which did not exceed over 150 μm, on the third pass. In contrast, zones of thermal damage greater than 500 μm are produced with one pass of a continuous wave CO₂ laser.

In a subsequent study, Kauver et al used the same model to investigate the tissue effects of the CPG used in conjunction with the UltraPulse laser (28). The scanning area of each pattern produced by this device is comprised of individual collimated 2.25 mm spots. These beams are then overlapped to varying degrees to produce a range of pulse energies with each laser scan. For this study, the square pattern #33 was tested at densities of 3, 6, and 9, corresponding to 10%, 35% and 60% overlap, respectively, of the collimated beams. Higher density settings resulted in deeper levels of tissue vaporization. Densities of 3, 6, and 9 produced approximate vaporization depths of 20, 40, and 60 μm, respectively. At a density setting of 3, partial epidermal vaporization was produced after one laser pass. In the gross tissue specimens, islands of intact epidermis were visible when the coagulated debris was wiped away following the first laser pass. Ablation through the dermal-epidermal junction occurred with subsequent laser passes at this density setting. One laser pass at a density setting of 6 resulted in full- thickness ablation of the epidermis, which was easily wiped away in the gross tissue specimens (Fig. 15.1). Even larger zones of tissue ablation were produced at a density of 9, resulting in ablation of the epidermis, as well as portions of the superficial papillary dermis. Larger zones of residual

FIGURE 15.1
Section of skin taken after 1 pass (A), 2 passes (B), and 3 passes (C) with the UltraPulse CO_2 laser used with the CPG at a density setting of 6.

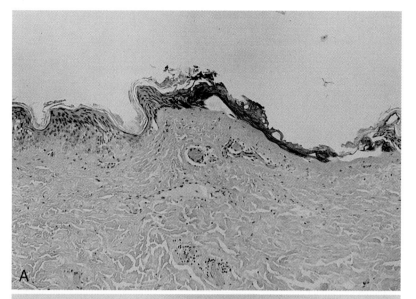

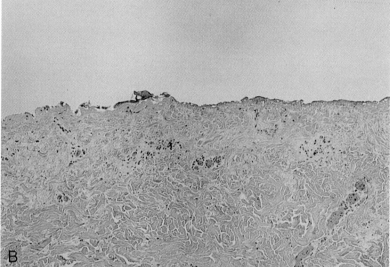

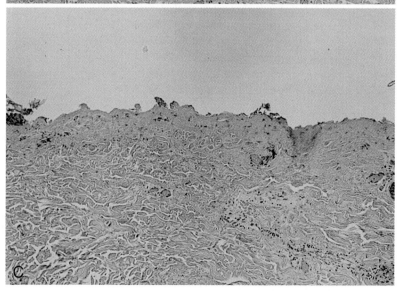

TABLE 15.3

IMMEDIATE TISSUE EFFECTS OF CO_2 LASERS

Model	Depth of Ablation (μm)	Residual thermal necrosis (μm)		
		1 pass	2 passes	3 passes
UltraPulse (3 mm)	20–30	20	40	60
CPG (density 3)	20	0	60	80
CPG (density 6)	40	20	80	120
CPG (density 9)	60	60	100	140
SilkTouch (6 mm)	50	30	80	150
SurgiPulse (3 mm)	50	30	100	150
FeatherTouch (6 mm)	20–30	20	40	90
TruPulse (3 mm)	20–30	—	—	50

thermal damage were produced at higher density settings on the CPG, but did not exceed 150 μm with each laser pass. The depths of ablation and zones of residual thermal necrosis produced by a variety of CO_2 resurfacing lasers are presented in Table 15.3. Appropriate treatment parameters and the number of laser passes necessary to achieve the desired depth of resurfacing with each laser system can be determined based upon these data.

We have also used this model to evaluate the immediate tissue effects of Er:YAG lasers. The higher water absorption coefficient at the 2,940 nm wavelength of this laser results in ablation of even thinner layers of tissue, with narrower zones of residual thermal damage compared to resurfacing CO_2 lasers. Using the Derma 20 laser (Energy Systems Corp., Needham, MA) with a 3.0 mm spot size and a pulse energy of 1 J, operating at 5 pulses per second, we found that approximately three laser passes were necessary to vaporize entirely through the epidermis (Fig. 15.2). Approximately 10 μm of tissue was vaporized with each pass, and the zone of residual thermal damage produced using the above parameters was approximately <10 μm. One pass ablated through the granular layer, two passes vaporized tissue to the level of the spinous layer, and a third pass was necessary to vaporize through the dermal-epidermal junction and produce a <10 μm layer of coagulation necrosis in the superficial papillary dermis. Clinically, when multiple laser passes are performed with the Er:YAG laser, pinpoint bleeding is evident because the <10 μm layer of thermal

necrosis is not sufficient to achieve hemostasis. A zone of thermally-coagulated tissue of greater than 50 μm is necessary to seal the superficial dermal capillaries.

Histologic studies of the effect of multiple passes with CO_2 resurfacing lasers on tissue have shown that, following the one to two passes that are necessary to achieve epidermal vaporization, progressively less tissue is ablated with each subsequent laser pass. As the water content of the skin is decreased following vaporization, the target chromophore for the CO_2 laser is reduced, and further ablation is less efficient. In addition, following multiple laser passes, the depths of residual thermal necrosis become constant for each laser system.

Histologic studies of the effects of overlapping scans or pulses during CO_2 laser resurfacing procedures have emphasized the importance of proper technique and training in this procedure. Ross et al used a pig model to examine the clinical and histological effects of multiple laser passes to one point of tissue without allowing the tissue time to cool between passes (29). In this study, tissue specimens were analyzed for the depth of residual thermal damage and the depths of cell death following laser treatment. Nitrotetrazolium blue staining was used to determine dermal cell visibility. These investigators found that the depth of thermal damage and cell death did not increase significantly with multiple laser passes. Double-pulsing or double-scanning individual skin sites, however, increased the depth of residual thermal damage and cell death by as much as 100% compared to treatment areas that received non-overlapping laser impacts. Clinically, scarring was increased focally in the areas treated with spot or scan overlap.

When a CO_2 laser is applied to skin with radiant exposures exceeding the vaporization threshold for tissue and tissue exposure times less than the 1 msec thermal relaxation time of skin, the majority of the laser energy is deposited in one optical penetration depth of the incident energy, which measures approximately 20 to 30 μm for CO_2 lasers. The fraction of light that is scattered results in heat diffusion and extension of collagen denaturization or residual thermal necrosis over a zone of 50 to 100 μm. If laser radiation is immediately repeated before the tissue has time to cool completely, tissue temperatures elevate additively, and thermal damage diffuses concentrically. Therefore, if repetitive pulsing with the CO_2 laser to one area of tissue is rapid enough, thermal diffusion will approximate that produced by a continuous wave laser. This study emphasizes the appropriate use of these lasers. Proper technique requires the administration of contiguous, but not overlapping laser pulses or scans. Inadvertent pulse or scan stacking will lead to excessive thermal damage and the potential for hypertrophic scarring.

FIGURE 15.2
Section of skin taken after 1 pass (A), 2 passes (B), and 3 passes (C) with the Derma 20 Erbium:YAG Laser.

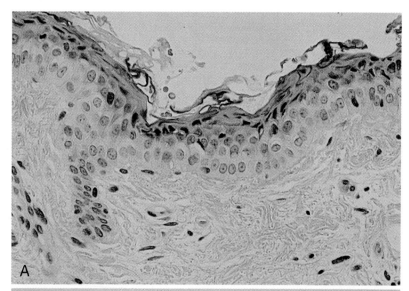

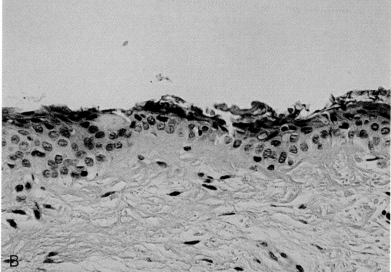

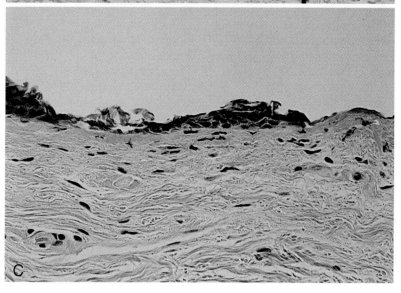

HISTOLOGY OF LASER RESURFACING: LONG TERM EFFECTS

Histologic studies following skin rejuvenation procedures have provided us with insight into the mechanisms whereby clinical improvement is achieved. Studies of skin specimens taken following chemical peeling and dermabrasion demonstrate a dermal repair zone with newly synthesized collagen comprised of thicker bundles. Similar subepidermal repair zones with neo-collagenesis and elastic fiber alteration have been described after CO_2 laser resurfacing procedures. New collagen I formation has been demonstrated in dermal repair zones following dermabrasion by means of western blot analysis and in situ hybridization.

Cotton et al examined the histologic changes occurring in human skin following treatment with a SurgiPulse XJ-150 laser (30). Test treatments were performed in the pre- and post-auricular skin in four patients who were scheduled to undergo elective rhytidectomy. Biopsy specimens were obtained at 1, 3 and 90 days after laser vaporization. Individual treatment sites were exposed to single laser passes at 250 mJ, 300 mJ and 400 mJ, and double laser passes at 400 mJ. The laser was operated at 10 watts with 0.33 second intervals between pulses. One day after laser treatment, extensive epidermal necrosis and coagulation necrosis of the superficial papillary dermis was observed, with a moderately dense mixed perivascular and interstitial upper dermal infiltrate. The depth of thermal wounding increased with increasing doses of laser energy. Partial or complete re-epithelialization occurred in 25 to 30 skin specimens by the third postoperative day. An intact epidermis was present in all biopsy specimens 3 months following laser irradiation, with half the specimens demonstrating a return of the normal rete ridge pattern. A subepidermal repair zone consisting of compact collagen bundles with parallel alignment to the skin surface was exhibited in most specimens by day 90. Beneath this repair zone, solar elastosis was evident in the dermis. Alterations in the density and distribution of elastic fibers were demonstrated by staining the specimens with acid Orcein-geimsa.

Similar observations were found in the Coherent UltraPulse multi-center trial (31). Skin biopsy specimens taken from patients 12 weeks following laser skin resurfacing of perioral and periorbital skin demonstrated a Grenz zone of new collagen and elastin formation in the superficial papillary dermis. In this study, the thickness of the new collagen layer did not correlate with the amount of photodamage present or the number of laser passes performed.

Based on these studies, it appears that the clinical improvement resulting from these skin rejuvenation procedures results from re-epithelialization and new collagen formation that occur in response to physically wounding the dermis and portions of the dermis. Un-like chemical peeling and dermabrasion, there may be additional beneficial, therapeutic effects that relate to heat induced collagen shrinkage following laser resurfacing procedures. Following epidermal vaporization, the application of each laser pulse or scan results in clinically evident skin contracture. This visibly evident tissue shrinkage is most likely a manifestation of heat induced shortening of collagen fibrils. Studies of corneal tissue have demonstrated that type I collagen fibrils shrink by as much as two-thirds lengthwise at temperatures of 55°C to 60°C. When temperatures exceed 70°C, collagen fibers undergo necrosis. It is possible that collagen shrinkage occurs within the thermally altered zone of dermal tissue that surrounds the zone of coagulation necrosis where irreversible cell death has occurred. This shrinkage of collagen may contribute to the persistent skin-tightening effect that has been observed following CO_2 laser resurfacing.

FUTURE DIRECTIONS

CO_2 laser resurfacing has been heralded as a major advance in our ability to rejuvenate photodamaged skin and improve facial scarring. Remarkable reproducibility and control are achievable with the modality compared to the traditional methods of chemical peeling and mechanical dermabrasion. Nonetheless, protracted healing times and long-lived erythema that develop following such procedures are deterring factors for many individuals. Following CO_2 laser resurfacing, re-epithelialization takes 7 to 10 days and is accompanied by intense erythema, edema, drainage and a burning discomfort. The erythema that is produced can last from 1 to 5 months and usually requires the use of camouflage concealers (make-up) for a period of time. Transient hyperpigmentation following laser resurfacing in individuals with type III skin or higher is not uncommon and post-treatment hypopigmentation occurs in 5 to 10% of patients undergoing this procedure (5). It is unknown whether these effects relate to the depth of tissue removal, the degree of thermal damage, or both. Novel approaches to laser skin resurfacing are now being sought, with attention particularly focused on techniques that will reduce re-epithelialization times, decrease the interval of postoperative erythema, and reduce the incidence of pigmentary change.

Research efforts are now being directed towards understanding the effects of Er:YAG laser resurfacing. If persistent erythema, prolonged re-epithelialization times, pigmentary alteration and scarring relate more to the degree of thermal damage produced than to the depth of tissue removal, this wavelength may have distinct advantages. If, on the other hand, an element of thermal damage and concomitant collagen shrinkage are necessary to achieve dramatic clinical improvement, equivalent depth laser resurfacing with the Er:YAG laser will produce less impressive clinical results. Based on early clinical experience, it appears that Er:YAG laser resurfacing is a useful modality for patients with minimal photodamage and rhytide formation (32).

Several other mid-infrared wavelengths are also being examined for the purpose of skin rejuvenation. Holmium:YAG lasers that emit at 2,100 nm and have water absorption coefficients lower than those of the CO_2 and Er:YAG lasers, are now being tested for skin resurfacing. Another interesting approach to skin rejuvenation is the use of nonablative laser technology. A 1,320 nm Neodymium:YAG laser used in conjunction with a cooling device has been shown to induce coagulation of the superficial papillary dermis without damaging the epidermis in histologic studies (33). It remains to be seen whether clinical improvement in photodamaged skin can be achieved by means of inducing thermal damage in the dermis without stripping the epidermis.

The development of pulsed and scanned resurfacing CO_2 lasers has revolutionized aesthetic skin surgery. Novel means of improving these techniques are now being sought. Histologic studies help provide us with a basis for determining the relative safety and efficacy of these new techniques and devices, and develop guidelines for their appropriate clinical use.

REFERENCES

1. Waldorf HA, Kauvar ANB, Geronemus RG. Skin resurfacing of fine to deep rhytides using a char free carbon dioxide laser in 47 patients. Dermatol Surg 1995;21:940-946.
2. Kauvar ANB, Bernstein LJ, Grossman MC, et al. Carbon dioxide laser resurfacing of scars. Lasers Surg Med 1996;8(Suppl):80.
3. Alster TS, West TB. Resurfacing of atrophic acne scars with a high-energy pulsed CO_2 laser. Dermatol Surg 1996;22:151-155.
4. Fitzpatrick RD, Goldman MP, Sator NM, et al. Pulsed carbon dioxide laser resurfacing of photoaged facial skin. Arch Dermatol 1996;132:395-402.
5. Bernstein LJ, Kauvar ANB, Grossman MC, et al. The short and long term side effects of carbon dioxide laser resurfacing. Dermatol Surg. 1997;23:519-525.
6. Apfelberg DB, Maser MR, Lash R, et al. Comparison of argon and carbon dioxide laser treatment of decorative tattoos: a preliminary report. Ann Plast Surg 1985;14:6-8.
7. Bailin PL, Ratz JL, Levine HL. Removal of tattoos by CO_2 Laser. J Dermatol Surg Oncol 1980;6:997-1001.
8. Friedman M, Gal D. Keloid scars as a result of CO_2 laser for molluscum contagiosum. Obstet Gynecol 1987;70;394-396.
9. Shapshay SM, Rebeiz EE, Bohigian RK, et al. Benign lesions of the larynx: Should the laser be used? Laryngoscope 1990;100:953-957.
10. Fitzpatrick RE, Ruiz-Esparza J, Goldman MP. The depth of thermal necrosis using the CO_2 laser: A comparison of the superpulsed mode and conventional mode. J Dermatol Surg Oncol 1991;17:340-344.
11. Flemming MG, Brody N. A new technique for laser treatment of cutaneous tumors. J Dermatol Surg Oncol 1986;12:1170-1175.
12. Ho C, Nguyen Q, Lowe NJ, et al. Laser resurfacing in pigmented skin. Dermatol Surg 1995;21:1035-1037.
13. Venugopalan V. Carbon dioxide laser ablation of biological tissue: Effect of pulse repetition rate on mass removal and thermal damage. MIT Archives Thesis, Sept 1990.
14. Walsh JJ, Flotte TJ, Anderson RR, et al. Pulsed CO_2 laser tissue ablation: effect of tissue type and pulse duration on thermal damage. Lasers Surg Med 1988;8:108-118.
15. Walsh JJ, Deutsch TF. Pulsed CO_2 laser tissue ablation: measurement of the ablation rate. Lasers Surg Med 1988;8:264-275.
16. Zweig AD, Meierhofer B, Muller OM, et al. Lateral thermal damage along pulsed laser incisions. Lasers Surg Med 1990;10:262-274.
17. Zweig AD, Weber HP. Mechanical and thermal parameters in pulsed laser cutting of tissue. IEEE J Quantum Electronics 1987;10:1787-1793.
18. Hobbs ER, Bailing PC, Wheeland RG, et al. Superpulsed lasers: minimizing thermal damage with short duration, high irradiance pulses. J Dermatol Surg Oncol 1987;13:955-964.
19. Lanzafame RJ, Naim JO, Rogert DW, et al. Comparisons of continuous-wave, chop-wave, and super-pulse laser wounds. Lasers Surg Med 1988;8:119-124.
20. McKenzie AL. How far does thermal damage extend beneath the surface of the CO_2 incisions? Phys Med Biol 1983;28:905-912.
21. Olbricht SM. Use of the carbon dioxide laser in dermatologic surgery: A clinically relevant update for 1993. J Dermatol Surg Oncol 1993;19:364-369.
22. Anderson RR, Parrish RR. Selective photothermolysis: precise microsurgery by selective absorption of pulsed radiation. Science 1983;220:524-527.
23. Green HA, Domankevitz Y, Nishioka NS. Pulsed carbon dioxide laser ablation of burned skin: in vitro and in vivo analysis. Lasers Surg Med 1990;10:476-484.
24. Green HA, Burd E, Nishioka NS, et al. Middermal wound healing: a comparison between dermatomal excision and pulsed carbon dioxide laser ablation. Arch Dermatol 1992;128:639-645.
25. Walsh JJ, Deutsch TF. Pulsed CO_2 laser tissue ablation: measurement of the ablation rate. Lasers Surg Med 1988;8:264-275.
26. Yang CC, Chai CY. Animal study of skin resurfacing using the UltraPulse carbon dioxide laser. Ann Plast Surg 1995;35:154-158.
27. Kauvar AN, Geronemus RG, Waldorf HA. Char-free tissue ablation: a comparative histopathological analysis of new carbon dioxide (CO_2) laser systems. Lasers Surg Med 1995;16(Suppl 7):50.
28. Kauvar ANB, Bernstein LJ, Grossman MC, Geronemus RG. Tissue effects of computerized scanners for char-free CO_2 lasers. Lasers Surg Med 1996;16(Suppl 8):34.
29. Ross EV, Glatter RD, Duke D, et al. Effects of overlap and pass number in CO_2 laser resurfacing: preliminary results of residual thermal damage, cell death and wound healing. SPIE Proceedings, San Jose, CA. 1997.

30. Cotton J, Hood AF, Gonin R, et al. Histologic evaluation of preauricular and postauricular human skin after high-energy, short-pulse carbon dioxide laser. Arch Dermatol 1996;132:425-428.

31. Fitzpatrick RE, Bernstein E. Histological findings associated with UltraPulse CO_2 laser resurfacing. Lasers Surg Med 1996;16(Suppl 8):34.

32. Khatri K, Ross V, Grevelink J, et al. Comparison of Erbium:YAG and CO_2 lasers in wrinkle removal. Lasers Surg Med 1997;9(Suppl):37.

33. Milner TE, Anvari B, Smithies DL, et al. Analysis of non-ablative skin resurfacing. SPIE Proceedings, San Jose, CA. 1997.

CHAPTER 16

Preoperative Preparation for CO$_2$ Laser Resurfacing

■ Tina S. Alster

The fact that the cosmetic laser industry is one of the fastest growing medical technologies, combined with the 76 million aging "baby boomers" in the United States who are eligible for cosmetic procedures, has prompted much attention on anti-aging or rejuvenation therapies. Carbon dioxide (CO$_2$) laser resurfacing has recently surpassed other currently available cosmetic treatments due to its increased availability and high degree of clinical effectiveness.

CUTANEOUS AGING: BACKGROUND

The cutaneous signs of aging occur as a result of both intrinsic and extrinsic processes. Intrinsic aging refers to the spontaneous process that results from the passage of time. Initially, subtle dermatologic manifestations become apparent in the fourth decade of life that gradually worsen with advancing age. Fine wrinkles with loss of skin elasticity and tissue sagging are evident clinically. Histologic tissue effects include thinning of the epidermis, hypocellularity of the dermis, and a decreased concentration of dermal blood vessels, collagen and elastin (1). Extrinsic aging is primarily a result of environmental exposure to ultraviolet light. Epidermologic and laboratory studies have conclusively demonstrated that cumulative sun exposure is the single-most important etiologic factor that leads to extrinsic skin aging (2, 3). Photoaging and photodamage are, thus, terms frequently used to describe the cutaneous changes observed after chronic ultraviolet light irradiation.

In addition to the eventual development of actinic keratoses and cutaneous malignancies, which are of medical significance, cumulative sun exposure can lead to developments that are indicative of extrinsic aging, including pigmentary irregularities, skin coarseness, sallowness, and wrinkling. As signs of facial aging occur (regardless of their intrinsic or extrinsic nature), and have been associated with negative views of body image, self-esteem and self-confidence, it is not surprising that patients are often "propelled" to seek medical evaluation (4, 5). Thus, reversal of photoaging has become a frequent goal pursued by the public and the medical profession alike. One of the purported strengths of cutaneous laser resurfacing is its ability to reverse photoaging, making patients' faces appear as their intrinsic biological destinies intended. For many patients, laser surgery offers an accessible middle ground between no treatment and conventional face lifting techniques.

PATIENT SELECTION AND EDUCATION

Proper patient selection and education are paramount to achieving the best postoperative clinical results. Because of the intense publicity that laser resurfacing has received in recent years, unrealistic expectations of the treatment have developed. Despite the positive results that can be achieved in many cases, sometimes the results from surgery are modest and subtle, disappointing those who have been led to expect the miraculous. In addition, the promise of a virtually pain-free experience with only a week of recovery time promoted by advertisements, magazine articles, or television reports is overly enthusiastic. Laser resurfacing may not involve incisions, but it is still a painful process with a prolonged postoperative course. Most patients are surprised at how much time is involved for healing and, thus, need strong

171

FIGURE 16.1

Patient receives preoperative instruction by laser nurse. Representative preoperative and postoperative photographs as well as the appropriate preoperative skin care regimen are reviewed.

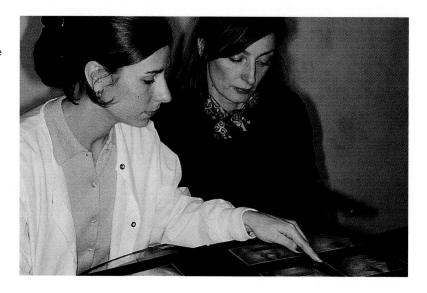

encouragement to schedule the appropriate time away from work or other obligations postoperatively. The importance of adequate preoperative patient preparation, therefore, cannot be overemphasized.

During a patient's initial consultation, several informative facts regarding the procedure should be provided and the patient should be evaluated thoroughly to determine whether he or she is a suitable candidate for resurfacing (Fig. 16.1). A preoperative patient checklist can be helpful to ensure that the patient is fully evaluated and educated on the specifics of laser treatment (Table 16.1).

To determine patient suitability for laser resurfacing a dermatologic evaluation as well as a complete medical history is required, the former evaluates the appropriateness of the lesions, and the latter identifies potential contraindications for treatment (e.g., concurrent isotretinoin use, scarring tendency, presence of collagen vascular or immunologic disease) (Table 16.2).

The use of a questionnaire as a preoperative screen can be helpful (Table 16.3).

1. *Does the patient have lesions that are amenable to laser resurfacing?* The facial areas that respond most favorably to laser treatment are non-movement-associated rhytides involving the perioral, cheek, and periorbital regions (6–13). Surgical procedures, such as facelifts or blepharoplasties, can improve skin laxity; however, they result in minimal improvement of perioral and periorbital rhytides. Similarly, chemical peels and dermabrasion have produced disappointing results in these regions due to the delicate nature of the periorbital area. Other lesions that improve with laser resurfacing include atrophic acne scars, actinic cheilitis, and various epidermal and dermal lesions (e.g., keratoses, verrucae, xanthelasma) (14, 15).

In general, full face resurfacing produces a better clinical result than treating isolated areas, as treatment of the entire cheek region results in further

TABLE 16.1

PREOPERATIVE PATIENT CHECKLIST

- ■ Perform complete patient medical history and dermatologic examination
- ■ Patient education
  - ■ video demonstration
  - ■ review brochure
  - ■ show representative photographs
  - ■ provide information sheet
- ■ Take preoperative patient photographs
- ■ Begin preoperative skin care regimen
- ■ Obtain informed consent for procedure

tightening of the nasolabial folds and lateral "crows feet" (6). Similarly, treatment of the forehead leads to additional improvement of glabellar creases and temporal lines. Diffuse facial dyspigmentation or mottling can also be substantially improved when the entire face is resurfaced (6). Lastly, from a practical standpoint, it is easier for patients to camouflage uniformly distributed erythema with makeup than with the "Kabuki mask" produced after perioral and periorbital regional treatment.

2. *Has previous treatment been received for the condition?* Many patients who have undergone chemical peels or dermabrasion exhibit demonstrable fibrosis in the treated skin. Because the fibrotic skin is more dense, less vaporization of the skin can be achieved with CO_2 laser resurfacing, which leads to a subsequent reduction in the desired clinical effect. In addition, underlying hypopigmentation from a previous dermabrasion or chemical peel may be unmasked or worsened after laser treatment (14). Patients who have had lower blepharoplasties are at a greater risk of ectropion formation due to the tissue tightening effect of laser resurfacing (6).

TABLE 16.2

CO_2 LASER RESURFACING INDICATIONS & CONTRAINDICATIONS

Primary Indications	Secondary Indications	Relative Contraindications	Absolute Contraindications
Light skin phototypes (I-II)	Darker skin phototypes (III-V)	Prior treatment with fibrosis or dyspigmentation	Concomitant isotretinoin use
Non-dynamic rhytides (perioral, cheek, periorbital)	Dynamic rhytides (glabella, forehead, nasolabial folds)	Collagen vascular, Koebnerizing, or immunologic disorder	Concurrent viral or bacterial superficial infection
Atrophic facial scars	Diffuse facial lentigines	Prior lower blepharoplasty	Presence of ectropion
Actinic cheilitis	Dermal lesions	Keloid or hypertrophic scar former	Unrealistic patient expectations or non-compliance
Epidermal lesions			

Modified from: Alster TS. *Manual of Cutaneous Laser Techniques*. Philadelphia: Lippincott-Raven Publishers, 1997.

TABLE 16.3

PREOPERATIVE PATIENT EVALUATION

Does the patient have lesions that are amenable to laser resurfacing?

Has previous treatment been received for the condition?

Is the patient taking isotretinoin or immunosuppressive medication?

What is the patient's skin type?

Does the patient have a history of cold sores?

Is there a history of collagen vascular disease or immunodeficiency?

Are other dermatologic conditions present which could spread after treatment?

Is the patient prone to acne breakouts?

Does the patient have a tendency to form hypertrophic scars or keloids?

Does the patient have realistic expectations of the procedure?

Will the patient be compliant with all preoperative and postoperative instructions?

Are there medical conditions that would interfere with using intravenous anesthesia?

3. *Is the patient taking isotretinoin or immunosuppressive medication?* Because poor wound healing and scar formation can occur up to 2 years following treatment with oral retinoids, it is best to avoid CO_2 laser resurfacing until several months have passed after cessation of drug use (16). Because the alteration in healing is idiosyncratic, a safe interval between the use of oral retinoids and resurfacing is impossible to delineate. Most laser experts wait 6 months to a year. Similarly, immunosuppressive medications may not only cause a delay in wound healing, but may also increase the risk of postoperative infections.

4. *What is the patient's skin type?* While patients with light skin phototypes (I-II) are the best candidates for CO_2 laser resurfacing, darker skin tones can also be treated. Because darker skin tones (III and higher) have a greater tendency to develop postoperative hyperpigmentation, proper preoperative and postoperative management is critical to ensure optimal results.

5. *Does the patient have a history of cold sores?* Reactivation of herpes simplex virus (HSV) following laser resurfacing is possible, even in patients with a remote history of herpes labialis. Patients with a positive history of oral HSV who undergo perioral resurfacing should receive a prophylactic course of antiherpetic medications. *Any* patient undergoing full face resurfacing should receive antiherpetic prophylaxis regardless of the herpetic history in order to limit the detrimental effect of reactivation or primary exposure on newly irradiated and granulating skin.

6. *Is there a history of collagen vascular disease or immunodeficiency?* The prolonged postoperative course associated with CO_2 laser resurfacing requires intact immunologic function and collagen repair mechanisms in order to optimize the tissue healing response. Thus, patients who have collagen vascular disorders (e.g., scleroderma or lupus erythematosus), or patients who are immunodeficient (e.g., having HIV or AIDS) should be forewarned of the possibility for slower or impaired postoperative healing as well as possible disease reactivation, recurrence, or worsening due to the stress of the procedure.

7. *Are other dermatologic conditions present which could possibly spread after treatment?* Autoimmune disorders (e.g., vitiligo) or Koebnerizing conditions (e.g., psoriasis, eczema, verrucae, molluscum) could conceivably worsen or spread after cutaneous laser vaporization. It is important that the skin being

treated is not affected with any of these conditions preoperatively.

8. *Is the patient prone to acne breakouts?* Inflammatory acneiform lesions may not only impair the operator's visibility during the laser procedure, but could conceivably lead to additional scarring postoperatively. Thus, individuals whose acne is flaring before laser resurfacing should receive appropriate preoperative anti-acne medications, such as topical or systemic antibiotics, until the condition clears.

9. *Does the patient have a tendency to form hypertrophic scars or keloids?* Patients with a scarring tendency will be at greater risk of scar formation following cutaneous laser resurfacing, regardless of the laser's specificity and the operator's skill. If unsure of a patient's propensity for scar formation, a test area can be lased in the cosmetic unit before determining whether laser treatment is a viable option for that particular individual.

10. *Does the patient have realistic expectations of the procedure and will he or she be compliant with all preoperative and postoperative instructions?* Patients who expect virtual elimination of their rhytides or scars will not be satisfied with the laser resurfacing procedure, regardless of the improvement obtained. Because clinical improvement varies based on the individual, the lesions present, and the skin regions affected, the actual amount of improvement expected is difficult to predict. Given the prolonged healing phase following laser treatment, it is imperative that the patient has a clear understanding of the postoperative course and importance of adhering to the postoperative regimen outlined. If a patient is hesitant to accept these facts or does not appear to understand what is entailed during the postoperative phase, then he or she is not a suitable candidate for treatment.

11. *Are there medical conditions present that would preclude the use of intravenous anesthesia?* Patients with a history of asthma, emphysema, and heart disease should receive medical clearance for the procedure from their primary care physicians. A review of current medications and known allergies should be documented and studied to exclude possible adverse drug interactions.

EXPLANATION OF BENEFITS AND RISKS

Simply identifying whether the patient is a suitable candidate for laser resurfacing is not sufficient preparation for the procedure. The patient needs to be fully informed of the benefits and risks of the surgery as well. The preoperative consultation is the best time to review with the patient the specifics of the laser procedure, including a summary of how the laser works on skin, what to anticipate in terms of risk, pain, recovery time

TABLE 16.4

CO$_2$ LASER RESURFACING: SIDE EFFECTS & RISKS

Swelling	Infection
Pain (burning and stinging)	Herpes reactivation
Skin oozing and crusting	Acne flareup
Prolonged erythema	Milia formation
Transient hyperpigmentation	Scarring
Long-lasting hypopigmentation	Ectropion development

and expense, and, above all, what results can realistically be achieved. Just as important as discussing with the patient the potential benefits of the procedure, is a frank review of the relative side effects and risks specific to the laser treatment so that the patient can make an informed decision about whether or not to proceed with surgery (Table 16.4). It is also helpful for patients to view representative postoperative photos of the most frequently seen side effects and complications (e.g., erythema, milia, hyperpigmentation).

Every patient who undergoes CO$_2$ laser resurfacing experiences immediate swelling, serous discharge and postoperative discomfort (stinging or burning). Because the erythema, swelling and exudate typically peak in 24 to 48 hours postoperatively, patients will not be prepared to face the public for several days. Even patients who think that they are "fast healers" will not heal expeditiously. Therefore, every patient should be prepared to take at least 1 week off from his or her regularly scheduled activities to allow sufficient time for healing. Even after the average 7 to 10-day reepithelialization phase, the patient's skin remains extremely erythematous, requiring the use of cosmetic camouflage (pancake or heavy base makeup). Patients will need to be prepared for prolonged postoperative erythema requiring not only more makeup coverage, but also ample sunscreen protection. The erythema typically persists for 3 to 4 months, but has been noted to last longer in some patients.

Even with sunscreen use and strict avoidance of ultraviolet light exposure, patients need to be aware that they could conceivably develop postoperative hyperpigmentation (seen in one-third of patients). While the hyperpigmentation is typically transient in nature and lasts a few months, it is even harder to camouflage and usually requires intervention to effect more rapid clearance. Hypopigmentation is permanent and fortunately, a rarity. Despite its rarity, the risks of hypopigmentation should be discussed with all patients, regardless of their skin type, as it appears to have no predilection for darker skin tones, as does the development of hyperpigmentation.

As with any resurfacing procedure, the possibility of infection should be addressed. Even in the absence of prophylactic antibiotics, the relative risk of bacterial infection is low. The risk of viral infection (HSV reactivation) is significantly higher, and thus, patients should be advised of this possibility even when prophylactic antiviral medications are prescribed.

Because of semiocclusive ointments and/or wound dressings used in the postoperative period and the cutaneous events associated with the re-epithelialization process, exacerbation of acne and/or the development of milia can occur in the postoperative period.

Certainly, the most severe (and distressing) risks associated with the CO₂ laser resurfacing procedure are scarring and ectropion formation. In addition to the possibility of a thermal burn by the laser, other potential contributing factors that can lead to scar or ectropion formations include poor wound care, concomitant cuta-

neous infection, and previous lower blepharoplasty. When proper lasing techniques are used, however, the risk of severe complications is minimal.

PREOPERATIVE PATIENT PREPARATION

Once a patient has been determined to be a suitable candidate for the laser resurfacing procedure, understands the benefits and risks of the procedure, and has given his or her consent, additional steps can be taken preoperatively to optimize the treatment results (Fig. 16.2). Certain topical therapies, including retinoic acid, alpha hydroxy acids (AHAs), and antioxidants, can improve the appearance of photodamaged skin; however, they

---

CO₂ LASER RESURFACING TREATMENT CONSENT FORM

Dr. _____ has explained to me that I am a good candidate for laser resurfacing treatment and that although laser surgery has been shown to be highly effective, no guarantees can be made that I will benefit from treatment. I understand that the most common side effects and complications of this laser treatment are:

1. PAIN.   The sharp, burning sensation of each laser pulse may produce a moderate to severe amount of discomfort. Anesthetic injection or intravenous sedation will be used to block the pain during the procedure. Oral pain medication will be prescribed for the postoperative period.

2. SWELLING AND OOZING.   Areas most likely to swell are around the eyes and neck. A clear fluid (serum) will also be present in the lased areas and may create a crust (or scab) if the areas are not kept moist. The swelling, crusting and oozing stage subsides within 5 to 7 days with regular application of ice and prescribed healing ointments.

3. PROLONGED SKIN REDNESS.   The laser-treated areas will initially appear bright red in color. After the first week, the redness can be camouflaged with opaque makeup. The redness fades to pink over the next several weeks and then to normal skin color in an average of 3 months.

4. SKIN DARKENING (HYPERPIGMENTATION).   This can occur in the treated areas and will eventually fade within 2 to 6 months. This reaction is more common in patients with olive or dark skin tones and can worsen if the laser-treated area is exposed to the sun.

5. SKIN LIGHTENING (HYPOPIGMENTATION).   This can occur in an area of skin which has already received prior treatment or can be a delayed response to the laser surgery. The light spots can darken or repigment in several months, but could be permanent. This is a very rare complication.

6. SCARRING.   The risk of this complication is minimal, but can potentially occur whenever there is disruption of the skin's surface. Strict adherence to all advised postoperative instructions will reduce the possibility of this occurrence.

7. INFECTION.   A skin infection in the postoperative period can result. This risk is minimized by the use of antibiotics and good skin care.

8. ALLERGIC REACTION.   It is possible that an allergic reaction to an anesthetic, topical cream, or oral medication can occur.

9. ECTROPION.   In rare instances, a downward pull of the eyelids can result after periorbital laser resurfacing.

10. ACNE OR MILIA FORMATION.   Flare-up of acne or formation of milia (tiny white bumps) can occur in the postoperative period.

By providing my signature below, I acknowledge that I have read and understood all of the information written above as well as that contained within the information sheet. I feel that I have been adequately informed of my alternative treatment option, the risks of the proposed laser surgery, and the risks of not treating my condition. I hereby freely consent to the laser surgery to be performed by Dr. _____ and authorized the taking of clinical photographs which will be used solely for my medical records unless my physician deems their anonymous use (in lectures or scientific publications) could benefit medical research and education. They will not be used for advertising without my written permission.

_____   _____   _____   _____
Patient's or Guardian's Signature   Date   Witness' Signature   Date

---

FIGURE 16.2
CO₂ Laser Resurfacing Treatment Consent Form.

are often unable to produce the result desired by patients when used alone. These products can be used prior to and following cutaneous laser resurfacing to reduce the risk of postoperative pigmentary changes and to enhance wound healing.

Tretinoin can stimulate proliferation of keratinocytes and fibroblasts, resulting in normalization of the epidermis and stimulation of new Type I collagen in the upper dermis as well as inhibiting ultraviolet B (UVB)-induced collagen degeneration (17, 18). In addition, angiogenesis, elastin formation, and redistribution of epidermal melanin has been demonstrated with tretinoin use (19). Because retinoic acid has been shown to enhance wound healing when used preoperatively for dermabrasion and chemical peels, many physicians now recommend its use with laser resurfacing (20).

AHAs, particularly glycolic acid, are beneficial in treating epidermal dyspigmentation as well as acne. AHAs can also increase epidermal and dermal thickness presumably by increasing glycosaminoglycan concentration and water binding. Their use before and after cutaneous laser resurfacing may help to reduce or even prevent the development of postoperative pigmentary irregularities.

Topical Vitamin C (ascorbic acid) preparations have been shown to act as antioxidants and to block UVA and UVB tissue damage (7). Vitamin C is known to be necessary for collagen metabolism, perhaps by acting as a cytokine that directly stimulates fibroblasts to produce collagen (21). The use of topical ascorbic acid following laser resurfacing has recently been shown to reduce the duration of postoperative erythema and serves as a potent photoprotectant in the postoperative healing phase (22, 23).

Based on their aforementioned effects, various topical agents can be used preoperatively (Table 16.5). Although a minimum of 2 weeks of preoperative treatment is often arbitrarily prescribed, additional benefit may be gained with a longer duration of preparation. On the other hand, some physicians do not advise *any* preoperative topical regimen, believing that topical products should be reserved for the postoperative period during which time postinflammatory hyperpigmentation is actually observed.

In addition to the preoperative use of topical preparations that enhance postoperative results, other adjunctive procedures include the use of BOTOX injections (Allergan, Inc., Irvine, CA) to block nerve transmission to the involved muscle groups (in particular, the procerus and corrugator muscles responsible for the production of frown lines) (Fig. 16.3) (24, 25). The injections can be performed 1 to 2 weeks preoperatively (or several months postoperatively) to prevent muscle motion in the treatment regions for 3 months or more following laser treatment during which time active collagenesis and collagen remodeling takes place. Potentially prolonged and enhanced clinical improvement may be obtained, especially if the injections are continued at regular intervals postoperatively.

As prophylaxis against HSV reactivation or dissemination after laser resurfacing, a 10-day course of oral antiviral medications (e.g., Zovirax [Burroughs Wellcome Co., Research Triangle Park, NC], Famvir [SmithKline Beecham Pharmaceuticals, Philadelphia, PA], Valtrex [Burroughs Wellcome Co.]) should be prescribed. In patients with a known history of herpes labialis, the course is started 24 to 48 hours preoperatively. All other patients begin the medication on the day of the procedure. The treatment should continue throughout the re-epithelialization healing phase (average, 7 to 10 days).

Prevention of postoperative bacterial infections can be achieved with the prophylactic use of systemic antibiotics with good gram-positive bacterial coverage (e.g., Zithromax [Pfizer Laboratories, Inc., New York, NY], dicloxacillin). The use of intravenous antibiotics during the laser resurfacing procedure, such as Ancef (SmithKline Beecham Pharmaceutical, Philadelphia, PA), can also provide excellent coverage during the postoperative re-epithelialization period. When a "closed" wound technique with semiocclusive dressings is used in the postoperative period, antibiotic coverage such as ciprofloxacin should be used to combat gram-negative organisms (e.g., *Pseudomonas aeruginosa*), since the moist dressing environment is ideal for bacterial growth when prophylactic gram-positive antibiotics are used.

IMMEDIATE PREOPERATIVE CONSIDERATIONS

The patient's skin should be rinsed thoroughly to remove all traces of makeup, lotions, and oils using mild soap and water (Fig. 16.4). Hair should be tied back and

TABLE 16.5

PREOPERATIVE SKIN CARE OPTIONS

Generic Name	Selected Trade Names	Administration
Retinoic acid	Retin A, Renova	Apply daily
Glycolic acid	GlyDerm, MD Forte	Apply 1-2 times/day
Ascorbic acid	Cellex-C	Apply daily
Azelaic acid	Azelex	Apply daily
Kojic acid	Therapeutic, Peter Thomas Roth	Apply 1-2 times/day
Hydroquinone	Solaquin, Eldoquin, Melanex	Apply 1-2 times/day

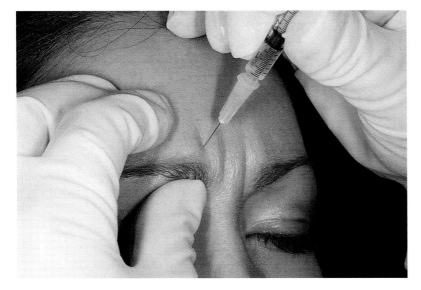

FIGURE 16.3
Botulinum toxin is administered intralesionally 2 weeks before the laser procedure to immobilize muscle groups that contribute to frown lines.

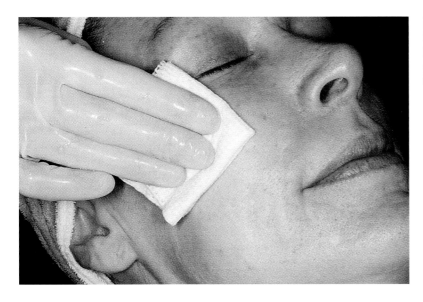

FIGURE 16.4
Patient's face is rinsed and cleaned with a nonflammable prepping solution in the immediate preoperative period. Wet drapes are secured around the patient's face and all hair is tied back.

secured with a headband. The periphery of the patient's face and neck should be draped with water-soaked cloth drapes. The skin should be further prepared with a nonflammable (nonalcohol-containing) solution, such as Septisol (Vestal Laboratories, Inc., St. Louis, MO) or Betadine (Purdue Fredrick Co., Norwalk, CT). Preparations such as chlorhexidine (Hibiclens [Stuart Pharmaceuticals, Inc., Wilmington, DE]) are not only flammable, but also are oculotoxic and therefore should be avoided.

Eye protection with sandblasted metallic eye shields carefully inserted on the patient's eyes after topical ophthalmic anesthesia is mandatory for full face and periorbital laser resurfacing (Fig. 16.5). If the periorbital regions are not being treated, external eye goggles and securely placed wet gauze can be used. Tooth enamel is similarly protected with wet gauze or placement of a metal shield between the lips and teeth.

PREOPERATIVE ANESTHETIC CONSIDERATIONS

When isolated facial regions such as the perioral or periorbital areas are treated, local field anesthesia and sensory nerve blocks can be used alone (Fig. 16.6). Because the sensory innervation of the face is complex, it is difficult to attain complete facial anesthesia with cutaneous nerve blocks even when perfect technique is used. Tumescent local anesthesia of the entire face is an option. Another option is intravenous sedation in conjunction with anesthetic nerve blocks. The use of various intravenous anesthetic agents such as propofol, midazolam, fentanyl, and ketamine, provide the patient with a comfortable and short-acting level of sedation, analgesia, and amnesia.

In addition to the supply of intraoperative anesthetics indicated, appropriate monitoring equipment is

FIGURE 16.5

Protective metal eye shields are carefully inserted with lubricant after anesthetic ophthalmic drops have taken effect.

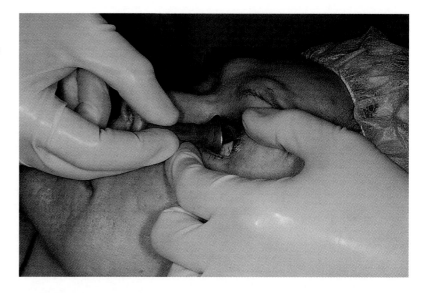

FIGURE 16.6

Intralesional anesthesia and trigeminal nerve blocks are placed immediately before the perioral CO_2 laser resurfacing procedure. The use of a topical anesthetic cream reduces the discomfort associated with the injections.

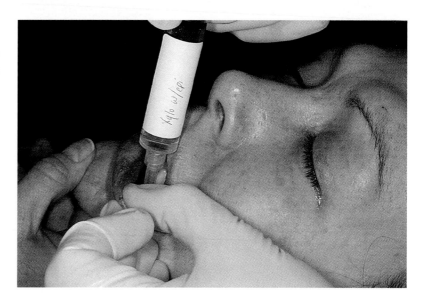

necessary. A blood pressure and ECG monitor, as well as a pulse oximeter and emergency resuscitation equipment (intubation supplies, oxygen delivery system, and defibrillator) should be present (26, 27). Because of the incendiary potential of oxygen, meticulous safety precautions should be followed when the laser apparatus is in use. Endotracheal tubes and masks should be fully protected with saline-soaked gauze or towels.

SUMMARY

While cutaneous laser resurfacing with high energy, pulsed and scanned CO_2 lasers provide a safe and effective alternative to conventional remedies for photodamaged and scarred skin, it is not usually the means to a flawless complexion. The common notion that the laser procedure is simplicity in itself (as easy as peeling a piece of fruit during laser workshops) is not only untrue, but leads to unrealistic patient expectations. These expectations are what physicians need to address during each patient's preoperative consultation.

In addition to providing the patients with basic laser education, it is important to determine the patient's suitability for treatment based on the medical and dermatologic history, previous and concurrent treatments, and actual lesions present. The relative benefits and risks of the laser procedure should be reviewed as well as the specifics of the postoperative healing period. The importance of close follow-up after the CO_2 laser resurfacing treatment should also be stressed in order to maximize the operative results. In general, when patients are properly and thoroughly prepared for the procedure, they are happier with the clinical results.

REFERENCES

1. Gilchrest BA. Skin aging and photoaging. Dermatol Nurs 1990;2:79-82.
2. Nicol NJ, Fenske NA. Photodamage: Cause, clinical manifestations and prevention. Dermatol Nurs 1993;5:263-277.
3. West MD. The cellular and molecular biology of skin aging. Arch Dermatol 1994;130:87-95.
4. Gupta MA, Schork NJ, Ellis CN. Psychosocial correlates of the treatment of photodamaged skin with topical retinoic acid: A prospective controlled study. J Am Acad Dermatol 1994;30:969-972.
5. Pearlman SF. Late mid-life astonishment: Disruptions to identity and self-esteem. Women Ther 1993;14:1-12.
6. Alster TS. Manual of Cutaneous Laser Techniques. Philadelphia: Lippincott-Raven, 1997.
7. Alster TS, Garg S. Treatment of facial rhytides with a high-energy, pulsed carbon dioxide laser. Plast Reconstr Surg 1996;98:791-794.
8. Fitzpatrick RE. Laser resurfacing of rhytides. Dermatol Clinics 1997.
9. Fitzpatrick RE, Goldman MP, Satur NM, et al. Pulsed carbon dioxide laser resurfacing of photoaged facial skin. Arch Dermatol 1996;132:395-402.
10. Lask G, Keller G, Lowe N, et al. Laser skin resurfacing with the SilkTouch flashscanner for facial rhytides. Dermatol Surg 1995;21:1021-1024.
11. Lowe NJ, Lask G, Griffin ME, et al. Skin resurfacing with the UltraPulse carbon dioxide laser: Observations of 100 patients. Dermatol Surg 1995;21:1025-1029.
12. Waldorf HA, Kauvar AN, Geronemus RG. Skin resurfacing of fine to deep rhytides using a char-free carbon dioxide laser in 47 patients. Dermatol Surg 1995;21:940-946.
13. Weinstein C, Alster TS. Skin resurfacing with high energy, pulsed carbon dioxide lasers. In: Alster TS, Apfelberg DB, eds. Cosmetic Laser Surgery. New York: John Wiley, 1996:9-28.
14. Alster TS, West TB. Resurfacing of atrophic acne scars with a high-energy, pulsed carbon dioxide laser. Dermatol Surg 1996;22:151-155.
15. Alster TS, West TB. Ultrapulse CO_2 laser ablation of xanthelasma. J Am Acad Dermatol 1996;34:848-849.
16. Katz B, MacFarlane D. Atypical facial scarring after isotretinoin therapy in a patient with previous dermabrasion. J Am Acad Dermatol 1994;30:852-853.
17. Griffiths CEM, Russman AN, Majmudar G, et al. Restoration of collagen formation in photodamaged human skin by tretinoin (retinoic acid). N Engl J Med 1993;329:530-535.
18. Kligman AM, Grove GL, Hirose R, et al. Topical tretinoin for photoaged skin. J Am Acad Dermatol 1986;15:836-839.
19. Hung VC, Lee JY, Zitelli JA, et al. Topical tretinoin and epithelial wound healing. Arch Dermatol 1989;125:65-69.
20. Mandy SH. Tretinoin in the preoperative and postoperative management of dermabrasion. J Am Acad Dermatol 1986;15:878-879.
21. Pinnell SR, Murad S, Darr D. Induction of collagen synthesis by ascorbic acid: A possible mechanism. Arch Dermatol 1987;123:1684-1686.
22. Darr D, Dunstan S, Faust H, et al. Effectiveness of antioxidants (Vitamins C and E) with and without sunscreens as topical photoprotectants. Acta Dermatol Venereol 1996;76:264-268.
23. Alster TS, West TB. Effect of topical vitamin C on post-CO_2 laser resurfacing erythema. Dermatol Surg 1997;23: (in press).
24. Carruthers JDA, Carruthers JA. Treatment of glabellar frown lines with botulinum-A exotoxin. J Dermatol Surg Oncol 1992;18:17-21.
25. Garcia A, Fulton JE. Cosmetic denervation of the muscles of facial expression with botulinum toxin: a dose-response study. Dermatol Surg 1996;22:39-43.
26. Fitzpatrick RE, Williams B, Goldman MP. Preoperative anesthesia and postoperative considerations in laser resurfacing. Seminars Cutaneous Med Surg 1996;15:170-176.
27. Formica K, Alster TS. Cutaneous laser resurfacing: A nursing guide. Dermatol Nurs 1997;9:19-22.

CHAPTER 17

Treatment Techniques of Laser Resurfacing Common to All Laser Systems

■ Richard E. Fitzpatrick
Stacy R. Smith
Mitchel P. Goldman

Modern laser systems intended for resurfacing are powerful tools. Like any other surgical device, they are capable of producing either dramatic results when used expertly or disastrous consequences when employed without proper knowledge and understanding. To achieve the desired results, it is paramount that the operator understands the principles of laser-tissue interaction. Beyond the basic physics of the carbon dioxide (CO_2) laser and its direct interaction with cutaneous tissue are the mechanisms by which the laser induces changes in the skin during laser resurfacing and the role played by subsequent wound healing. While the operative technique appears deceptively simple at first, careful consideration of mechanical and physical principles, combined with subtle variations in technique and attention to detail during the resurfacing procedure can yield spectacular improvement in photoaged skin.

Using the principles of selective thermolysis, discussed in Chapter 14, superficial photodamaged tissue can be heated and ablated with appropriately pulsed CO_2 lasers, leaving only a small layer of residual thermal injury to the underlying tissue (1). Initially, single pulse ablation with removal of the outermost photoaged portions of the upper dermis was felt to be the primary mechanism by which laser resurfacing improved aging facial skin. It is now known that several other mechanisms are also at work during laser resurfacing. These include collagen shrinkage, new collagen formation and collagen remodeling as well as the effects of multiple pulse vaporization.

MECHANISMS OF ACTION

Single Pulse Vaporization

The most important principle underlying CO_2 laser resurfacing is that of single pulse tissue vaporization. Resurfacing lasers that are commonly used today employ high-pulse energies and short pulse widths (<1 msec) and deliver fluences to tissue which allows complete vaporization in one pulse. If adequate energy is delivered to tissue in a single pulse (>5 J/cm²) and results in vaporization, then the energy of vaporization is released in the plume of steam that forms and the residual thermal injury approaches the theoretical minimum. This residual thermal injury generally is less than 100 μm, and is often in the 30 to 50 μm range, adequate for capillary hemostasis, but limited enough to avoid interference with wound healing (2).

When single pulse vaporization occurs, pulse width is irrelevant, as sub-vaporization tissue heating does not occur. When vaporization is attempted using a train of sub-threshold pulses to reach a cumulative threshold, thermal diffusion occurs during the inter-pulse intervals and control of the residual thermal injury is lost.

181

Tissue experiments and calculations have determined that energies >250 mJ per pulse using a 3 mm collimated beam are necessary for single-pulse, complete vaporization of the epidermis (3). Some laser systems deliver a Gaussian beam profile and overlap of pulses may be necessary to achieve complete vaporization at the edges of each pulse. Scanners can be adjusted or free hand movement of the beam can be altered to achieve consistent minimal overlap of each spot. This allows the surface to be treated in a confluent manner resulting in a desiccated epidermis that can be wiped away easily with a saline soaked gauze pad after a single laser pass. Systems with non-Gaussian "top hat" beam profiles result in uniform fluence across the beam and, therefore, should use little or no overlap since there is no attenuation of the pulse energy at the beam perimeter because overlap may result in excessive tissue heating.

Once the epidermis is removed, the physical parameters of the skin change. The dermis normally contains substantially less water than the epidermis and mostly in an extracellular state (4). As further passes are made, more water is vaporized from the tissue leaving a progressively increasing layer of desiccated tissue comprising the layer of thermal necrosis. Since the pulse energies necessary to vaporize collagen are much greater than are necessary for water, the result is significantly higher ablation thresholds for the remaining dermal tissue. Thus, each pass of the laser will ablate successively less dermal tissue than the 75 to 100 μm of epidermis removed. In this situation of nonablative tissue heating, the laser pulse width becomes critical, as it must be less than the thermal relaxation time of the target tissue in order to avoid increasing residual thermal necrosis (5). Tissue studies with single pulse vaporization using a pulse width of less than 1 msec and standard operative technique demonstrate that 10 consecutive passes of the laser with saline wiping between passes results in two important phenomena. The first is that the depth of vaporization per pass progressively decreases and plateaus at laser pass number four corresponding to a depth of approximately 250 μm (Fig. 17.1). An additional six passes results in a negligible increase in depth of vaporization. Second, residual thermal damage gradually increases from one to ten passes, but does not exceed 100 μm (6). The 1 msec pulse allows heated, nonablated tissue to cool prior to the time necessary for thermal diffusion to occur. Thus, single pulse vaporization creates a safety mechanism preventing an injury deep enough to interfere with normal wound healing.

Collagen Shrinkage

The contraction of collagen due to heat has been noted for many years. It was used clinically over 100 years ago for corneal reshaping (7). This shrinking effect occurs when Type I collagen is heated between 55°C and 62°C, at which point the fibrils may shorten by as much as one

third (8). The fact that this phenomenon occurs in skin and contributes to the success of laser resurfacing was unanticipated. The success of the laser procedure in areas where results were not expected (nasolabial folds, deep lines/folds of cheeks, loose eye lid tissue), combined with the dramatic tissue contraction that is immediately visible with laser interaction of the dermis led to investigation of a possible role regarding collagen shrinkage as a mechanism.

Collagen shrinkage can be seen intraoperatively as a general sudden contraction of the skin immediately following a single laser pulse or series of laser pulses (as occurs with programmable scanners). Some have argued that this represents only a temporary desiccation of collagen that rapidly returns to normal after rehydration. Recent animal work and ex vivo studies with human skin (with careful attention to hydration) have demonstrated persistent shrinkage of dermal tissue after pulsed CO_2 laser irradiation, which concurs with clinical observation (9).

New Collagen Formation

Data from chemical peeling and dermabrasion studies have shown the formation of new collagen during wound healing plays an important role in photoaging improvement (10). Similar processes occur after laser resurfacing. After reepithelialization is complete, the skin synthesizes and remodels 200 μm or more of new collagen for up to 6 months after the procedure. This synthesis is represented histologically as a band of new collagen separating the previously elastotic papillary dermis and the newly reformed epidermis (Fig. 17.2). Clinically, new collagen formation is seen when patients undergo resurfacing only to have the edema resolve and are left with persistent deep rhytides or acne scars. As time progresses, more collagen is deposited with gradual improvement in the wrinkled or acne scarred areas (Fig. 17.3). Most importantly, this new collagen is synthesized on a contracted dermis, thus stabilizing the remaining contracted collagen fibrils in their shortened state. The added collagen is composed of fine bundles parallel to the surface, having the overall architectural structure and microscopic appearance of normal dermal collagen, not that of scar tissue.

Multiple Pulse Vaporization

The theory of selective photothermolysis and single pulse vaporization is the foundation of pulsed CO_2 laser ablation and laser resurfacing. Multiple pulse vaporization can be defined as repetitive pulses delivered to the same tissue site with a rapidity that exceeds the tissue's ability to dissipate heat. The critical frequency of 5 Hz has been measured and calculated as the pulse delivery frequency that, if exceeded, causes accumulation of thermal energy and a subsequent increase in residual thermal damage (11). This accumulation of residual

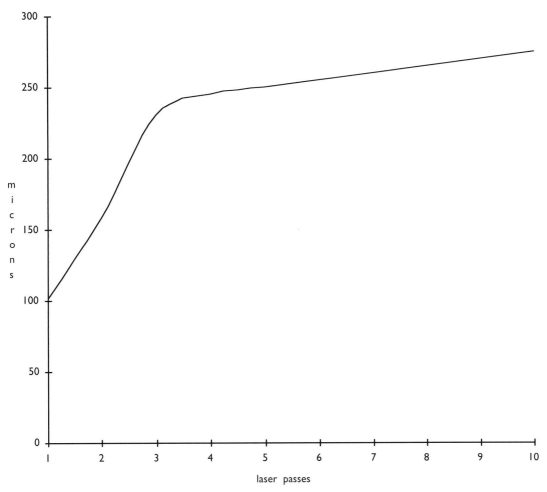

FIGURE 17.1
Depth of single pulse vaporization with increasing number of laser passes.

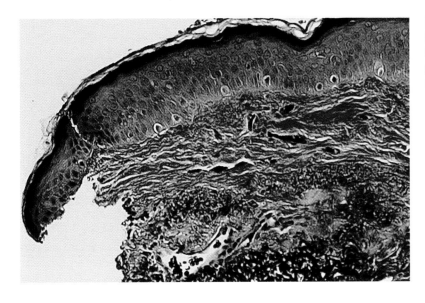

FIGURE 17.2
Photomicrograph of specimen taken 6 months after laser resurfacing. Note thick layer of new collagen deposition and fibroplasia superficial to elastotic material. Original magnification ×400. Trichrome stain.

FIGURE 17.3
A, Preoperative photograph. B, Same patient 3 months
after resurfacing. C, Same patient 6 months after resurfacing. Notice subtle improvement in facial and perioral rhytides between 3 and 6 months, consistent with
further collagen deposition and remodeling.

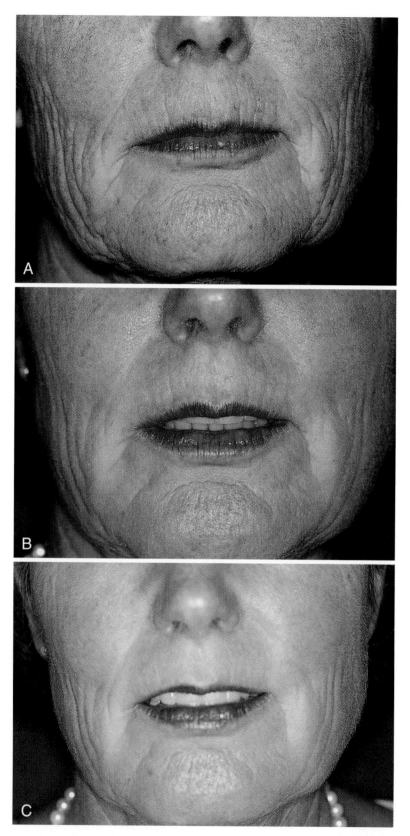

thermal necrosis can exceed 300 μm and is not accompanied by significant increases in tissue ablation unless
the number of pulses impacting the same site exceeds
three. When this pulse-stacking occurs during resurfac-

ing, a yellow-brown discoloration of the tissue is seen
that persists after wiping with saline. This discoloration
is a sign of thermal injury to the dermis, and identifies
tissue that will slough during the healing process.

Multiple pulse vaporization or pulse stacking can be used intentionally to remove excessive tissue found in keratoses, verruca or thickened scars. Unfortunately, more often, pulse stacking occurs inadvertently when the handpiece is moved too slowly or high overlap/density settings are used (>40%) in scanning devices. The multiple pulse vaporization technique can be hazardous as it is difficult to estimate the degree of accumulating thermal injury. The result of pulse stacking can be tissue necrosis, delayed wound healing and potentially scarring. Experience in CO_2 laser resurfacing with close observation of wound healing is required to use this technique safely. Otherwise, it is best to discontinue treatment as soon as tissue yellowing, indicative of thermal injury, occurs.

Endpoints of Treatment

While treating any tissue in resurfacing, it is critical to pay close attention to the laser tissue interaction to identify the endpoints of treatment. Three identifiable endpoints exist:

1. Elimination of the photodamage, rhytides, wrinkles or growths being treated
2. No further tissue tightening occurs
3. A yellow-brown discoloration of tissue, indicative of thermal injury, is visible

When any of these three endpoints is reached, treatment in that area should be discontinued.

TECHNIQUE

Substantial improvement in photoaging can be achieved with simple, complete passes over the entire face or individual cosmetic units using the CO_2 laser. Superior results occur when techniques are varied for the different facial regions. In addition, techniques should be altered when treating conditions other than photoaging such as acne scarring.

Periorbital Area

Generally, the eyelids are treated with pulse energies lower than that used on the remainder of the face, because of the thinner character of this skin. Densities generated by scanners or computer pattern generators are likewise decreased. Though obtaining excellent results in this area is relatively easy, safety should be of paramount concern. Eye shields of metal, not plastic, construction should be in place for any resurfacing procedure of the upper half of the face. Significant ectropion can result if overly aggressive treatment is pursued on the lower eyelids, particularly in patients with prior blepharoplasties. A single laser pass should first be performed over each upper and lower eyelid and surrounding periorbital region to the lateral and inferior extent of the visible wrinkle lines. Doing so removes the epidermis and, due to the thin, lax nature of the skin in

this area, gives modest skin tightening not seen in other areas. A second pass on the skin between the eyebrow and the fold of the upper lid and the skin of the lower lid can be performed (with consideration to reducing the density or pulse overlap), provided the skin has enough excessive tissue to compensate for the skin tightening that can occur on this pass. The interaction of the laser with the tissue must be watched closely during this pass and any subsequent pass, carefully observing for any signs of retraction of the lid margin or incomplete closure of the lids. Further passes directly over the upper and lower lids should be done with the utmost care and are best carried out with a single beam directed at the highest point along the folds of the eyelid skin. Additional passes *can* be performed at the lateral orbital rim and beyond as needed for deeper rhytides with little fear of ectropion.

When the periorbital area is treated as part of a full-face treatment, it is recommended that it be the last area treated so that the tightening effects on the lids by treated cheeks and adjacent areas are visible prior to treatment of the lids. Once the lids have been completely treated, check that the epidermis just adjacent to the lash line has been resurfaced as well, since this will leave a visible line if not treated.

Perioral Area

One of the most popular single cosmetic units for laser resurfacing is the perioral area. No other surgical technique has shown as much promise for consistently improving perioral rhytides. This area is often the most photodamaged location on the facial skin in women (12). In rare cases, only the upper lip, from the vermilion border to the nasolabial folds, may need resurfacing. In the vast majority of individuals, the entire upper and lower lip area extending out to the crescent lines of the medial lower cheek just lateral to the mouth and down the chin across the jawline should be lased. During the procedure, the usual anatomic border of the perioral "unit," the nasolabial fold, is crossed. For this reason, careful feathering of the periphery by decreasing the depth and surface density of resurfacing is necessary. Anesthesia in perioral cases can be easily accomplished by nerve blocks and local infiltration.

Originally, it was recommended to cross the vermilion border and completely resurface the lips. However, unless actinic cheilitis is present, complete lip resurfacing should probably not be done as it tends to cause a flattening of the vermilion surface and blurring of the vermilion border. In addition, this area is by far, the slowest surface to heal. It is preferable to treat up to the vermilion border as the tightening of the skin directly adjacent to the lips may cause the lips to appear fuller. After completing treatment of the cutaneous surface, individual deep lines may be traced on the vermilion surface to stop lipstick from "bleeding" into these lines. Three passes with the Coherent UltraPulse laser (Coherent Laser Corp., Palo Alto, CA) are routinely performed in this area as this area is generally treated more aggressively than others. If substantial photodamage or uneven texture remains, a fourth pass may be performed provided the yellow-brown discoloration associated with excessive residual thermal necrosis is not seen.

Generally, after the second or third pass with the computer pattern generator (CPG), an individual spot handpiece is used to treat the remaining lines and surface irregularities by tracing along the shoulders of the rhytides and the highest points of surface irregularities. One pass with the individual spot handpiece is made along the cutaneous surface of each vermilion border as this is the most common area of persistent lines. These passes with the individual spot handpiece may be done with a pulse-stacking technique to intentionally induce deeper thermal necrosis and tissue slough, if experience with this technique is adequate.

Full Face Resurfacing

Unless the patient desires improvement in only a single cosmetic unit, full face resurfacing is recommended. A substantial increase in tightening of nasolabial lines, lateral crow's feet and medial cheek creases can be obtained by full resurfacing of the face. One of the primary benefits of full facial resurfacing is epidermal renewal with smoothing of texture and evened pigmentation. Even with skilled feathering, patchwork treatment of selected areas can appear cosmetically inferior to resurfacing the whole face. Long-term follow-up has revealed that isolated treatment areas tend to heal with a visible border at the juncture with nontreated photodamaged skin. Postoperative redness after full face resurfacing is often likened to a "rosy glow" that is much preferable to focal erythema of individual cosmetic unit procedures as well. Although feasibly done with regional nerve blocks and infiltrative local anesthesia, full face resurfacing under IV sedation is a much more comfortable procedure for both patient and physician.

Two passes are routinely performed over the entire face because a single pass does not tighten the skin and, in general, does not significantly improve wrinkle appearance. A third pass is often done for moderate or severe photodamage and may be used selectively in these areas only. If difficult areas remain and skin tightening is still seen with each pulse or scan, a fourth pass can be undertaken. The perioral and periorbital areas are treated as previously described. The collimated single pulse handpiece may be judiciously used to treat residual seborrheic keratoses, actinic keratoses, lesions of sebaceous hyperplasia, thickened scars or other surface irregularities.

Feathering

Whether treating a single cosmetic unit or the full face, careful feathering of the treatment periphery is critical.

Sharp demarcations between treated and untreated areas persist as differences in pigmentation, texture and degree of photoaging after healing is complete. Originally, peeling agents such as trichloroacetic acid or Jessner's solution were used to blend the treatment edges but better transitions are now achieved with use of the laser for feathering.

The key principle to feathering is to decrease the depth of ablation *and* thermal damage gradually at the periphery. The simplest way to do this is to decrease the pulse energy delivered. With the Coherent UltraPulse laser the pulse energy can be adjusted directly while on the Sharplan systems (Sharplan Laser, Inc., Allendale, NJ), a decrease in the overall power reduces the energy per scan/pulse. Angling the beam to an incidence angle less than 90° is another method of feathering. By angling the beam, the spot is elongated, and the effective fluence is decreased which results in less ablation and thermal injury. On adjustable scanners, such as the Coherent CPG, the density or overlap can also be reduced, while on other systems the individual pulse handpiece can be moved more quickly so that the number of pulses per treatment area is reduced.

Feathering should be carried approximately 1 cm into the hairline, 3 to 5 cm below the jawline and onto the external ear. Creased earlobes can be improved with multiple passes. A band of widely spaced (2 to 5 mm apart), random individual pulses 1 to 2 cm wide at the periphery also helps to achieve a more gradual transition.

Other Body Sites

Now successfully employed for facial skin, application of laser resurfacing to other body sites seems like a natural progression. Unfortunately, facial skin, rich in adnexal structures and blood supply, is more tolerant of thermal injury than nonfacial skin (13, 14).

With the popularity of submental liposuction and surgical neck lift procedures, resurfacing of the neck is the next progression in overall rejuvenation. Results to date, however are poor. Even with a single pass and low pulse densities, unacceptable rates of scarring, hypopigmentation and prolonged healing are noted (15). The upper neck is more tolerant of resurfacing and may be treated if necessary. However, the lower half of the neck is very problematic. It is possible that the lower neck area could be treated using feathering techniques, although this would be considered investigational work. It is also possible that the Erbium:YAG (Er:YAG) laser may be used more superficially in this location. However, if laser resurfacing of the neck proves to be successful, the treatment goals will need to be limited. Improvement in pigmentation appears possible while improvement in texture may be a greater challenge, but tightening of skin and improvement in wrinkling do not appear to be realistic goals.

Treatment of widespread actinic keratoses of the hands and arms has been done with CO_2 and Er:YAG lasers successfully. These areas are slower to heal and are more painful, but the initial cases have not resulted in the same problems as in treatment of the neck.

Acne Scarring

Although all patients undergoing facial resurfacing should undergo thorough preoperative counseling and preparation, those with acne scarring may require special attention. Of primary importance is that acne should be in prolonged remission before resurfacing. Exacerbations of acne are frequent in resurfacing patients either from shock injury to adnexal structures, or due to the prolonged occlusion during the postoperative period (16). If oral isotretinoin has been used, an absolute minimum of 6 months (12 months may be even safer) should elapse from the patients' last dose prior to resurfacing. Depth of scarring should be assessed, and small, sharply marginated so-called "ice-pick" scars should be excised. Scarred areas of substantial depth should be filled by dermal grafting, autologous fat or synthetic substances. Resurfacing can then take place 6 to 12 weeks after any facial surgery or injections of filler materials. Multiple passes should be performed as is done for photoaging. Less attention can be paid to the upper lip and periorbital areas unless photaging is present.

Individual scars can be "sculpted" at their edges using individual spot handpieces. When treating soft, atrophic acne scars, the primary benefit from resurfacing is tightening of the skin adjacent to scars, as well as at the depth of the scar, in order to pull up the base of the soft, depressed scar. When treating sharply defined fibrotic scars, the laser is used to ablate the sharp edges of the scars in an attempt to soften and smooth the cutaneous surface of these scars. These areas are generally treated more aggressively than rhytides, commonly receiving 4 to 6 laser passes.

It is generally true that a single procedure does not produce the degree of improvement desired by most patients with acne scars. Multiple excisions of small scars, dermal grafting, fat transfer preceding laser resurfacing and possibly more than one resurfacing procedure may be necessary to achieve the desired result. It is critical that the patient understand this point and the expected outcome of each stage in this process. In some patients, this may be a lengthy process, requiring 2 to 3 years to complete with a minimum of 6 months between resurfacing procedures to allow adequate time for new collagen formation, collagen remodeling and normalization of pigment.

NEW DEVICES AND TECHNIQUES

The development of the CO_2 laser for medical use began in the 1960s and has culminated with the short pulse or short dwell time devices used in resurfacing today (17). Newer devices or treatments that will further enhance this procedure are the Er:YAG laser, botulinum toxin and epidermal cooling devices.

The Er:YAG laser, already in clinical use, delivers energy at a wavelength of 2940 nm. This corresponds nearly exactly to the maximal absorption peak of water. The resultant higher coefficient of absorption when compared with CO_2 laser output leads to more efficient energy absorption and decreased depths of residual thermal damage (18). Early clinical results show less postoperative erythema and marginally faster healing, but little intraoperative tightening and less clinical improvement with more superficial treatment. Refinements in parameters and outputs may make the Er:YAG laser a superior tool for resurfacing of some areas such as the neck and hands.

Botulinum toxin (BOTOX [Allergan Corporation, Irvine CA]), originally approved by the FDA for blepharospasm and the treatment of extraocular muscle disorders, has shown considerable efficacy in treating "hyperdynamic lines" of facial expression. Recent studies of pre- and postresurfacing use of BOTOX have shown added benefit. This may become a standard adjunct to resurfacing.

The predominate value of laser resurfacing is remodeling of the dermis and improvement in rhytid appearance. Much of the discomfort, annoyance, and healing time of resurfacing comes from the need for epidermal regeneration. Techniques recently devised to cool the epidermis are now being paired with various lasers with parameters specifically chosen to penetrate to the upper dermal layers and cause thermal injury. The result is nonablative resurfacing, tightening of facial skin without loss of the epidermis. This is an exciting area of clinical research.

Facial resurfacing using pulsed CO_2 lasers has rapidly become a widely used, routine procedure. Currently available devices are easy to use and capable of delivering excellent results. Understanding the mechanisms of laser wounding and healing, combined with careful observation during the procedure and techniques gleaned from the experience of others leads to effective, safe, repeatable results in facial resurfacing.

REFERENCES

1. Fitzpatrick RE, Goldman MP, Satur NM, et al. Pulsed carbon dioxide laser resurfacing of photoaged facial skin. Arch Dermatol 1996;132:395-402.
2. Fitzpatrick RE, Goldman MP, Satur NM, et al. Trichloroacetic acid, Baker-Gordon phenol and dermabrasion: A comparative clinical and histologic study of cutaneous resurfacing in a porcine model. Arch Dermatol 1996;132: 469-471.

3. Green HA, Domankevitz Y, Nishioka NS. Pulsed carbon dioxide laser ablation of burned skin: in vitro and in vivo analysis. Lasers Surg Med 1990;10:476-484.

4. Rothman S. Physiology and Biochemistry of the Skin. Chicago: University of Chicago Press, 1954:494.

5. Walsh JJ, Flotte TJ, Anderson RR, et al. Pulsed CO_2 laser tissue ablation: effect of tissue type and pulse duration on thermal damage. Lasers Surg Med 1988;8:108-118.

6. Fitzpatrick RE, Smith SR. Depth of vaporization and residual thermal damage using multiple passes of the Ultrapulse CO_2 laser. SPIE Proceedings 1997.

7. Tans LJ. Experimentelle Untersuchungen über Entstehung von astigmatismus durch nicht- perforirende Corneawunden. Graefes Arch Ophthalmol 1898;45:117-152.

8. Stringer H, Parr J. Shrinkage temperature of eye collagen. Nature 1964;204:1307.

9. Gardner ES, Reinisch L, Stricklin GP, et al. In vitro changes in non-facial human skin following CO_2 laser resurfacing: a comparison study. Lasers Surg Med 1996;19:379-387.

10. Nelson BR, Majmudar G, Griffiths EM, et al. Clinical improvement following dermabrasion of photoaged skin correlates with synthesis of collagen! Arch Dermatol 1994; 130:1136-1142.

11. Brugmans MJP, Kemper J, Gijsbers GHM, et al. Temperature response of biological materials to pulsed nonablative CO_2 laser irradiation. Lasers Surg Med 1991;11: 587-591.

12. Gilchrest BA. Skin aging and photoaging: an overview. J Am Acad Dermatol 1989;21:610-613.

13. Moretti G, et al. Vascular patterns in the skin of the face. J Invest Dermatol 1959;33:103.

14. Benfenati A, Brillanti F. Sulla distribuzione delle ghiandole sebacee nella cute del corpo umano. Arch Ital Dermatol 1939;15:33.

15. Fitzpatrick RE, Goldman MP. Resurfacing of photodamage of the neck using the ultrapulse CO_2 laser [abstract]. Lasers Surg Med 1997;(Suppl 9):33.

16. Sriprachya-Anunt S, Fittzpatrick RE, Goldman MP, et al. Infections complicating pulsed carbon dioxide laser resurfacing for photoaged facial skin. Dermatol Surg 1997;23: 527-536.

17. Polanyi TG, Bredemeier HC, Davis TJ Jr. CO_2 laser for surgical research and medical and biological engineering. New York: Pergamon Press, 1970.

18. Walsh JJ, Flotte TJ, Deutsch TF. Er:YAG laser ablation of tissue: effect of pulse duration and tissue type on thermal damage. Lasers Surg Med 1989;9:314-326.

CHAPTER 18

Postoperative Care After Laser Resurfacing

■ Naomi Lawrence
William P. Coleman III

A carbon dioxide (CO_2) laser that is modified to deliver high peak power and short pulses with the duration less than the thermal relaxation of skin (325 to 695 msec) provides precise tissue ablation with minimal thermal damage (1, 2). The UltraPulse 5000 (Coherent Laser Corp., Palo Alto, CA) is the prototype laser of this technology. The SilkTouch (Sharplan Laser Inc., Allendale, NJ) also provides precise tissue vaporization through a microprocessor-controlled miniature optomechanical flashscanner that is compatible with any continuous wave CO_2 laser (3). Many new CO_2 lasers are entering the market. Erbium:YAG lasers create a much shallower injury and consequently have rapid, less complex healing. The wound care described in this chapter is relevant to the two widely used pulsed CO_2 lasers and lasers similar to these.

THE WOUND

There are two components of a pulsed CO_2 laser wound: a zone of vaporization and a zone of thermal necrosis. The optimal zone of thermal necrosis (30 to 150 μm) provides adequate hemostasis while minimizing the risk of scarring. Kauvar et al compared the zones of ablation and thermal damage for each pass with the SilkTouch laser and the UltraPulse 5000 laser (4). For the SilkTouch laser, one pass caused complete ablation of the epidermis (30 to 50 μm) into the superficial and deeper papillary dermis. For the UltraPulse 5000 laser, one pass ablated 20 to 30 μm with incomplete epidermal ablation. Only after a second pass with the Ultra-Pulse 5000 laser did ablation into the papillary dermis

occur. The SilkTouch laser also had a greater zone of thermal necrosis for each pass (30 μm, 100 μm, 150 μm) than the UltraPulse 5000 (20 μm, 50 μm, 70 μm).

IMMEDIATE POSTOPERATIVE PAIN

For immediate postoperative pain, gauze soaked in 2% plain xylocaine provides quick relief. Postoperative swelling can be lessened with a short-acting intramuscular steroid or a tapered regimen of oral corticosteroids. Important to proper postoperative care are explicit day by day written instructions. For most patients, acyclovir is prescribed preoperatively, which is continued 7 to 10 days postoperatively until full re-epithelialization occurs. Resurfacing patients need constant encouragement, and should be seen every 2 to 3 days until re-epithelialization is complete and the patients are ready to wear makeup. All patients are shown one or more series of postoperative pictures during their consultation to prepare them for their postoperative appearance. In spite of honest and diligent preparation, many patients still become slightly depressed during their healing period. This depression can become worse if healing is delayed. Close follow up in the early postoperative period also ensures that a complication, such as herpes simplex virus, bacterial or yeast infection or contact dermatitis, is detected at its earliest possible stage.

CLOSED POSTOPERATIVE TREATMENT

Dermabrasion results in a wound that is bloody, produces copious exudate, and requires patients to leave

189

the office with a mask to cover the exudative wound. Patients are often repulsed and intimidated by the bleeding and by the mask. Because the resurfacing laser results in a dry wound, occlusion may be desirable for better wound healing, but is not essential for wound management.

Biologic dressings reduce postoperative discomfort and time to re-epithelialization (5, 6). The dressing preferred for dermabrasion is Vigilon (Bard Inc., Murray Hill, NJ) (6). Vigilon is a polyethylene film that can retain a significant amount of exudate. It is not adhesive and must be held in place with a mask or tape.

Silon-TSR (Biomed Science Inc., Bethlehem PA) is a silicone with a polytetrafluoroethylene interpenetrating polymer network (7). It is supplied as a very thin single sheet with handles and can be tied around the head to secure in place. Slits for the eyes, nose, and mouth must be cut. It is recommended that a gauze dressing be wrapped around the Silon-TSR dressing to collect wound exudate (8). This dressing is left in place for 1 to 2 days postoperatively and then the area is cleansed. If a second Silon-TSR dressing is put on the face, it can be left in place for remainder of the re-epithelialization process (5 to 7 days).

Flexzan (Dow B. Hickon Inc., Sugarland, TX) is a polyurethane foam laminated with a pressure sensitive adhesive (9). It has a porous wound contact surface that allows uptake of wound exudate through the cross hatching pattern of the adhesive into the inner conical voids until it evaporates. The vapor transport rate (permeability) of Flexzan is greater than $5000g/m^2/24$ hrs. This vapor transport rate is much more efficient than that of thin films ($400-1500g/m^2/24$ hr) and hydrocolloids ($100g/m^2/24$ hr) (9). The risk of maceration is decreased because exudate pooling is minimal. The external surface of Flexzan is nanoporous (pores 10^{-3} μm) and forms a barrier to exogenous microbial contamination (9, 10). It is permeable to moisture vapor and air. Flexzan has greater conformability than thin films or hydrocolloids and has elasticity superior to hydrocolloids and analogous to thin films (9). One problem with Flexan is that it is opaque. If left on as long as recommended, the wound cannot be monitored during the crucial first postoperative week. The signs of infection after laser resurfacing can be very subtle and a completely covered wound risks delaying appropriate and timely antibacterial and antiviral intervention. Another concern is anecdotal reports of inadvertent skin stripping or imprinting of skin when the Flexzan is removed.

N-terface (Winfield Laboratories Inc., Richardson, TX) is a thin, pliable porous, polyethylene sheeting (11). It must be covered by an absorptive layer in an exudative wound (12). Salasche et al looked at several different regimens of use and found that leaving the N-terface sheeting in place for 4 to 6 days was optimal

for allowing progression of reepithelialization and a decrease in exudate (12). Fulton also indicated that 5 days is ideal to allow adequate epithelial regrowth (11). N-terface sheeting provides an excellent contact layer for open wounds (13).

OPEN POSTOPERATIVE TREATMENT USING OINTMENT

During the reepithelialization period we use a modified open technique for healing. While reclining, or sleeping the patient uses Vigilon, Aquaphor gauze (Beiersdorf, Norwalk, CT) or SecondSkin (Bionet Inc., Little Rock, AR) which is stored in the refrigerator to enhance the soothing effect. When the patient is ambulatory, frequent soaks with a dilute vinegar in water solution (1:16) followed by copious application of Vaseline (Chesebrough-Ponds, Inc., Greenwich, CT) or Aquaphor ointments provide adequate occlusion. The exudate combined from oils in the topicals can result in a yellow film that patients are often afraid to clean. We instruct patients to soak 4×4 gauze pads in a vinegar/water solution and place it on the affected area to hydrate for 5 minutes or longer.

Removing the gauze causes a gentle debridement of the yellow film. It may also be necessary to gently wipe some areas with gauze to remove debris. Copious amounts of ointment are reapplied and this cleansing is repeated 4 to 5 times daily until re-epithelialization is complete. It is important to see the patient the day after surgery and 2 to 3 days postoperatively to be certain he or she understands how to properly remove this film and prevent crusts which could delay healing.

One intangible advantage to the open care method is psychological. Many patients enjoy being actively involved in their wound care. They feel empowered and have a sense of accomplishment when their wound is healed. The wound care also gives them a positive focal point which helps distract them from their appearance. Conversely, other patients do not like the responsibility of wound care and find it a difficult and unappealing task. These patients require closer physician observation and psychological support.

During the immediate postresurfacing period, occlusive topical creams and ointments facilitate epithelial cell migration (14-18). Petroleum jelly (Vaseline), Aquaphor, and Elta (Swiss-American Products, Inc., Dallas, TX) are all fragrance-free products with low irritation potential that work well in the immediate postoperative care of the laser patient. Some products have been promoted particularly for resurfacing. Catrix (Donell Den Medex, New York, NY) contains a protein mucopolysaccharide complex derived from bovine tracheal cartilage (19). In a study conducted to measure the effects of Catrix on tretinoin-treated skin, data showed a statistically significant decrease in skin temperature by thermography when treated with Catrix (19). The mechanism for skin cooling caused by Catrix is thought to be an anti-inflammatory effect. In a small blinded, unpublished study (7 patients after a 35% trichloroacetic acid peel) Rubin compared 70% Catrix ointment to 1% hydrocortisone ointment in a split face design (20). He noted faster healing, less sensitivity, itching and erythema on the Catrix side in 6 of 7 patients. One drawback of using this particular product is that the manufacturer requires the physician to "train" to use the product.

Vitamin A & E ointment (Professional Solutions, Boca Raton, FL) is another product that has been marketed for the post laser resurfacing patient. The concern with this product is that it contains Vitamin E, which has been reported to cause irritant and contact dermatitis after facial resurfacing. Hunter et al reported four cases of adverse reactions to aloe vera and topical Vitamin E after skin resurfacing (21). Aloe vera and topical Vitamin E are commonly used by the public and are perceived as natural healing promoting skin products. Even if the physician does not recommend these products, the patient may self administer them because they are considered harmless. Aloe is a complex mixture of aloin and anthraquinone (which may cross react with balsam of Peru and benzoin) (21, 22). Vitamin E is a form of di-alpha-tocopherol of which there are four racemic pairs of stereoisomer (which makes it difficult to patch test). Vitamin E contact dermatitis is not uncommon (21, 23, 24). The cases reported by Hunter had several features in common. The application of the topicals caused a severe immediate reaction (indicating probable irritant contact dermatitis). One report related a severe inflammatory reaction and scarring when Vitamin E came into direct contact with the dermis (21, 25). One patient was able to subsequently use Vitamin E on healthy skin which may mean that intact skin is less susceptible to the irritant effect. In this case, healing was delayed and persistent erythema resulted. We did experience one case of chemical conjunctivitis from Vitamin A & E ointment and have since switched to Lacrilube (Allergan Inc., Irvine, CA) in the periocular area. Since this change in protocol, we have had no problems with chemical conjunctivitis.

Once reepithelialization is complete (7 to 10 days after the procedure) the patient is placed on a moisturizing cream, such as Cetaphil (Galderma Lab Inc., Fort Worth, TX) or Eucerin (Biersdorf, Norwalk, CT). Patients can progress to moisturizing lotions as tolerated which are more compatible with makeup. During the second postoperative week, depending on the depth of the original pathology, there are often areas that still need frequent cleaning and ointment-based topicals. Thus portions of the face require ointments while other areas are ready for creams. The earlier occlusive ointments can be discontinued the less likely acne will occur. We

hold off the use of makeup until 10 to 14 days postoperatively. Patients can be provided a corrective green color pot (Dermatologic Cosmetic Labs, North Homer, CT) in their postoperative kit that can be used under an oil-based makeup. Some patients prefer a heavier correction makeup such as Dermablend (Dermablend Corrective Cosmetics, Chicago, IL). The use of postoperative cosmetics is discussed more completely in Chapter 26.

It is very important to watch for signs of complications during the postoperative period. Any inexplicable reversal in healing, increase in discomfort, or delay in re-epithelialization beyond 2 weeks should stimulate prompt investigation for infection. Once re-epithelialization occurs, blotchy erythema particularly along a bony prominence, such as the jawline, is cause for close observation and early intervention to prevent an incipient scar. The recognition and management of resurfacing complications are discussed more completely in Chapter 26. Once re-epithelialization is complete, a number of topical products are used postoperatively to decrease complications and maintain skin rejuvenation.

MAINTENANCE OF SKIN POST RESURFACING

Tretinoin

We use tretinoin for at least 2 weeks preoperatively in a concentration of 0.025% or 0.05% to ensure rapid re-epithelialization (26, 27). Many laser patients have used tretinoin for years. Some laser experts do not recommend preoperative tretinoin because of concern over the high incidence of retinoid reaction and its potential effect on resurfacing (28).

Tretinoin can usually be reinstituted 1 to 4 weeks after re-epithelialization of a peel or dermabrasion, depending on the depth of wounding. After laser resurfacing, however, most patients require a 4 to 6-week period after re-epithelialization before they can tolerate tretinoin. Creams are better tolerated than gels. Tretinoin (0.05% or 0.1%) decreases clinical actinic damage such as actinic keratoses, actinic dyschromia, and rhytides (29, 30). At the cellular level there is increased collagen formation and increased fibroblasts resulting in a widened papillary dermal Grenz zone (between epidermis and amorphous solar elastosis). Telangiectatic blood vessels are also dilated and the epidermis shows compaction of the stratum corneum, normalization of melanocyte number and size, and reversal of global epidermal dysplasia (31). These benefits help to maintain and refine the effects of laser resurfacing.

Sunscreens

Sunscreens are an important part of the patient's postoperative regimen. We prefer a physical sunscreen such as micronized titanium dioxide because it blocks ultraviolet A (UVA) and UVB rays and is less sensitizing than chemical sunscreens. Sunscreens protect the post-resurfacing skin from melanocyte stimulation (resulting in hyperpigmentation). They also protect the newly resurfaced patient from sunburn and further photo-damage. Patients should be counseled to avoid direct sun for several months after laser resurfacing. Once tolerated, broad-spectrum, waterproof, high sun protection factor (SPF) lotions are cosmetically more appealing than physical blocking agents.

Topical Vitamin C

Topical vitamin C (Cellex-C [Cellex-C Cosmaceuticals, Toronto, Canada]) is a 10% aqueous solution with an acid pH. This solution is promoted as able to deliver 20 times the Vitamin C found in normal skin. This amount of Vitamin C cannot be delivered by oral administration or diet. Vitamin C also apparently provides photoprotection from UVA and UVB rays. This is theoretically thought to occur, not through blocking the irradiation, but as an antioxidant. Topical Vitamin C is promoted for its ability to quench reactive oxygen species (free radicals) created by UV damage. Free radical molecules play a role in skin carcinogenesis, photoaging, and inflammation (32-37). Topical vitamin C may be useful after laser resurfacing, both as an anti-inflammatory (possibly decreasing erythema through sun protection effect) and as an anti-aging agent. A hindrance to the widespread prescription of topical Vitamin C is the cost (approximately $50.00 per bottle cost to the physician). Other topical Vitamin C compounds are becoming available at much less cost. Unfortunately, there is no sound scientific evidence to promote the claims of companies that market topical Vitamin C. All information to date is anecdotal.

Hydroquinones

Hyperpigmentation is a relatively common adverse reaction after laser resurfacing (38). It is estimated to occur in 20% to 30% of patients with Fitzpatrick skin type III and in almost 100% of patients with skin type IV (39). The pigment becomes visible 3 to 4 weeks after the procedure as a slight brownish tinge. It usually resolves in 2 to 6 months with appropriate topical therapy. This incidence and clinical course of hyperpigmentation after laser resurfacing is consistent with other forms of deep skin resurfacing (40).

The biologic mechanisms of postinflammatory hyperpigmentation have been investigated (41, 42). Tomita et al identified the arachidonic acid metabolite, LTC4, as the most potent stimulator of tyrosinase activity (41). LTC4 also stimulates the growth of cultured melanocytes. Histologic and ultrastructural studies of postinflammatory hyperpigmentation show increases in dopa-positive melanocytes per area of skin, in tyrosi-

nase, in melanocyte activity, in melanocyte dendricity and cell body size, and increases in dermal melanosis (42).

Hydroquinone is hypothesized to have depigmentation activity through three mechanisms (43). First, it acts as an alternative substrate for the enzyme tyrosinase, preventing tyrosine oxidation. Second, hydroquinone causes an increase in formation of reactive oxygen species within the pigment cell leading to damage of the lipid membrane. Finally, hydroquinone can cause vacuolation of the cytoplasm and destruction of the melanocyte. It takes about 8 weeks of therapy for hydroquinone to shut down the melanocytes maximally (44). Tretinoin is adjunctive in the treatment of hyperpigmentation (30). Hydroquinones should be employed preoperatively to gauge any sensitivity. Postoperatively, hydroquinone cream formulations can usually be tolerated 3 weeks postoperatively. The more potent gels can be introduced later once skin sensitivity decreases, Tretinoin is also reintroduced as tolerated. This regimen may be required for several months in darker skin types.

As discussed in Chapter 22, the use of botulinum exotoxin-A (BTX-A) not only maximizes initial laser treatment but probably helps to maintain the result. BTX-A is thought to accomplish this by eliminating the dynamic component for rhytides in the forehead, glabellar, and periocular area. As the skin ages, the traction/counter-traction between the skin and underlying facial muscles becomes unbalanced (45). The elastic network in the dermis degenerates with age and the collagen becomes stiffer (45). Repetitive muscular contractions etch defects into the dermis resulting clinically in lines and wrinkles. The muscles of the upper third of the face are not necessary for functional eating and talking, so paralysis of these muscles is safe with few untoward effects. Maintaining paralysis of key facial muscles allows the laser resurfaced skin to form new collagen in the wrinkled areas, without dynamic muscle activity causing recurrent rhytides.

Alpha hydroxy acids (AHAs)

Alpha hydroxy acids (AHAs) loosen epidermal corneocytes causing exfoliation of the stratum corneum (46-48). AHAs reduce hydrogen bonding and lead to decreased interaction among polar groups on keratin chains, increasing skin flexibility (48, 49). It is also thought that AHAs may increase skin extensibility by occupying binding sites for water in the stratum corneum (48, 49). Kligman proposed that dilute glycolic acid solutions (5% to 10%) act on the stratum corneum, but higher concentration solutions (>50%) also cause epidermolysis and stimulate dermal macrophages and fibroblasts (47, 48). A new group of AHA skin products use a nonphospholiposomal delivery system and may

TABLE 18.1

HOW TO PROTECT YOUR SKIN FROM THE SUN

1. Sunburning rays (UVB) are strongest between the hours of 10 A.M. and 3 P.M.
2. Geographic factors affect sun exposure.
   The closer one lives (or vacations) to the equator, the stronger the sun's rays.
   The sun is stronger at higher altitudes.
3. A tan is the body's defense against the sun. There is no healthy tan. A tan is always a sign of sun damage.
4. Tanning booths are not safe. Studies have shown an increase in the risk of skin cancer in young people who use tanning booths.
5. Sunscreen must be applied thickly and reapplied hourly. Water, wind, and sweat all cause sunscreen to be less effective.
   For a complete sun block, both the sunburning rays (UVB) and the suntanning rays (UVA) must be blocked. Some chemical sunscreens can do this. If they block UVA and UVB, it should be indicated on the label. Physical sunscreens (zinc oxide and micronized titanium dioxide) also block UVA and UVB and have the additional advantage of being relatively nonirritating. The main disadvantage of physical sunscreens is their increased thickness and are thus more difficult to apply smoothly.
6. Snow, sand, and water reflect the sun's rays and greatly increase their intensity. Clouds do not completely block UVB rays and it is possible to get a sunburn on a cloudy day.
7. Additional clothing provides further protection from the sun. Broad rimmed hats protect the ears (particularly important for those with short hair). A tightly woven cotton fabric is also useful for people who are sun sensitive.

have the advantage of prolonged release and reduced the irritation of glycolic acid (47). AHA lotions should be added to a regimen of tretinoin and hydroquinones to maintain the long term effects of laser resurfacing. Higher concentrations of glycolic acid, such as 70%, may be used in monthly pulse treatments to further these benefits.

LONG-TERM SKIN CARE MAINTENANCE

The laser procedure is costly and has significant morbidity. Because of the dramatic results, most patients are very pleased with the improvement in their skin. It is in the patient's best interest to maintain these results as long as possible. Education on sun protection to prevent further photodamage is essential (See Table 18.1). Topicals such as tretinoin and AHA lotions help maintain good skin quality. In a newly resurfaced patient, these are used at the lowest concentration (0.025% tretinoin, 8% AHAs). In time the concentrations are increased as the patient tolerates it. After complete healing for resurfacing adding periodic light peels to the skin care main-

tenance program will help to ensure the best results and maintain physician-patient continuity.

REFERENCES

1. Hruza GJ, Geronemus RG, Dover JS, Arndt KA. Lasers in dermatology—1993 [editorial]. Arch Dermatol 1993;129(8):1026-1035.
2. Fitzpatrick RE, Ruiz-Esparza J, Goldman MP. The depth of thermal necrosis using the CO_2 laser: a comparison of the superpulsed mode and conventional mode. J Dermatol Surg Oncol 1991;17(4):340-344.
3. Waldorf HA, Kauvar AN, Geronemus RG. Skin resurfacing of fine to deep rhytides using a char-free carbon dioxide laser in 47 patients. Derm Surg 1995;21(11):940-946.
4. Kauvar AN, Waldorf HA, Geronemus RG. A histopathological comparison of "char-free" carbon dioxide lasers. Derm Surg 1996;22(4):343-348.
5. Fazio JF, Zitelli JA, Goslen JB. Wound Healing. In: Coleman WP, Hanke CW, Alt TH, Asken S, eds. Cosmetic surgery of the skin: principles and techniques. 2nd ed. St Louis: Mosby Inc., 1997:18-38.
6. Pinski JB. Dressings for dermabrasion:new aspects. J Dermatol Surg Oncol 1987;13:673.
7. Weiss RA, Weiss MA. Promising results found with new interpenetrating polymer network. Cosmet Dermatol 1995;8(10):31-32.
8. Silon-TSR Instruction sheet Bio Med Sciences, Inc. 101 Technology Drive, Bethlehem PA 18015
9. Barr, JE. Product Notebook: Multi-center evaluation of a new wound dressing. Ostomy Wound Manage 1993;39(9):60-67.
10. Ives CL, Reed AM, Szycher M. Spyroflex: a tryptosorbent wound dressing and wound closure. J Biomat Appl 1992;6:341.
11. Fulton, Jr JE. Dermabrasion, chemabrasion, and laserabrasion. J Dermatol Surg 1996;22:619-628.
12. Salasche SJ, Winton GB. Clinical evaluation of a nonadhering wound dressing. J Dermatol Surg Oncol 1986;12(11):1220-1222.
13. Weller K. Achieving compliance and consistency: avoidance of wound bed trauma utilizing a wound contact layer material in chronic and post-surgical (open) wounds. Presented as an abstract at the 6th Annual Clinical Symposium on Pressure Sore & Wound Management. St. Charles, IL September 12-13 1991.
14. Eaglstein WH, Mertz PM. "Inert" Vehicles do affect wound healing. J Invest Dermotol 1980;74:90.
15. Geronemus RG, Mertz PM, Eaglstein WH. Wound healing: The effects of topical antimicrobial agents. Arch Dermatol 1979;115:1311.
16. Winter GD. Formation of the scab and the rate of epithelialization of superficial wounds of the skin of the young domestic pig. Nature 1962;193:293.
17. Winter GD, Scales JT. Effect of air drying and dressing on the surface of a wound. Nature 1963;197:91.
18. Hinman CD, Maibach HI. Effect of air exposure and occlusion on experimental human wounds. Nature 1963;200:377.

19. Schwartz SR, Davis GF. Thermographic assay: the action of bovine tracheal cartilage mucopolysaccharide after topical application of tretinoin. Cosmet Toilet 1993;108(8):67.
20. Rubin MG. Catrix quickens wound healing of TCA peels. Dermatology Times 1992 Jul;13(7):1.
21. Hunter D, Frumkin A. Adverse reactions to vitamin E and aloe vera preparations after dermabrasion and chemical peel. Cutis. Mar 1991;47(3):193-196.
22. Fisher AA. Aloe vera. In: Fisher AA, ed. Contact Dermatitis. 3rd ed. Philadelphia: Lea & Febiger, 1986;174.
23. Goldman MP, Rapaport M. Contact dermatitis to vitamin E oil. J Am Acad Dermatol 1986;14:133-134.
24. Brodkin RH, Bleiberg J. Sensitivity to topically applied vitamin E. Arch Dermatol 1965;92:76-77.
25. Peters CR, Shaw TE, Raju DR. The influence of vitamin E on capsule formation and contracture around silicone implants. Ann Plast Surg 1979;5:347-353.
26. Hevia O, Nemeth AJ, Taylor JR. Tretinoin accelerates healing after trichloroacetic acid chemical peel. Arch Dermatol 1991;127:678-682.
27. Hung VC, Lee JY, Zitelli JA, et al. Topical tretinoin and epithelial wound healing. Arch Dermatol 1989;125:65-69.
28. Weinstein C, Alster TS. Skin resurfacing with high energy pulsed carbon dioxide lasers. In: Alster TS, Apfelberg DB, eds. Cosmetic laser surgery. New York: Wiley-Liss 1996: 9-25.
29. Kligman AM, Grove GL, Hirose R, et al. Topical tretinoin for photoaged skin. J Am Acad Dermatol 1986;15:836-859.
30. Weiss J, Ellis CN, Headington JT, et al. Topical tretinoin improves photoaged skin: a double-blind vehicle controlled study. JAMA 1988;259:527.
31. Weiss JS, Ellis CN, Goldfarb MT, et al. Tretinoin treatment of photodamaged skin: cosmesis through medical therapy. Dermatol Clin 1991;9:123-129.
32. Cloven RM, Pinnell SR. Topical Vitamin C in aging. Clin Dermatol 1996;14:227-234.
33. Brash DE, Rudolph JA, Simon JA et al. A role for sunlight skin cancer: UV-induced p53 mutations in squamous cell carcinoma. Proc Natl Acad Sci USA 1991;88:10124-10128.
34. Ziegler A, Leffell DJ, Kunala S, et al. Mutation hotspots due to sunlight in the p53 gene of nonmelanoma skin cancers. Proc Natl Acad Sci USA 1993;90:4216-4220.
35. Trenan CW, Dabbagh AJ et al. Skin inflammation induced by reactive oxygen species. Br J Dermatol 1991;125: 325-329.
36. Bissett DL, Hannon DP, Orr TV. An animal model of solar-aged skin: histological, physical and visible changes in UV-irradiated hairless mouse skin. Photochem Photobiol 1987;46:367-378.
37. Darr D, Combs S, Dunston S, Manning T, Pinnell S. Topical vitamin C protects porcine skin from ultraviolet radiation-induced damage. Br J Dermatol 1992;127:247-253.
38. Weinstein C. Carbon dioxide laser resurfacing In: Coleman WP III, Hanke CS, Alt TH, Asken S, eds. Cosmetic Surgery of the Skin: Principles and Techniques. 2nd ed. St Louis: Mosby, 1997:152-177.
39. Roberts TL III, Lettieri JT, Ellis LB. CO2 laser resurfacing: recognizing and minimizing complications. Aesthetic Surg Quart 1996;16(2):142-148.
40. Lawrence N, Brody HG, Alt TN. Chemical peeling In: Coleman WP III, Hanke CW, Alt TH, Asker S, eds. Cosmetic surgery of the skin: principle and techniques. 2nd ed. St Louis: Mosby 1997;85-111.
41. Tomita Y, Maeda K, Tagami H. Melanocyte-stimulating properties of arachidonic acid metabolites: possible role in postinflammatory pigmentation. Pigment Cell Research 1992;5(5 Pt 2):357-361.
42. Farooqui JZ, Auclair BW, Robb F, Sarkisian E, Cooper C, Alexander JW, Warden G, Biossy RE, Nordlund J. Histological, biochemical, and ultrastructural studies on hyperpigmented human skin xenografts. Pigment Cell Research 1993;6(4 Pt 1):226-233.
43. Bolognia JL, Sodi SA, Osber MP, Pawelek JM. Enhancement of the depigmenting effect of hydroquinone by cystamine and buthionine sulfoximine. Br J Dermatol 1995; 133(3):349-357.
44. Yi K, Hart LL. Use of hydroquinone as a bleaching cream. Annals of Pharmacotherapy 1993;27(5):592-593.
45. Dzubow L. The aging face. In: Coleman WP III, Hanke CW, Alt TH, Asken S, eds. Cosmetic surgery of the skin: principles and techniques. 2nd ed. St. Louis: Mosby 1997, 7-17.
46. Kligman A. Results of a pilot study evaluating the compatibility of topical tretinoin in combination with glycolic acid. Cosmet Dermatol 1993;6(10):28-32.
47. Alfieri DR. Alphahydroxy acids and nonphospholipid liposomes. Cosmet Dermatol 1997;10(3):42-52.
48. Hill JC, White RH, Barrett MD, Mignini E. The skin plasticization effect of a medium chain 2-hydroxy acid and the use of potentiators. J Appl Cosmetol 1988;6:53-68.
49. Takahashi M, Machida Y, Tsuda Y. The influence of hydroxy acids on the rheological properties of the stratum corneum. J Soc Cosmet Chem 1985;36:177-187.

CHAPTER 19

The Future of Laser Resurfacing

■ Ronald G. Wheeland

Since its original creation in 1964, the carbon dioxide (CO_2) laser has been successfully used to treat a variety of sun-related conditions, including actinic cheilitis, actinic keratoses and even basal cell carcinomas. A new group of highly modified CO_2 lasers has recently been developed that delivers short-pulses of high energy infrared light. These lasers ablate tissue with greater precision, safety and effectiveness than was possible with the older CO_2 laser technology (1-4). This new and revolutionary laser procedure for managing aged or photodamaged skin has been termed *laser resurfacing* (3). The anticipated advances in laser technology are described in this chapter. Any improvement in technology is dependent on a better understanding of the nature of the laser-tissue interaction and laser wound management. These innovations should help to refine the resurfacing operative technique and improve the ability to care for patients who have clinical evidence of cutaneous aging or solar damage.

DEFINING THE LASER-TISSUE INTERACTION

In the current laser resurfacing procedure, thin layers of damaged epidermis and upper dermis can be precisely ablated in a layer-by-layer fashion with successive passes of a CO_2 laser using either a freehand technique or a robotic scanning device attached to the laser (5, 6). The short pulses of light produced by the new lasers reduce the amount of residual collateral thermal injury that could otherwise result in permanent scarring or unwanted textural changes (7, 8). In addition, the minimal residual thermal damage also permits re-epithelialization to occur quickly.

The clinical improvement seen in wrinkles and photodamaged skin is partially due to the removal of the most severely sun-damaged portions of the dermis. However,

studies have also shown that the energy from the CO_2 laser also produces immediate contraction and shrinkage of the dermal collagen fibers. This shrinkage presumably accounts for the immediate tightening of the skin that occurs during the tissue ablation process (9). In spite of recognizing this effect, the mechanism responsible for producing collagen shrinkage has not been fully defined and the longevity of the effect is also unknown. The combination of tissue ablation, collagen contraction, and synthesis of new collagen and elastic fibers, which occurs during the subsequent phases of wound healing, improves the clinical appearance of both wrinkles and folds, while reducing skin sagging and rejuvenating the skin to provide a more youthful appearance. However, the relative roles played by each of these different components in providing the clinical improvement remains unclear and further basic research is required.

In spite of the dramatic clinical successes and wide public acceptance that has been achieved in treating aged or photodamaged skin over the past 4 to 5 years with short-pulsed, high-energy CO_2 lasers, the mechanisms involved in laser resurfacing remain poorly defined. The relative roles that the ablation process, thermal effect, inflammation, and growth factors play in determining the outcome have not been established. Furthermore, the ideal pulse duration and pulse energy for using the CO_2 laser to treat aged or photodamaged skin is still undefined. As a result, some anatomic areas, like the neck and dorsal aspect of the hands, remain at risk for the development of unwanted scarring or permanent skin texture changes.

IMPROVING LASER WOUND MANAGEMENT

The safety, speed, precision, and effectiveness of short-pulsed, high energy CO_2 laser skin resurfacing has resulted in widespread patient interest in this high technology therapy for improvement or correction of the commonest cutaneous signs of aging and solar damage. One manifestation of the expanding indications for laser resurfacing is that more individuals are now considered appropriate candidates for this procedure and include those who once might have been excluded from having treatment with one of the older resurfacing techniques, such as dermabrasion or chemical peels. In view of the number of older individuals or those with preexisting health problems who now routinely undergo laser resurfacing, additional research must be performed to evaluate the effect on wound healing of both general nutrition and skin preparation (the preoperative use of vitamin and mineral supplements and topical skin preparation using retinoids, emollients or growth factors) (10-12).

The ideal postoperative regimen that takes maximal advantage of the precision offered by lasers and permits the most rapid wound healing possible has not, as yet, been clearly established (13). While not strictly related to the newer laser resurfacing procedures, the number of different wound management techniques in common use today may be a function of a failure to understand the complex nature of the interrelated events that occur during the various phases of wound healing. It is also important to consider the important role played by the multitude of recently identified growth factors that can stimulate or inhibit various components of the early exudative and proliferative phases of wound healing as well as the later repair and remodeling phases (14-16). To achieve the most rapid healing possible, more basic molecular biology research is required to better understand the relative roles played by the various peptide growth factors, fibronectin, and the fibrin clot in the early phases of wound healing. The obvious purpose and benefit of improving both the preoperative and postoperative care of patients undergoing laser skin resurfacing is to maximize the rate and quality of wound healing while reducing the risk of complications, such as hypertrophic or textural scarring and irregular pigmentation.

It is well established that open wound healing following partial thickness wounding is slowed if dressings, ointments or lotions are not applied postoperatively. Whenever an epidermal defect has been created, keratinocytes at the margins of the wound as well as within adjacent hair follicles and sweat ducts flatten and begin migrating into the wound. Increased mitotic figures are detected at the edges of the wound (17). If the wound is kept moist and protected from desiccation, re-epithelialization occurs more rapidly than in a dry wound since there is no impediment to the migrating epithelial cells (18). During the past decade, various occlusive dressings have been successfully introduced into routine clinical practice. The positive effect of occlusion on the rate of epidermal resurfacing in noninfected superficial wounds has been proven multiple times with various types of synthetic surgical dressings.

The emergence of biosynthetic occlusive or semi-occlusive dressings have provided the cutaneous surgeon with many superior alternatives in treating various types of ulcers, abrasions, burns, or wounds (19-22). The occlusive dressings can be divided into films of polyurethane and polyethylene, hydrogels of cross-linked polyethylene oxide or polyvinyl-pyrrolidone, composite polymers, and hydrocolloids of gelatin, pectin and carboxymethyl cellulose. In controlled situations, these dressings speed re-epithelialization, decrease pain, and absorb water, serum, or blood through expansion of the dressing matrix. Adhesives are not used in all of these dressing formulations, but when present may consist of acrylics, latex, or other components. Contact dermatitis resulting from the use of these synthetic surgical dressings has been rarely reported (23).

CONTACT DERMATITIS FOLLOWING LASER SKIN RESURFACING

Clinical experience has shown that patients undergoing laser skin resurfacing are at an apparent increased risk for developing contact dermatitis (4, 5, 13, 24). Not only can this complication contribute significantly to postoperative morbidity, it may also result in increased pain and swelling, delayed healing, prolonged erythema, and in some severe cases permanent textural changes or hypertrophic scarring. Although relatively common, the factors predisposing patients who undergo laser skin resurfacing to this reaction have not been clearly defined with meticulous patch testing or allergen challenge tests (25). Therefore, consideration of the potential causes of these reactions must include preoperative scrubs or antiseptics, topical or local anesthetics, and postoperative topical antibiotics, adhesives or dressings (26-37). Because of the apparent increased incidence of allergic reactions to many of the standard postoperative dressings and topical agents, a minimalistic approach to healing following laser resurfacing has been promulgated by some in which no topical lotions or ointments are applied and the wound is left open to the air to heal by second intention. Obviously, more clinical research is required to first determine the cause of these allergic reactions and then develop an effective hydrating topical preparation or synthetic surgical dressing that can be safely used in patients undergoing laser skin resurfacing without difficulty.

ADVANCES IN CO_2 LASER TECHNOLOGY

Understanding the Mechanism of the Laser-Tissue Interaction

To properly use short-pulsed, high energy CO_2 lasers, an improved understanding of the laser-tissue interaction is necessary (38-40). Currently, the mechanism of action for these devices is poorly understood and the duration of the effects produced is unclear. One question that must be answered is the relative role played by each of the various components of the laser resurfacing process: ablation, residual collateral thermal damage, postoperative erythema, and inflammation.

Since the ideal pulse duration and pulse energy have also not yet been fully defined, it remains possible that perhaps even shorter pulse durations might prove to be more effective in skin resurfacing. At least one of the current CO_2 lasers (TruPulse, Tissue Technologies, Inc., Albuquerque, NM) operates in the 60 to 90 msec domain, and can even be operated in the nanosecond domain (7). However, without a clear understanding of the role that pulse duration and collateral injury play in producing skin rejuvenation, it remains speculative whether or not shorter pulses would be helpful in improving the cosmetic result (40, 41). With reports now currently appearing of hypopigmentation developing in patients 2 to 3 years following laser resurfacing, it also seems reasonable to investigate the apparent increased susceptibility of melanocytes to infrared light at different pulse durations.

Additionally, with limited follow-up of 4 to 5 years duration, more research must be performed to satisfactorily answer the question as to how long the beneficial effects of laser resurfacing persist. Also, even though collagen shrinkage following laser resurfacing has now been adequately documented, there is little information as to the length of time this effect persists and what role it plays in determining the final cosmetic appearance of the resurfaced patient (9).

New Robotic Scanners for CO_2 Lasers

At present, a large number of robotic scanners exist that permit safe and rapid treatment of large areas with highly reproducible results (1, 4). Future developments in robotic technology could allow use of larger scan sizes providing more sophisticated programming to reduce, or even potentially eliminate, the surgeon's role in actually performing the procedure while simultaneously providing ideal reproducibility and safety. Three-dimensional models are currently under development to deal with the difficulty in treating a complex surface like the human face.

Higher Power CO_2 Laser Systems

The speed with which CO_2 laser skin resurfacing can currently be performed is determined by peak energies, pulse duration, pulse energies and repetition rates of each individual device. Higher peak energies would permit the delivery of larger beam diameters at a faster repetition rate and thus reduce the operating time for the treatment of large surface areas. The two biggest problems associated with the development of lasers that can deliver higher peak energies and faster

repetition rates are the size of the instrument and the greater production cost. It remains to be determined if the benefits in laser skin resurfacing that might occur from the development of larger, more powerful CO_2 lasers would outweigh the additional cost and bulk of the instrument. However, many laser companies continue to perform significant amounts of research and development to provide smaller, less expensive, more powerful and user-friendly devices for laser skin resurfacing.

ERBIUM:YAG LASER

The Erbium:YAG (Er:YAG) laser emits infrared light at a wavelength of 2940 nm, which is the highest absorptive peak for water. As a result, this source of light can provide extremely precise ablation of soft tissue, including skin, by operating at 4 to 5 J/cm^2 at a pulse duration of 250 to 350 msec with a 5-mm spot size.

Soft tissue ablation is possible with the Er:YAG laser because it does not char the skin surface and limits the collateral thermal damage to less than 50 μm (42). These user friendly devices can provide an effective form of treatment for fine to medium coarse wrinkles, especially periorally, where no topical or local anesthetic is typically required (43). When treating periorbital rhytides, however, sedation and local anesthetics are often required to obtain optimal patient compliance during the procedure. Some bleeding can be anticipated with the Er:YAG laser as the ablation proceeds deeper into tissue because hemostasis is poor with the laser. This complication limits the potential usefulness of the device to superficial Class I and Class II rhytides only as the blood will absorb the Er:YAG laser energy and prevent deeper treatment. However, this may also be viewed as a safety feature since it may prevent deeper penetration and subsequent scarring if the light is held too long in one place. The poor hemostatic capabilities of the Er:YAG laser does, however, substantially increase the risk of transmission of infectious blood borne pathogens to members of the operative team.

The benefits of precise Er:YAG laser ablation with minimal thermal effects is seen as rapid healing, less postoperative pigmentary alteration and reduced erythema. However, the biggest concern about using the Er:YAG laser for resurfacing is that the mechanism of action remains undefined. In view of this fact, it remains at least possible that there is insufficient residual thermal damage following Er:YAG laser ablation to stimulate the production of new collagen and elastic fibers and to provide a rejuvenating effect. Also, the lack of clear clinical signs of penetration depth make endpoints difficult to discern. For these reasons, much additional research with longer follow-up periods is required to determine the potential role that Er:YAG lasers may play in the future of laser resurfacing.

HOLMIUM:YAG LASER

Very little is currently known about the potential usefulness of the Holmium:YAG (Ho:YAG) laser for skin resurfacing. However, its prior use in orthopedic surgery indicates that it can precisely ablate tissue while producing minimal collateral thermal damage (44, 45). This capability is due to its emission at 2,100 nm, which is a substantial absorptive peak for water. For that reason, it is anticipated that light from the Ho:YAG laser could be delivered via fiberoptics to ablate skin while causing only limited collateral thermal damage. Also, since the Ho:YAG laser's absorption profile indicates high intracellular and extracellular water absorption, hemostasis following exposure to this wavelength of light is likely to be good.

Obviously, much additional clinical and basic research is required with the Ho:YAG laser before the appropriate clinical indications and laser parameters can be determined. In addition, the two biggest disadvantages of this system are the high cost of the device and the undesirable mechanical damage produced by the photoacoustic wave from this system, similar to the Q-switched lasers, that might be expected at the shorter pulse durations produced by the device.

DIODE LASER

High-energy laser diode arrays (LDAs) are capable of delivering sufficient energy at a wavelength of 805 nm to cut or ablate soft tissue. However, since this wavelength of light is poorly absorbed by living tissue, thermal coagulation is only possible by first applying a topical solution of indocyanine green dye (46, 47).

The low cost, small size, and portability of the diode laser make it a potentially attractive system for practitioners with multiple medical offices. Too little information currently exists to know if the combination of topical dye and laser light offer sufficient precision and effectiveness to allow this device to be advantageously used for skin resurfacing. More research into this area should help define the potential for this category of lasers.

NEODYMIUM:YAG LASER (1320 nm)

Recently, the Neodymium:YAG (Nd:YAG) laser has been employed in clinical trials as a nonablative recontouring device. Operating at a wavelength of 1320 nm, a macropulse of infrared light is delivered to the skin surface overlying fine periorbital rhytides (48). This technique allows thermal energy to be delivered with one or more passes of laser energy using a pulse waveform of three 200 msec pulses at 100 Hz, and energy fluences of 10 to 25 J/cm^2 with a 5- mm spot size delivered by a fiberoptic cable to the dermal structures. To prevent thermal damage to the epithelium, a short burst of cryogen is sprayed on the skin surface preceding the pulse of laser light. This process, known as dynamic cooling, serves to cool and protect the epidermis while not lowering the temperature of the dermis (49).

It is assumed that the thermal energy presumably stimulates collagen synthesis by fibroblasts to produce an improvement in the clinical appearance of the wrinkle. However, the mechanism has not been defined at this point and extended clinical studies are currently underway to evaluate the potential benefit of performing a series of treatments at 7 to 10-day intervals in an attempt to further augment the stimulatory effects of this infrared light.

LOW ENERGY LASERS

One potential future laser application is the use of nonablative low-energy lasers (LELs) to noninvasively modify wound healing or rejuvenate aged or photodamaged skin by stimulating changes in the composition and structure of the dermis (50-58). An LEL is defined as one that, upon exposure, produces a minimal temperature elevation in tissue of less than 0.1°C to 0.5°C (33). The most commonly used LEL systems are the helium-neon (HeNe) laser, the gallium-arsenide (GaA) laser and the gallium-aluminum-arsenide (GaAlA) laser (Table 19.1). All of these devices produce red light that can be delivered by fiber optics through the skin surface without requiring the creation of a surgical wound or incision.

Through basic cellular and molecular biology research the mechanisms by which LELs can stimulate various cell functions have been identified (Table 19.2). This research has demonstrated a number of photobiologic effects produced by LELs in a variety of different cell types (59). For cultured human fibroblasts, low energy light from a HeNe laser was capable of stimulating the attachment of fibroblasts to a substrate, increasing collagen synthesis and fibroblast proliferation (60, 61). It

TABLE 19.1

TYPES OF LOW ENERGY LASERS

Laser	Wavelength	Color of Emission
Helium-Neon (HeNe)	632.8 nm	Red
Gallium-Arsenide (GaAs)	904 nm	Near-Infrared
Gallium-Aluminum-Arsenide (GaAlAs)	805 nm	Near-Infrared
Neodymium:Yttrium-aluminum-garnet (Nd:YAG)	1,064 nm	Near-Infrared

TABLE 19.2

EFFECTS OF LOW ENERGY LASERS ON HEALING

Stimulatory Effects	Laser
Keratinocytes	
Cell motility	HeNe
RNA synthesis	HeNe & GaAs
DNA synthesis	HeNe & GaAs
Fibroblasts	
Cell proliferation	HeNe
Cell binding ability	HeNe
Collagen synthesis	HeNe & GaAs
Membrane potential	HeNe

was suggested that the mechanism by which LELs might produce these changes included stimulation of the co-enzyme nicotinamide adenine dehydrogenase (NADH) (62), photoactivation of catalase (a porphyrin-containing enzyme), or increase the transmembrane electrical potential in mitochondria to stimulate the synthesis of adenosine triphosphate. For keratinocytes, both the proliferation and motility can be stimulated by exposure to LELs (63, 64). The mechanism for this observed effect might be a local increase in the production of plasminogen activator, a protease that can stimulate keratinocyte migration (65).

In wound healing it has also been shown that light from LELs can stimulate the closure rate of open wounds and the rate of tensile strength development in incised wounds (52, 66). The mechanism for this effect, was a significant increase in the collagen synthesis as a result of increases in both type I and type III procollagen mRNA suggesting an enhancement of gene expression (57). However, it has been proposed that the myofibroblast, the cell responsible for most of the wound contraction that occurs during full thickness wound healing, may be responsive to LEL light. Light from a LEL is also capable of promoting neovascularization as determined by measuring blood flow through microangiography. This neovascularization might be partially responsible for producing some of the beneficial effects seen in rejuvenating aged or photodamaged skin (67). It is apparent from both human and animal research that LELs can stimulate various aspects of wound healing and that these effects might also prove useful in modifying the epidermal and dermal damage produced by aging or chronic sunlight exposure. These effects are produced in cell cultures by regulating the biosynthesis of various proteins, growth factors, DNA and RNA. Since the physiologic conditions under which these changes occur have not been fully defined and the ideal laser parameters to use in each clinical situation have not been established, it is anticipated that additional re-

search will be required before these devices will become an integral part of the rejuvenation process.

LASER CONCEPTS OF RELEVANCE TO SKIN RESURFACING—PHOTOABLATIVE DECOMPOSITION

Photoablative decomposition is a nonthermal form of tissue ablation that occurs when high energy photons are generated by a laser that produces a physical plasma. These photons are of sufficiently high energy to break molecular bonds, thus generating photoacoustic shock waves, producing cavitation bubbles that fragment the targeted tissue and eject the skin pieces from the impact site with a result of precise tissue ablation. The depth of the sharply defined and smooth-walled ablation crater can be optimized by the pulse threshold, which typically has an intensity of 2.5 terawatts/cm^2. Both subthreshold and suprathreshold pulses do not produce tissue ablation. Typical ablation depths are 0.1 μm at 2 mJ and 100 μm at 36 mJ.

Tissue ablation must be performed in a helium atmosphere to reduce the distortion of the pulse and prevent the nonlinear breakdown of air that could otherwise occur. Tissue ablation by plasmas from either the excimer or titanium sapphire (Ti:Al$_2$O$_3$) lasers is incredibly precise as the control is determined by both the number and energy of pulses. As an example, the epidermis can be precisely removed by delivering one pulse from the Ti:Al$_2$O$_3$ laser at 22 mJ, ten pulses at 9 mJ, or 100 pulses at 2 mJ. Although the precise cellular effects remain unknown following exposure to the light from either titanium-sapphire or excimer lasers, there is minimal nonthermal collateral damage varying in width from 0 to 30 μm.

The potential clinical uses for photoablative decomposition in skin resurfacing include the precise treatment of superficial lesions without scarring caused by unwanted thermal injury. This would likely speed wound healing and improve the cosmetic result.

TITANIUM:SAPPHIRE LASER

The titanium:sapphire (Ti:Al$_2$O$_3$) laser is an experimental solid state device that consists of a titanium-doped sapphire rod (Al$_2$O$_3$). It is a tunable system that is capable of operating at wavelengths from 695 to 905 nm at peak intensities of up to 10 terawatts (10^{12}), and pulse durations of less than 120 femtoseconds (10^{-15}). Because of these features, the titanium:sapphire laser is capable of producing photoablative decomposition (68). These experimental lasers are extremely expensive to operate and have a potential for unwanted photomechanical effects when they are used at higher energy fluences.

EXCIMER LASERS = *EXCITED DIMER*

The excimer lasers are a group of rare earth-halide medium lasers and are characterized by the argon-fluoride, krypton-fluoride, xenon-chloride and xenon-chloride lasers. These devices produce light at wavelengths of 193 nm, 248 nm, 308 nm and 351 nm, respectively. This emission spectrum produced by these lasers is of concern because of the potential mutagenic effects that may be induced by the lasers' ultraviolet light. Due to difficulty in achieving and preserving a homogeneous beam profile, there are high operational costs associated with the operation of these lasers. In addition, these systems contain highly toxic gases that require special handling and precautions. The excimer lasers share many features with the titanium:sapphire laser and can produce precise photoablative decomposition (69). At present, the excimer lasers have been approved for correcting visual refractive errors by performing precise corneal sculpting (70).

CONCLUSION

At the present time, laser skin resurfacing using the new short-pulse, high-energy CO_2 lasers are primarily indicated for rejuvenating photodamaged skin seen as fine to medium-coarse periorbital and perioral rhytides, extensive solar elastosis, atrophy with mottled pigmentation and a leathery texture with excess skin laxity. Local and extensive actinic damage with actinic keratoses, actinic cheilitis and lentigines can also be effectively corrected with this new technique. In addition, the revision of atrophic acne scars, broad or spread traumatic and surgical scars are also possible with current techniques (71). It is anticipated that future developments will broaden the scope of skin resurfacing to include a wider range of patients and clinical conditions with the added benefits of more rapid healing and a reduction in the risks and complications that can occur with the current procedure. In order for any significant advances in laser skin resurfacing to be accomplished in the future, a substantial amount of basic research must be done to understand and subsequently control the mechanisms involved in the laser-rejuvenation process. Only then can new surgical techniques, dressings and better equipment be developed to provide patients with better clinical results. In addition, it is anticipated that, in the future, techniques employing the nonablative Nd:YAG laser and low energy diode lasers will be sufficiently refined to allow effective nonsurgical treatment of fine rhytides and other signs of photodamage. Also in the future, the mechanism of the laser-tissue interaction associated with photoablative decomposition will likely provide much useful information that can help to further modify the current laser resurfacing techniques and reduce the risks of hypertrophic scarring, textural and pigmentary changes.

REFERENCES

1. Weinstein C. UltraPulse carbon dioxide laser removal of periocular wrinkles in association with laser blepharoplasty. J Clin Laser Med Surg 1994;12:205-209.
2. Fitzpatrick RE, Goldman MP. Advances in carbon dioxide laser surgery. Clin Dermatol 1995;13:35-47.
3. Hruza GJ, Dover JS. Laser skin resurfacing. Arch Dermatol 1996;132:451-455.
4. Fitzpatrick RE, Goldman MP, Satur NM, Tope WD. Pulsed carbon dioxide laser resurfacing of photoaged facial skin. Arch Dermatol 1996;132:395-402.
5. Trelles MA, David LM, Rigau J. Penetration depth of UltraPulse carbon dioxide laser in human skin. Dermatol Surg 1996;22:863-865.
6. Alster TS. Comparison of two high-energy, pulsed carbon dioxide lasers in the treatment of periorbital rhytides. Dermatol Surg 1996;22:541-545.
7. Smith KJ, Graham JS, Hamilton TA, et al. Additional observations using a pulsed carbon dioxide laser with a fixed pulse duration. Arch Dermatol 1997;133:105-107.
8. Fitzpatrick RE, Tope WD, Goldman MP, et al. Pulsed carbon dioxide laser, trichloroacetic acid, Baker-Gordon phenol, and dermabrasion: a comparative clinical and histologic study of cutaneous resurfacing in a porcine model. Arch Dermatol 1996;132:469-471.
9. Gardner ES, Reinisch L, Stricklin GP, et al. In vitro changes in non-facial human skin following CO_2 laser resurfacing: a comparison study. Lasers Surg Med 1996;19:379-387.
10. Reynolds RD. Vitamin supplements: current controversies. J Am Coll Nutr 1994;13:118-126.
11. Goldfarb MT, Ellis CN, Weiss JS, et al. Topical tretinoin therapy: its use in photoaged skin. J Am Acad Dermatol 1989;21:645-650.
12. Griffiths CEM, Russman AN, Majmudar G, et al. Restoration of collagen formation in photodamaged human skin by tretinoin (retinoic acid). New Engl J Med 1993;329:530-535.
13. Lowe NJ, Lask G, Griffin ME. Laser skin resurfacing: pre- and posttreatment guidelines. Dermatol Surg 1995;21:1017-1019.
14. Brown GL, Curtsinger L, Brightwell JR, et al. Enhancement of epidermal regeneration by biosynthetic epidermal growth factor. J Exp Med 1986;163:1319-1324.
15. Brown GL, Nanney LB, Griffen J, et al. Enhancement of wound healing by topical treatment with epidermal growth factor. New Engl J Med 1989;321:76-79.
16. Nanney LB. Epidermal and dermal effects of epidermal growth factor during wound repair. J Invest Dermatol 1990;94:624-629.
17. Winter GD. Effects of air drying and dressings on the surface of a wound. Nature 1963;197:91-92.
18. Eaglstein WH, Davis SC, Mehle AL, et al. Optimal use of an occlusive dressing to enhance healing: Effect of delayed application and early removal on wound healing. Arch Dermatol 1988;124:392-395.

19. Curreri W, Desai M, Bartlett R, et al. Safety and efficacy of a new synthetic burn dressing. Arch Surg 1980;115:925-927.

20. Barnett A, Berkowitz R, Mills R, Bistnes L. Comparison of synthetic adhesive moisture vapor permeable and fine-mesh gauze dressings for split-thickness skin graft donor sites. Am J Surg 1983;145:379-381.

21. Eaglstein W. Experiences with biosynthetic dressings. J Am Acad Dermatol 1985;12:434-440.

22. Young JR, Terwoord BA. Stasis ulcer treatment with compression dressing. Cleve Clin J Med 1990;57:529-531.

23. Helland S, Nyfors A, Utne L. Contact dermatitis to Synthaderm™. Contact Derm 1983;9:504-506.

24. Waldorf HA, Kauvar ANB, Geronemus RG. Skin resurfacing of fine to deep rhytides using a char-free carbon dioxide laser in forty-seven patients. Dermatol Surg 1995;21:940-946.

25. Wilhelm K, Maibach H. Factors predisposing to cutaneous irritation. Dermatol Clin 1990;8:17-22.

26. Marks J, Rainey M. Cutaneous reactions to surgical preparations and dressings. Contact Derm 1984;10:1-5.

27. Fernandes deCorres L, Leanizbarrutia I. Dermatitis from lignocaine. Contact Derm 1985;12:114-115.

28. Curley R, Macfarlane A, King C. Contact sensitivity to the amide anesthetics lidocaine, prilocaine, and mepivacaine. Arch Dermatol 1986;122:924-926.

29. Ashinoff R, Geronemus R. Effect of the topical anesthetic EMLA on the efficacy of pulse dye laser treatment of port-wine stains. J Dermatol Surg Oncol 1990;16:1008-1011.

30. Glinert RJ, Zachary CB. Local anesthetic allergy. J Dermatol Surg Oncol 1991;17:491-496.

31. Taylor JS, Cassettari J, Wagner W, Helm T. Contact urticaria and anaphylaxis to latex. J Am Acad Dermatol 1989;21:874-877.

32. Turjanmaa K, Reunala T, Alenius H, et al. Allergens in latex surgical gloves and glove powder. Lancet 1990;336:1588.

33. Prystowsky S, Nonomura J, Smith R, et al. Allergic hypersensitivity to neomycin. Arch Dermatol 1979;115:713-715.

34. Held JL, Kalb RE, Ruszkowski AM, DeLeo V. Allergic contact dermatitis from bacitracin. J Am Acad Dermatol 1987;17:592-594.

35. Fisher A. Topical medicaments which are common sensitizers. Ann Allergy 1982;49:97-100.

36. Bryant RA. Saving the skin from tape injuries. Am J Nurs 1988;88:189-191.

37. Norris P, Storrs FJ. Allergic contact dermatitis to adhesive bandages. Dermatol Clin 1990;8:147-152.

38. Fulton JE Jr. Dermabrasion, chemabrasion, and laserabrasion: Historical perspectives, modern dermabrasion techniques, and future trends. Dermatol Surg 1996;22:619-628.

39. Alster TS, Lewis AB. Dermatologic laser surgery: a review. Dermatol Surg 1996;22:797-805.

40. Cotton J, Hood AF, Gonin R, et al. Histologic evaluation of preauricular and postauricular human skin after high-energy, short-pulse carbon dioxide laser. Arch Dermatol 1996;132:425-428.

41. Ross EV, Domankevitz Y, Skrobal M, Anderson RR. Effects of CO_2 laser pulse duration in ablation and residual thermal damage: implications for skin resurfacing. Laser Surg Med 1996;19:123-129.

42. Kaufman R, Hibst R. Pulsed 2.94 micron erbium-YAG laser skin ablation: experimental results and first clinical application. Clin Exp Dermatol 1990;15:389-393.

43. Kaufmann R, Hibst R. Pulsed erbium:YAG laser ablation in cutaneous surgery. Lasers Surg Med 1996;19:324-330.

44. Soffa AJ, Markel MD, Converse LJ, et al. Treatment of inflammatory arthritis by synovial ablation: a comparison of the holmium:YAG laser, electrocautery, and mechanical ablation in a rabbit model. Lasers Surg Med 1996;19:143-151.

45. Domankevitz Y, McMillan K, Nishioka NS. Characterization of tissue ablation with a continuous wave holmium laser. Lasers Surg Med 1996;19:97-102.

46. Diven DG, Pohl J, Motamedi M. Dye-enhanced diode laser photothermal ablation of skin. J Am Acad Dermatol 1996;35:211-215.

47. Cromeens DM, Johnson DE, Stephens LC, Gray KN. Visual laser ablation of the canine prostate with a diffusing fiber and an 805-nanometer diode laser. Lasers Surg Med 1996;19:135-142.

48. Nelson JS, Milner TE, Dave D, et al. Clinical study of non-ablative laser treatment of facial rhytides. Lasers Surg Med 1997;9(Suppl):32-33.

49. Milner TE, Dave D, Anvari B, et al. Pulsed photothermal radiometry measurements of skin irradiated under non-ablative laser wrinkle reduction conditions. Lasers Surg Med 1997;9(Suppl):44.

50. Mester E, Spiry T, Szende B, Tota JG. Effect of laser rays on wound healing. Am J Surg 1971;122:532-535.

51. Kana JS, Hutschenreiter G, Haina D, Waidelich W. Effect of low-power density laser radiation on healing of open skin wounds in rats. Arch Surg 1981;116:293-296.

52. Surinchak JS, Alago ML, Bellamy RF, et al. Effects of low-level energy lasers on the healing of full-thickness skin defects. Lasers Surg Med 1983;2:267-274.

53. Hunter J, Leonard L, Wilson R, et al. Effects of low energy laser on wound healing in a porcine model. Lasers Surg Med 1984;3:285-290.

54. Abergel RP, Meeker CA, Lam TS, et al. Control of connective tissue metabolism by lasers: recent developments and future prospects. J Am Acad Dermatol 1984;11:1142-1150.

55. Mester E, Ludani G, Selyei M, et al. The stimulating effect of low power laser rays on biological systems. Laser Rev 1986;1:3-8.

56. Lyons RF, Abergel RP, White RA, et al. Biostimulation of wound healing in vivo by a helium-neon laser. Ann Plast Surg 1987;18:47-50.

57. Abergel RP, Lyons RF, Castel JC, et al. Biostimulation of wound healing by lasers: experimental approaches in animal models and in fibroblast cultures. J Dermatol Surg Oncol 1987;13:127-133.

58. Braverman B, McCarthy RJ, Ivankovich AD, et al. Effect of helium-neon and infrared laser irradiation on wound healing in rabbits. Lasers Surg Med 1989;9:50-58.

59. Basford JR. Low-energy laser therapy: controversies and new research findings. Lasers Surg Med 1989;9:1-5.

60. Boulton M, Marshall J. He-Ne laser stimulation of human fibroblast proliferation and attachment in vitro. Lasers Life Sci 1986;1:125-134.

61. Lam TS, Abergel RP, Meeker CA, et al. Laser stimulation of collagen synthesis in human skin fibroblast cultures. Lasers Life Sci 1986;1:61-77.

62. Pasarella S, Dechecchi MS, Quagliariello E, et al. Optical and biochemical properties of NADH irradiated by high peak power Q-switched ruby laser or by low power CW He-Ne laser. Bioelectrochem Bioenerg 1981;8:315-319.

63. Haas AF, Isseroff RR, Wheeland RG, et al. Low-energy helium-neon laser irradiation increases the motility of cultured human keratinocytes. J Invest Dermatol 1990;94: 822-826.

64. Rood PA, Haas AF, Graves PJ, et al. Low-energy helium neon laser irradiation does not alter human keratinocyte differentiation. J Invest Dermatol 1992;99:445-448.

65. Morioka S, Lazarus GS, Baud JL, Jensen PJ. Migrating keratinocytes express urokinase-type plasminogen activator. J Invest Dermatol 1987;88:418-423.

66. Wheeland RG. Lasers for the stimulation or inhibition of wound healing. J Dermatol Surg Oncol 1993;19:747-752.

67. Namenyi J, Mester E, Foldes I, et al. Effect of laser irradiation and immunosuppressive treatment on survival of mouse skin allotransplants. Acta Chir Acad Sci Hung 1975;16:327-335.

68. Frederickson KS, White WE, Wheeland RG, et al. Precise ablation of skin with reduced collateral damage using the femtosecond-pulsed, terawatt titanium-sapphire laser. Arch Dermatol 1993;129:989-993.

69. Parrish JA. Ultraviolet-laser ablation. Arch Dermatol 1985; 121:599-600.

70. Watenebe S, Flotte TJ, McAuliffe DJ, et al. Putative photoacoustic damage in skin induced by pulsed ArF excimer laser. J Invest Dermatol 1988;90:761-766.

71. Alster TS, West TB. Resurfacing of atrophic facial acne scars with a high-energy, pulsed carbon dioxide laser. Dermatol Surg 1996;22:151-155.

SECTION V

Combination Approaches

CHAPTER 20

Combining Skin Resurfacing Modalities

■ Naomi Lawrence
William P. Coleman III

There are marked interfacial variations in the signs of intrinsic and extrinsic (photo) aging. Each cosmetic unit ages on its own timetable (1). The periocular region is usually the first to show lines and wrinkles especially in the lateral canthal (crow's feet) area. This is usually due to a combination of a thinning skin envelope in association with repeated contraction of the relatively powerful orbicularis oculi muscle. Smiling also "crinkles" the lower lid and gradually leads to a network of fine rhytides. In people with very expressive faces, horizontal forehead lines and parallel smile lines lateral to the angles of the mouth also appear early. Next, the glabella frown lines show in people predisposed to squinting or frowning. Vertical lip lines show up later and are almost exclusively seen in women, especially in those who smoke or purse their lips. Curvilinear wrinkles in the substance of the cheek are seen with advanced aging or earlier in those who have sun-damaged skin.

Conventional cosmetic wisdom is to treat the cosmetic units of the face as separate entities and match the level of resurfacing to the changes in that unit. For years segmental combinations of dermabrasion with peeling and deep peeling with medium depth peeling have been used for facial rejuvenation. With the arrival of laser resurfacing the wisdom of combining different modalities has come into question. One reason for this questioning is the intense postoperative erythema seen in most patients after laser treatment. Some experts feel that this erythema gives a very unnatural appearance and is more difficult to disguise with makeup unless the full face has been treated (Fig. 20.1).

Another reason for questioning the wisdom of combining modalities is the "skin tightening" seen with laser resurfacing. The belief is that more advantage can be made of this pseudo lifting if the whole face is treated. For instance, laser resurfacing in the nasolabial region on both sides of the furrow tightens from two directions achieving more softening of this area (Fig 20.2). Although these are two excellent reasons to use full face laser resurfacing, there are equally compelling reasons to combine modalities or use laser resurfacing more sparingly.

Many patients require conscious sedation or general anesthesia for full face resurfacing. Laser resurfacing of the periocular and perioral areas combined with a medium depth peel of the rest of the face can be done easily with local anesthesia and oral sedation (and sometimes with intramuscular analgesics). This results in less cost. Also, as the number of units resurfaced with laser increases, the infection rate increases (2). Certainly deeper resurfacing (laser, dermabrasion, phenol peel) has a greater complication rate than a medium depth peel. Finally, one risks patient misperception of motives (i.e., "I only came in to get my eyes done and he/she convinced me to do more"). This is a particularly sensitive issue. It becomes even more difficult if the patient experiences a complication (such as hypo- or hyperpigmentation, or persistent erythema) in a location remote from their area of chief concern.

DEEP RESURFACING MODALITIES

Each technique has inherent advantages and disadvantages (Table 20.1). These must be carefully considered

by the physician as a custom plan for care is formulated. When in doubt, do not use techniques with as many disadvantages as advantages for that patient. The first rule is "do no harm."

INDICATIONS FOR DEEP RESURFACING IN A SINGLE COSMETIC UNIT

Acne Scars

Some areas are very appropriately treated in isolation. In a young patient who is fair skinned with acne scaring confined to the cheeks and temple region, "blending"of the nose and forehead cosmetic units is not necessary if there is little evidence of photodamage. Also, some erythema in the cheek area has an acceptable cosmetic appearance. Laser resurfacing or dermabrasion both work well on acne scars (Fig. 20.3). The choice between these two modalities is operator dependent. However, dermabrasion allows simultaneous excision and repair of deep scars. Also, there are vastly larger clinical experience and proven long-term results with this technique.

Scarabrasion

A surgical or traumatic scar is also an indication for treatment of a single area. Studies show that scars are

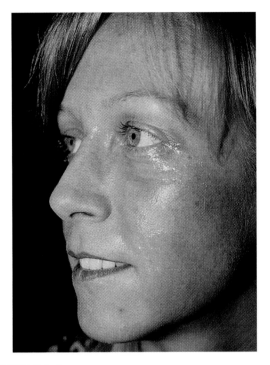

FIGURE 20.1

Appearance 1 week after laser resurfacing in the periocular and smile line areas.

FIGURE 20.2

A, Appearance before softening of nasolabial folds with full face laser. B, Appearance 1 month postoperatively.

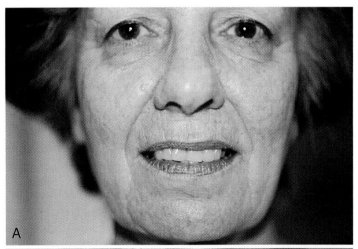

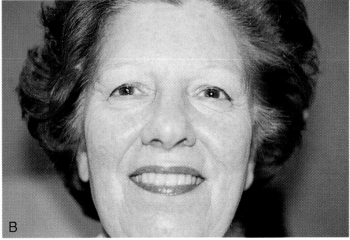

TABLE 20.1

COMPARING DEEP RESURFACING MODALITIES

	Dermabrasion	Laser Resurfacing	Phenol Peels
Blood, aerosol exposure	++	+	0
Degree of manual dexterity required	High	Low	Low
Cost of equipment	Low	High	Low
Postoperative hypopigmentation	Low	Low	High
Postoperative hyperpigmentation	Low	High	Low
Scar	Low	Low	Low
Infection	Low	Moderate	Low

optimally resurfaced 6 to 8 weeks after wounding (3, 4). If it is not possible to treat the scar this soon, it can still reorganize and improve when older, but results are better if done less than 1 year after trauma or surgery. Although there are no studies that prove the efficacy of laser resurfacing for improving surgical or traumatic scars, it is probable that the depth of destruction caused by the laser is sufficient to cause scar reorganization. The authors still prefer dermabrasion because the postoperative erythema is less intense and fades much quicker (Fig. 20.4).

Actinically Damaged Scalp (and Forehead)

It is common for men with early onset androgenic alopecia to have a severely actinically damaged scalp and forehead. This is often disproportionate to the actinic damage on the rest of the face. Therefore, deep resurfacing in the affected unit may be indicated in these patients. All three resurfacing modalities are treatment options in these patients: deep or aggressive medium depth peel, dermabrasion, or laser resurfacing. Medium depth peeling has been studied in the

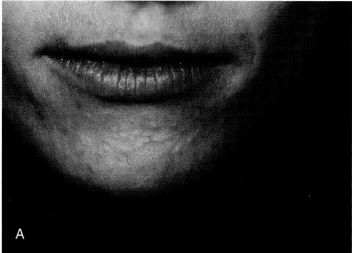

FIGURE 20.3

A, Appearance of the chin before laser resurfacing for acne scarring. B, Appearance 4 months after laser treatment. (Figure courtesy of Sue Ellen Cox, MD.)

FIGURE 20.4
A, 6 weeks after bilobed flap operation (pre-dermabrasion). B, Bilobed flap 4 months post-dermabrasion.

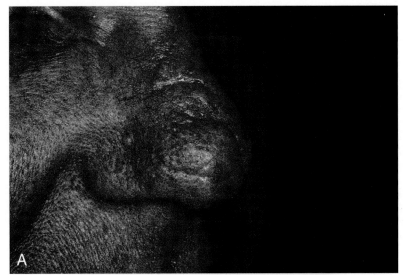

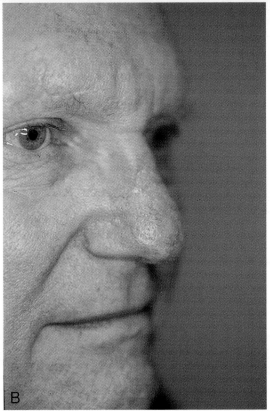

treatment of widespread actinic damage and was found to be equally effective as 3 weeks of topical 5 fluorouracil (5-FU) application (5). The effect of 5-FU and medium depth peels lasted at least 1 year but usually requires retreatment in 3 years. The advantage of the medium depth peel is that morbidity is lower than 5-FU. Patients in the study preferred the medium depth peel. Dermabrasion has also been studied in the treatment of widespread actinic damage (Fig. 20.5). Dermabrasion has greater morbidity than the medium depth peel but is longer lasting (5 to 15 years) (6, 7).

Resurfacing lasers should theoretically work similarly to dermabrasion because of the depth of destruction. Again, the intense erythema postoperatively in this location is not as cosmetically acceptable. Also, this is a patient population (males) who cannot camouflage with make up. Finally, the laser would require anesthetic blocks, local anesthesia, and possibly sedation. Medium depth peels are tolerated with no local or sedation. Dermabrasion of the scalp and forehead is well tolerated with the cryogen refrigerant sprays or tumescent local anesthesia.

Nose: Actinic Damage, Rhinophyma, Acne Scarring

Often skin pathology is found only on the nose when the rest of the face is relatively undamaged. Actinic degeneration often occurs preferentially on the nose because of its prominent facial location in relation to the sun above. Patients are sometimes seen with recurrent actinic keratoses of the dorsum and lateral aspects of the nose. These patients are more prone to the development of cutaneous malignancies on the nose. Chemical peeling, dermabrasion, or laser resurfacing may be employed on the entire nasal cosmetic unit to eliminate these precancerous changes. Sometimes a resurfacing procedure is done in combination with reconstruction after flap or graft surgery to blur the margins of the repair. Local anesthesia is all that is required for dermabrasion or laser resurfacing of the nose. The tumescent anesthetic technique using 0.1% lidocaine and 1:500,000 epinephrine is particularly appropriate for these modalities.

Rhinophyma may occur with or without accompanying rosacea. Some patients are genetically prone to gradual thickening of the nasal skin. This can become quite exuberant creating a distracting deformity. Rhinophyma of the skin may be planed down by dermabrasion or laser. These two approaches are preferred to electrosurgery, which creates a great deal of thermal damage and the potential for scarring or alar retraction. The resurfacing should be performed three-dimensionally to resculpt the original shape of the nose. Tumescent local anesthesia also works well here omitting the need for significant sedation.

Acne scarring may also occur preferentially on the nose. Often these scars are deeply pitted and respond only moderately well to resurfacing with dermabrasion or laser. Although punch grafting may be employed, it is difficult to match the thick sebaceous skin of the nose with a retro-auricular graft. The thicker skin near the inferior posterior auricular area usually matches better than the thinner skin above. Alternatively, excision and repair of these pits can be performed prior to dermabrasion or laser resurfacing. However, the sebaceous skin often found accompanying this type of scarring heals poorly and there is a possibility of creating an even worse defect using excisional surgery. Often the best approach is to simply resurface the skin as far down as feasible, and to inform the patient that only partial improvement may be obtained. Additional resurfacing procedures can be performed at one year intervals to achieve improved results.

Lower Eyelid Rhytides

In many younger individuals there are significant rhytides of the lower lid and crow's feet area even though the rest of the face is mildly wrinkled. The lower lids can be resurfaced by laser or deep chemical peeling

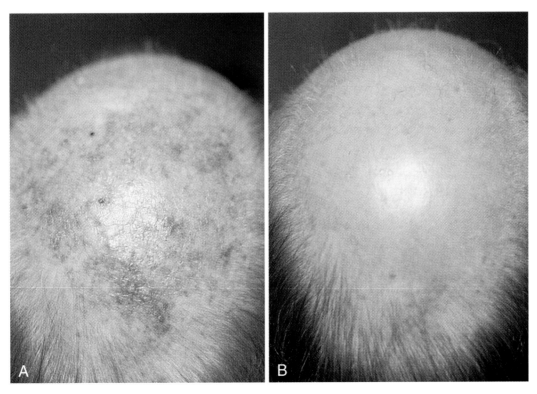

FIGURE 20.5
A, Appearance of scalp before dermabrasion. B, Appearance 3 months postoperatively.

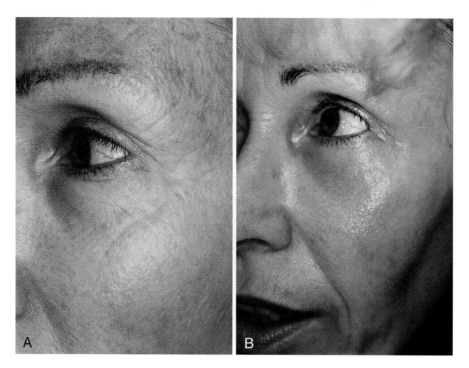

FIGURE 20.6
A, Appearance before laser abrasion of periocular skin. B, Appearance 5 weeks postoperatively, only erythema remains.

with or without treating the rest of the face. In these cases, it is important to feather the edges of the more deeply resurfaced lids (Fig. 20.6). Using the laser in a defocused mode or at an angle helps to blend the margins of the resurfacing in with the surrounding untreated skin. Alternatively, manual dermasanding may be employed at the margins of the lased tissue to create a feathered junction zone.

Upper Lip Rhytides

Some individuals desire improvement of vertical rhytides of the upper lip but are not interested in significant resurfacing of the rest of the face. In many cases, they only have mild photodamage elsewhere and are correctly focused on improving the more significant defect of the upper lip. Deep resurfacing techniques including dermabrasion, laser resurfacing, or deep chemical peeling can all be employed with great success in this location. All resurfacing should be extended up to the vermillion border to smooth out the fine wrinkles that often extend over the mucocutaneous junction. Often these deeper resurfacing approaches are combined with medium depth chemical peeling over the rest of the face.

STRATEGIES FOR COMBINING RESURFACING MODALITIES

Laser, chemical, and abrasive resurfacing can be combined *simultaneously*, *segmentally*, or *sequentially*. Almost

any imaginable combination of these various techniques can be used to give the physician the utmost flexibility in approaching wrinkles, photodamage, and scars (8).

Simultaneous resurfacing is employed when the physician uses two or more resurfacing modalities at the same time and on the same tissue. Stagnone used the term "chemabrasion" to describe application of 50% trichloroacetic acid (TCA) followed by dermabrasion with topical cryoanesthesia (9). This technique made the dermabrasion more efficient because it involved the abrasion of coagulated tissue and there was a bloodless field, which allowed better visualization. Although chemabrasion was never widely accepted, Spira recommended another combination of these two modalities (10). His technique involved dermabrasion of more severely damaged cosmetic units with chemical peeling of the surrounding areas, overlapping the dermabraded portions with the chemical peel solution to avoid lines of demarcation. Brody and Alt have demonstrated using chemical peeling to blend in unabraded skin during repeat partial dermabrasion (11).

More recently, Harris has described dermasanding after peeling with 25% to 35% TCA (12). Likewise, dermasanding may be used to blend in and feather the edges of cosmetic units treated with laser resurfacing. When the surgeon is uncomfortable with preceding with another pass during laser resurfacing, additional depth can be obtained by focal dermasanding of more pronounced scars or wrinkles. This provides deeper penetration without additional thermal damage, perhaps even removing some residual thermally damaged tissue.

Segmental resurfacing can be employed as well. This involves using one resurfacing approach on one cosmetic unit and another on other cosmetic units. Sometimes all three forms of skin resurfacing are employed on the same patient. In some cases, one cosmetic unit may be better treated by one skin resurfacing approach while the adjacent one would respond better to another approach. A common combination includes laser resurfacing of the lower eyelids and perioral areas with medium depth chemical peeling of the rest of the face. Likewise, laser resurfacing, dermabrasion, or deep chemical peeling can be used on the upper lip with medium depth chemical peeling to blend in the rest of the face. Dermabrasion may be used for severe actinic damage of the forehead and medium depth peeling performed over the remainder of the less damaged face. In many acne patients, dermabrasion is discontinued at the malar rim because lower lid tissue is difficult to abrade. In these cases medium depth chemical peeling or laser resurfacing may be used on the lower eyelids. Countless combinations of these segmental approaches to resurfacing can be employed.

Sequential resurfacing is used when different techniques are employed at different times. Once the skin is fully healed from one resurfacing treatment, there may be an indication for using another approach to fine tune

residual abnormalities. For instance, after laser resurfacing, some mottled areas of pigmentary dyschromia may remain. These may be treated by medium depth chemical peeling or repeated superficial chemical peels in conjunction with a home care program of hydroquinones and tretinoin. Chemical peeling may also be used to blend in lines of demarcation remaining after dermabrasion or laser resurfacing. This may be necessary at the mandibular margin where the newly resurfaced skin may have a significantly different color than the untreated neck. Superficial chemical peeling or very light medium depth chemical peeling may be useful here to blur the color differences. In a contrasting situation, dermabrasion or laser resurfacing may be used after medium depth chemical peeling in which the rhytides did not respond sufficiently. Sometimes, fine lines of the lower eyelids persist after medium depth combination chemical peeling. Laser resurfacing may be employed 3 to 6 months after the peel to further improve these lines.

APPROACHES TO FOUR COMMON RESURFACING SCENARIOS

Full Face Photoaging Glogau Type III or IV Skin With Perioral and Periocular Rhytides (Fig. 20.7).

These patients require deeper resurfacing in the periocular and perioral areas. Around the eyes, lasers give the

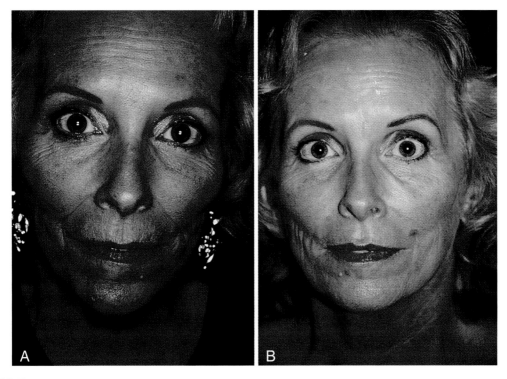

FIGURE 20.7
A, Appearance of perioral area before laser abrasion combined with Jessner's solution with TCA peel to the face. B, Appearance of the perioral area 6 weeks postoperatively. (Figure courtesy of Sue Ellen Cox, MD.)

best results of the resurfacing modalities. The contraction of the orbicularis oculis muscle contributes variably to the periocular rhytides. Although this is sometimes easily assessed clinically, other patients who appear to have little muscular contribution to their rhytides will have less than optimal results because of the orbicularis action. If possible, a single treatment with BOTOX (botulinum A toxin) (Allergan, Inc., Irvine, CA) before laser resurfacing can help with assessment of the muscular component of the rhytides, make the skin more amenable to the resurfacing, and help long range planning for maintenance with BOTOX.

The perioral area responds well to laser, dermabrasion or phenol peel. Perioral rhytides are divided more clearly along two separate types. The first (type I) has actinic damage as the primary cause and these patients respond very well to deep resurfacing (Fig. 20.8). Type II is almost completely secondary to orbicularis oris contraction (as seen with smokers or those who purse their lips) and can show some improvement with resur-

facing but not nearly as dramatic as in type 1 (Fig. 20.9). Type II patients must be prepared for a much more modest improvement or the possibility of complete resistance to treatment. The rest of the patient's face in these cases requires less aggressive resurfacing. A medium depth peel (combination Jessner's solution or 70% glycolic acid with 35% TCA) can blend these other areas nicely. In transition zones between cosmetic units, manual dermasanding can be used to fine tune these and other minor problem areas.

Acne Scarring With Actinic Damage

The approach to this patient depends on the extent of actinic damage and rhytides in the perioral and periocular area. The acne scarring is usually most severe on the cheeks, temples, and chin. These areas can be treated with laser or dermabrasion and the remaining areas blended with a 35% TCA peel or combination medium depth peel. If there are significant rhytides in the periocular and perioral area, it is often best to use the resur-

FIGURE 20.8

A, Appearance before upper lip dermabrasion with 70% glycolic acid and 35% TCA peel on the rest of the face. B, Appearance 6 months postoperatively there is good improvement without an obvious junction zone.

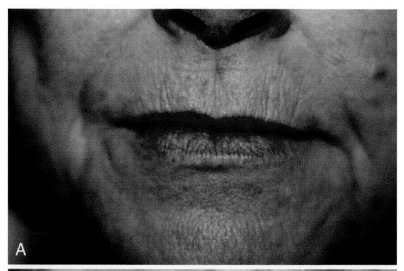

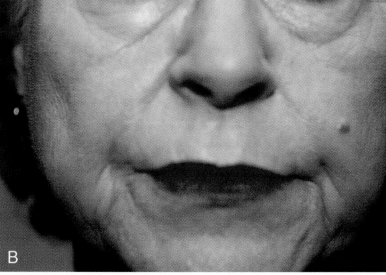

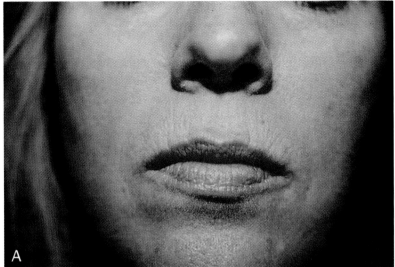

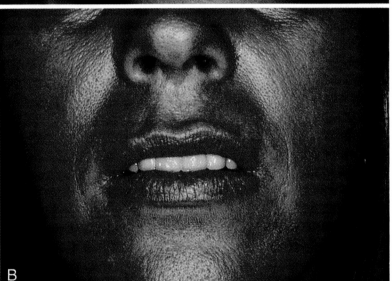

FIGURE 20.9
A, Upper lip rhytides secondary to muscular contraction. B, 6 weeks after laser abrasion shows resistant upper lip rhytides. (Figure courtesy of Sue Ellen Cox, MD.)

facing laser. Acne scars often extend into the jawline area. This area has a propensity for hypopigmentation and hypertrophic scarring. In this area dermabrasion and laser should be used more superficially. It is best to err on the side of caution when treating deeper scars in this area. Prepare the patient for a possible touch up rather than being overly aggressive with passes in this area.

Young Patient, Single Cosmetic Unit Rhytides, Periocular or Perioral, with mild actinic damage elsewhere (Fig. 20.10).

In these patients we first do a full face medium depth peel, excluding the area to be treated with a laser. The periocular unit is usually treated with a laser. The perioral unit may be approached with dermabrasion or laser. If the perioral or periocular area is lased, the zone between the peel and lasered areas can be lightly dermasanded for blending. These combination resurfacing patients do very well but do have to wear more cover up in the lased area. The advantage, of course, is that the procedure is easily done with local anesthesia and the risk profile is decreased by doing a less aggressive procedure in the areas that do not need deeper resurfacing.

Advanced to Severe Actinic Damage (Fig 20.11)

These patients have extensive rhytides and solar damage. They also usually have considerable skin laxity. It is possible to use a combined method approach in these patients, but it must be kept consistent within each unit. Because of economic concerns or systemic disease, simpler local anesthetic techniques may be preferable. These concerns may tilt the scale toward segmental laser or abrasive resurfacing. Phenol peels should also be considered in these patients, either full face or combined with medium depth peels in some cosmetic units.

FIGURE 20.10
A, Preoperative appearance of lower eyelids before laser resurfacing and 70% glycolic acid 35% TCA peel of the rest of the face. B, Appearance immediately following laser resurfacing and peel. C, Appearance 6 months postoperatively.

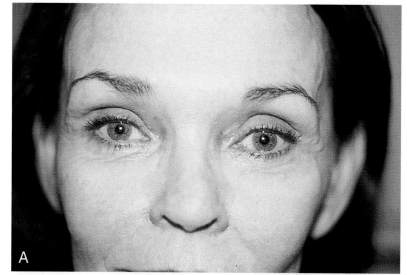

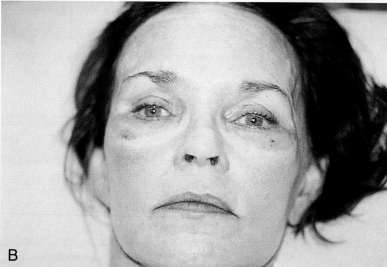

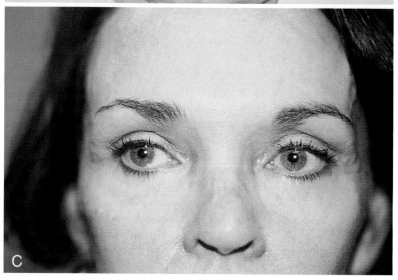

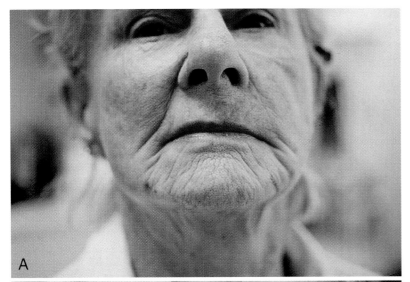

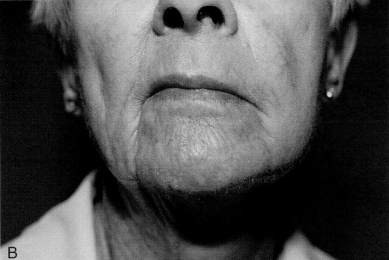

FIGURE 20.11

A, Appearance of the perioral area before laser resurfacing combined with Jessner's solution and TCA peel to rest of face for severe actinic damage. B, Appearance 4½ months after combined laser abrasion and chemical peel.

If a laser is used, one must be particularly careful in the substance of the cheek. Lasered areas retract more than those areas resurfaced with a medium depth peel causing "pouching out" between wrinkles. The full face laser abrasion can provide skin tightening which is an advantage to a patient who has skin laxity but does not want to undergo a facelift.

CONCLUSION

The cosmetic surgeon who can offer the full range of the resurfacing armamentarium has the ability to best match the treatment to the patient's needs. The development of new techniques and new tools makes skin resurfacing an exciting, challenging field of practice. However, this should not make us forget the benefits of older techniques. We should always look to controlled studies with objective means of evaluation to assess new techniques. This will allow us to rationally choose what is best for our patients.

REFERENCES

1. Dzubow L. The aging face. In: Cosmetic surgery of the skin. Coleman WP III, Hanke CW, Alt TN, Asken S, eds. 2nd Ed. St Louis: Mosby, 1997:7-17.
2. Sripachya-Aruht S, Fitzpatrick RE, Goldman MP, et al. Infections complicating pulsed CO_2 laser resurfacing for photoaged skin. J Dermatol Surg 1997;23:527-536.
3. Yarborough JM. Ablation of facial scars by programmed dermabrasion. J Dermatol Surg Oncol 1988:14:292-294.
4. Katz BE, Oca AG. A controlled study of the effectiveness of spot dermabrasion ("scarabrasion") on the appearance of surgical scars. J Am Acad Dermatol 1991;24:462-466.
5. Lawrence C, Cox SE, Cockerell CJ, et al. A comparison of the efficiency of Jessner's solution and 35% trichloracetic acid vs 5% fluorouracil in the treatment of widespread facial actinic keratoses. Arch Dermatol 1995;131:176-181.
6. Benedetto AV, Griffin TD, Benedetto EA, et al. Dermabrasion: therapy and prophylaxis of the photoaged face. J Am Acad Dermatol 1992;27(3):439-437.
7. Coleman WP III, Yarborough JM, Mandy SH. Dermabrasion for prophylaxic and treatment of actinic keratoses. Derm Surg 1996;22(1):17-21.

8. Coleman WP III, Narris RS. Combining surgical methods for skin resurfacing. Semin Cutan Med Surg 1991;15:194-199.

9. Stagnone JJ. Chemabrasion. A combined technique of chemical peeling and dermabrasion. J Dermatol Surg Oncol 1977;3:217.

10. Spira M. Treatment of acne scarring by combined dermabrasion and chemical peel. Plast Reconstr Surg 1977;60:38.

11. Brody H, Alt TN. Dermabrasion. In: Cosmetic surgery of the skin. Coleman WP III, Hanke CW, Alt TN, Asken S, eds. St Louis: Mosby 1997;85-111.

12. Harris DR, Noodleman FR. Combining manual dermasanding with low strength trichloroacetic acid to improve actinically injured skin. J Dermatol Surg Oncol 1994;20: 436-442.

CHAPTER 21

Combining Skin Resurfacing With Soft Tissue Augmentation

■ William P. Coleman III
Gregory Goodman
Naomi Lawrence

All forms of skin resurfacing are effective in improving wrinkles and scars. The degree of improvement, however, varies with the aggressiveness of the resurfacing modality. Deep resurfacing, whether chemical, abrasive, or laser, can lead to permanent hypopigmentation and/or scars. The eternal paradox of all surgery is that more aggressive approaches may yield higher dividends but at greater risks.

Instead of using one modality aggressively, a combination of approaches will often yield the desired benefits with fewer potential complications. Combining skin resurfacing with soft tissue augmentation is an example of this approach. Skin resurfacing is used to eliminate surface defects while soft tissue augmentation is employed to correct deeper abnormalities.

Many forms of soft tissue augmentation are best performed after skin resurfacing. Often these augmentations are minor procedures that do not cause substantial morbidity and are best timed to allow accurate assessment of the full effects of the resurfacing procedure. Augmentation occurs as late as 3 to 6 months after resurfacing. Many forms (but not all) of soft tissue augmentation are short-lived and should be regarded as fine tuning to further enhance the results of the resurfacing procedure. Skin resurfacing and soft tissue augmentation should be thought of as complementary and not competing technologies. The use of collagen, whether autologous or nonautologous, should wait until all collagen remodeling from the resurfacing procedure with its host of reparative enzymes, including col-

lagenases, has settled. This period is at least 3 months after the resurfacing procedure.

Patients who desire skin resurfacing but cannot schedule the required recovery time can undergo soft tissue augmentation as a temporary method for improving wrinkles or scars until the time is right for a resurfacing procedure. There are a small number of soft tissue augmentation procedures, mainly autologous, that carry a certain degree of morbidity and may be more conveniently timed to coincide with the resurfacing procedure, especially dermabrasion and laser resurfacing. These include autologous fat transfer, dermal grafting, and harvesting the skin for autologous collagen therapy. Punch grafts, which may be thought of as another form of an autologous filling agent, may also be performed at the time of resurfacing surgery. For these autologous procedures, exact timing with the resurfacing is important.

The conditions that require augmentation as well as resurfacing are logically those in which soft tissue augmentation is usually indicated and for which resurfacing procedures have little or inadequate effect. These include expression lines and deeper scarring or aging changes. In general, these indications can be thought of as static versus dynamic change and deep versus superficial disease.

STATIC VERSUS DYNAMIC CHANGES

Resurfacing procedures remove minor changes produced primarily by movement in areas such as perioral lines and other minor rhytides visible at rest. However, these procedures only have a modifying or temporary effect on other expression lines such as periorbital, glabella and horizontal forehead lines. They have almost no effect on nasolabial furrows.

Two possible ways of dealing with these muscle-induced changes exist. Either one may fill the offending defect and not allow the muscular action to recreate the line, or one may paralyze the muscle action that produces the line using botulinum toxin. Either method is practical and acceptable, and the choice depends on the defect and the patient's wishes.

DEEP VERSUS SUPERFICIAL DISEASE

Deep disease may occur as a result of various disease states or as part of the aging process. Diseases such as discoid lupus erythematosus, scleroderma, past radiotherapy and Romberg's facial atrophy may require soft tissue augmentation. In these diseases, resurfacing may be insufficient, not required, or contraindicated and soft tissue augmentation becomes the prime therapy. However, scarring from surgery and acne is a major indication for combining resurfacing and soft tissue augmentation. Complex cicatricial patterns may involve epidermis, dermis, and subcutis with both bound down scars and loss of structure necessitating a combination of several techniques. The choice of treatment depends on the severity and depth of the tissue loss and the choice of timing depends on the treatment chosen.

Aging changes add another group of patients that require composite correction of deep and superficial disease. Superficial rhytides and sun damage are well handled with resurfacing, but the deeper changes are not. As the face ages, the skeleton loses density and fat is lost. Patients often deliberately increase their body weight as they age to offset this loss of facial fullness. As thin people age, they look gaunt and tired due to this resorption. These changes often require soft tissue augmentation such as fat transfer in addition to whatever resurfacing procedure is employed. Rhytidectomy for these patients is often not the treatment of choice as it can leave patients looking even more gaunt, worsening their appearance.

SILICONE

Silicone fluid was used widely for soft tissue augmentation in the middle of the 20th Century. Clinical studies confirmed an excellent record of safety (1). However, the United States Food & Drug Administration (FDA) never approved the use of this substance. Recently, the FDA and similar ministries in other countries have become increasing aggressive about restricting the use of silicone products. Until governmental policy changes, silicone will be used by only a very small number of physicians. Therefore, the technique of micro-droplet silicone injection will not be discussed in this chapter.

Since silicone is a permanent substance, physicians may encounter patients who have had silicone implanted with resulting chronic dermal granulomas due to a type IV hypersensitivity reaction. Although these reactions are rare, they are long lasting and patients become frustrated, often seeking a variety of physician options about improvement of their condition. Skin resurfacing approaches, especially dermabrasion, have been employed in an attempt to eliminate the implanted silicone. Most of these attempts fail. Excision of the offending silicone granuloma appears to be the only long lasting solution but does result in a permanent scar.

BOVINE COLLAGEN

Zyderm I collagen was approved for marketing by the FDA in the 1981. Zyderm II followed in 1983 and Zyplast in 1985. Produced by the Collagen Corporation (Palo Alto, CA) these materials have become the most widely used substances for soft tissue augmentation (2). Zyderm is derived from cow collagen that has been chemically digested and sterilized. Potential antigenicity is reduced by hydrolyzation of the telopeptide end-regions of the collagen molecule. Zyderm is packaged as fibrils of collagen suspended in buffered saline with 0.3% lidocaine. Zyderm I contains 35 mg/ml of collagen, 95% of which is type I and 1.5% type III. Zyderm II contains 65 mg/ml of collagen. Zyplast contains 35 mg/ml of collagen which is cross linked with glutaraldehyde (3).

In a refrigerated state, Zyderm and Zyplast are composed of molecules in suspension. Injection of the collagen into human skin increases the material to body temperature, which then stimulates the molecules to reform into fibers. The material is shipped in a refrigerated package and is designed for storage in a refrigerator until used. It is prepackaged in syringes containing 0.5 to 2 ml of collagen. For precise injection into the dermis, 30-gauge needles are supplied. Recently, the ADG (Adjustable Depth Gauge, Collagen Corp., Palo Alto, CA) needle has been supplied with the collagen syringes (Fig. 21.1). This device features an adjustable wheel around the needle that can be dialed forward or backward to expose different lengths of the needle. This feature has been shown to increase the precision of dermal augmentation, especially with physicians inexperienced in using this material (4).

Zyderm collagen is not recommended in patients with autoimmune diseases, especially lupus erythematosus, dermatomyositis, and rheumatoid arthritis. Zyderm collagen is also contraindicated in patients with hypersensitivity to lidocaine or a history of anaphylaxis. Patients with a strong allergic history should be carefully evaluated before collagen is employed (5).

One of the chief complications of Zyderm and Zyplast is an allergic reaction. These granulomatous hypersensitivity reactions may persist for several months up to years (Fig. 21.2). Therefore, patients with the

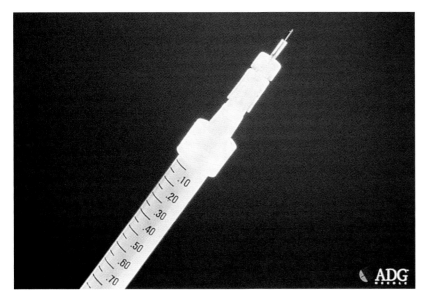

FIGURE 21.1
The ADG (Adjustable Depth Gauge) needle with an adjustable wheel to increase the precision of Zyderm collagen injections.

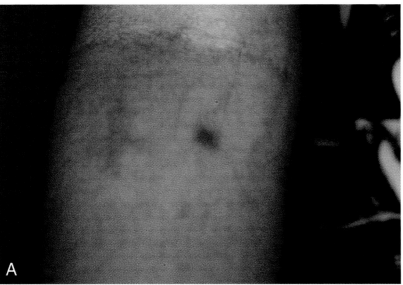

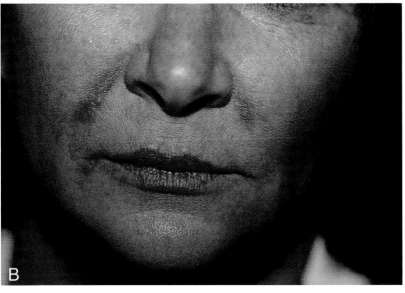

FIGURE 21.2
A, A positive skin test to Zyderm in the volar forearm. B, A rare granulomatous reaction in a patient who previously demonstrated two negative skin tests to Zyderm.

potential for allergy to Zyderm or Zyplast should be excluded. Identifying patients allergic to Zyplast or Zyderm is accomplished with a series of two skin tests. A small amount of Zyderm I (0.1 ml) is injected into the dermis of the flexor forearm. If the first skin test is negative, a second test is highly recommended 2 to 4 weeks later. The second test is designed to eliminate those who would become sensitized to Zyderm or Zyplast after the first skin test. A positive skin test response is defined as any change (even a minor one) in the original Zyderm welt (such as increased erythema, induration, tenderness or swelling) with or without accompanying pruritus, which persists for more than 6 hours or appears after 24 hours after implantation. Any rash, arthralgia or myalgia in the post test patch period should be evaluated carefully for its relationship to the test implantation. Needle punctures may produce mild erythema during the first day, but these should fade spontaneously. A positive reaction at the test site is usually present within 72 hours. Some physicians prefer to read these skin tests in all patients at 72 hours. Others rely on patient history or the appearance of the site at 2 weeks, at which time a second test is administered if the first was negative. Treatment should not be begun until at least 4 weeks after a first negative skin test (6). Some physicians administer the second test at 4 weeks and do not treat until 8 weeks after the first test. Other physicians prefer a second test on the face near the hairline. These second tests largely eliminate the patients who may develop a reaction after an initial negative skin test. After two negative skin tests the likelihood of an allergic reaction is dramatically decreased (less than 0.01%).

THE TECHNIQUE OF AUGMENTATION

Wrinkles and scars are better appreciated with the patient seated and illuminated from the side. All make up should be removed and the skin cleansed with an antibacterial agent such as chlorhexidine. Loops for magnification help the physician to detect subtle details. Some physicians prefer to mark the deepest portion of each rhytid or scar with a sterile marking pen prior to augmentation.

Because Zyderm and Zyplast are injected through a 30-gauge needle, local anesthesia is usually not required. Furthermore, the suspension contains 0.3% lidocaine resulting in partial anesthesia within 60 seconds after injection. EMLA topical anesthetic cream or ice can be used to diminish the sting of injection. Some patients are extremely intolerant of needles and require regional nerve blocks or field anesthesia with 1% or 2% lidocaine. The physician must be careful not to distort the contours of the depressed scars or rhytides with the local anesthetic.

Zyderm I should be injected into the papillary dermis. This requires an acute angled insertion of the needle (approximately 15°). The ADG needle allows the physician to reveal only a small portion of the needle shaft to decrease the depth of penetration and maintain a superficial position. Zyderm I is usually injected into superficial wrinkles such as the crow's feet or upper lip lines. Some material may leak through pores in the skin surface. Occasionally, visible beads of the implant are apparent through the skin surface. These can be smoothed out by digital massage immediately after implantation (Fig. 21.3). If these beads persist for more than 24 hours, they may take several weeks to resolve. Some patients' skin is more prone to beading than others (Fig. 21.4).

Zyderm II is twice the concentration of Zyderm I. This material is used slightly deeper in the dermis and with less over correction. Excessive over correction may leave a yellow discoloration to the skin for several weeks. Zyplast is injected into the deep dermis. Implantation that is too superficial will result in beads that may take months to resolve. Some experienced Zyplast users

FIGURE 21.3

After Zyderm I is injected into superficial wrinkles of the forehead, a visible wheal results. These can be smoothed out by digital massage immediately after implantation.

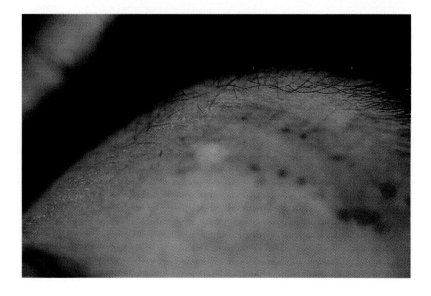

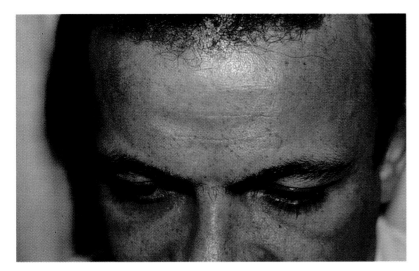

FIGURE 21.4
Persistent beading due to Zyplast augmentation of superficial forehead rhytides.

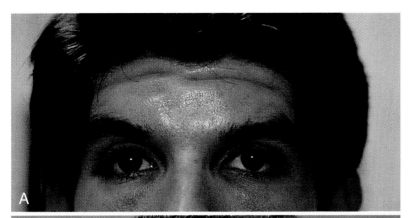

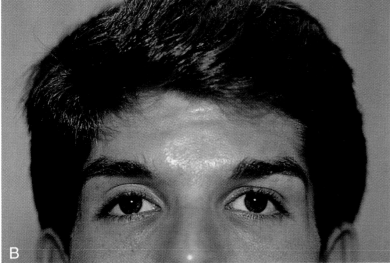

FIGURE 21.5
A, Before augmentation of a deep furrow of the forehead. B, One month after two augmentations with Zyderm II there is excellent improvement.

employ the "linear threading technique." This involves injecting the Zyplast while the needle is withdrawn. In some rhytides, better correction can be achieved by layering Zyderm in the superficial dermis over Zyplast, which is injected into the deeper dermis.

Full correction with Zyderm or Zyplast may take two or three treatment sessions. Patients should be warned that an aggressive first treatment may result in over correction that is unattractive and takes months to even out. Instead, it is more appropriate to fill the wrinkle or scar until a pleasing contour is achieved. Additional treatments can be performed at 2-week intervals until the patient and physician are satisfied (Fig. 21.5).

The major complaint from patients who have undergone Zyderm or Zyplast augmentation is that the correction does not last long enough. The longevity varies considerably from patient to patient. Studies in both animals and humans have shown that Zyplast lasts longer (7). This may be the result of colonization by fibroblasts and stimulation of new collagen. In most wrinkles, the correction has completely faded by 12 months. Many patients return for touch-up treatments at 9 month intervals, others are able to detect some loss of correction as early as 3 or 4 months and return for touch ups much more often. Clinical studies have demonstrated that both Zyderm and Zyplast are still present in the dermis 9 months after augmentation (7).

FIBREL

The use of fibrin foam to treat depressed scars was first reported by Spangler in 1957 (8). He continued to modify his technique reporting good results in 80% of 700 scars treated by 1975. Gottlieb developed a modification of this technique in which porcine gelatin powder was mixed with the patients' plasma and ϵ-amino caproic acid (9). This was designed to stimulate collagen production at the injection site. His approach was patented as Fibrel and approved for treatment of scars by the FDA in 1988 and later for wrinkles in 1990. Originally marketed by the Serano Corporation, it was later acquired by the Mentor Corporation (Santa Barbara, CA).

Fibrel is supplied from the manufacturer as a sterile kit containing all the needed components except for the patient's plasma. 100 mg of the porcine gelatin powder and 125 mg of ϵ-amino caproic acid are combined with 0.5 ml of sterile saline and 0.5 ml of the patient's plasma. These components are mixed by pushing them back and forth between two syringes joined by a biluer lock adaptor. The physician or assistant must be careful not to inadvertently spray the material onto their skin if the syringes become loose. The risk of contact with blood-borne pathogens is a disadvantage of this technique. Clinical experience indicates that Fibrel may work as well without the addition of plasma, eliminating this problem.

Although allergic reactions to Fibrel are rare, a skin test is recommended using 0.05 ml of Fibrel in normal saline injected into the dermis of flexor forearm. Second testing is normally not performed although 1.8% of patients may be allergic to Fibrel (10). As with Zyderm and Zyplast, Fibrel is contraindicated in patients with autoimmune diseases or an allergy to any component of the kit. Fibrel must be injected through a larger gauge needle than Zyderm or Zyplast. The 27-gauge needle supplied and used with the kit results in more pain and local anesthesia is preferred by most patients. Usually, a small amount of 1% lidocaine with 1:100,000 epinephrine is carefully employed as a field

block so as to not distort the contour of the scar or wrinkle. The Fibrel kit also contains a spade-shaped 20-gauge cutting needle that is designed to lyse the fibrotic base of depressed scars. This allows the skin at the bottom of the scar to be freed up prior to augmentation with Fibrel.

Fibrel usually results in more induration at the treatment site than does Zyderm or Zyplast. Erythema and swelling may last for several days after implantation. Usually two or three treatments are required to improve pliable acne scars. Fibrotic or ice pick scars respond less favorably, but may be improved using the cutting needle. Fibrel, however, is less effective on wrinkles than Zyderm or Zyplast. Furthermore, Fibrel is more viscous and difficult to use than Zyderm or Zyplast in thin wrinkles such as the crow's feet. Deeper wrinkles or furrows may be augmented using a linear threading technique similar to Zyplast. Although nasolabial furrows can be improved nicely with Fibrel, this product has not achieved popularity with physicians for soft tissue augmentation of wrinkles.

In acne scars, Fibrel may achieve longer correction than Zyderm or Zyplast. By 90 days after correction, the Fibrel is replaced by host collagen. This improvement has been shown to persist for 1 to 2 years. In one study, 87 patients followed for 5 years demonstrated over 50% persistent correction (11).

AUTOLOGOUS FAT TRANSPLANTATION

Fat has been used for over a century to correct subcutaneous defects. Until the development of liposuction, Fat transplantation was achieved by en-bloc resection at a donor site and implantation through an incision (12). This resulted in scars of both the recipient and donor sites. Liposuction techniques provided a new way of obtaining fat grafts (13). Using a syringe and a small cannula, fat is aspirated and then reinjected leaving only small punctures at the donor and recipient sites.

Many patients seek fat transplantation in conjunction with formal liposuction. In these cases, the fat is harvested with syringes prior to machine aspiration of the remainder of the localized adiposity. Other patients who seek soft tissue augmentation can only undergo fat transplantation as a minor outpatient procedure using only local anesthesia.

The tumescent anesthetic technique has been demonstrated to provide excellent anesthesia and vasoconstriction for liposuction. This approach also works well for fat transplantation (14). Using a solution of 0.1% lidocaine with 1:1,000,000 epinephrine, a suitable donor area is tumesced until firm. No bicarbonate, steroids or other additives should be used in the tumescent fluid. The donor area should be marked before infiltration of the anesthetic with the patient standing. Usually an area of asymmetry is chosen so that the harvesting will give the patient a more harmonious appearance.

Ten minutes after tumescing, the overlying skin will reveal a consistent blanch indicating vasoconstriction. At this time, a small puncture is made in the skin and a 12- to 14-gauge blunt cannula is advanced into the subcutaneous tissue. Tissue harvesting is accomplished using 10 ml syringes attached to the cannula by a Luer lock (Fig. 21.6). The surgeon pulls out the plunger and moves the cannula to and fro through the subcutaneous tissue until the syringe is filled with fat. The assistant then provides the surgeon with an empty syringe and the process continues until enough fat is harvested for the anticipated series of augmentations. These syringes are left standing upright (plunger up) in a test tube rack until the fat separates from an infranate of anesthetic fluid. The anesthetic fluid is then discarded and the material is ready for implantation. Other surgeons centrifuge the fat to more fully and quickly separate the layers. This may risk damaging the fat and should be performed at low speeds (2500 to 3500 revolutions per minute) and for only 2 to 3 minutes.

Using the tumescent technique, there is usually no need for washing the fat or other preparations. There is no scientific evidence that washing provides better graft integration. Only if significant amount of blood is present in the harvested fat should gentle washing be employed by drawing 0.9% saline or Ringer's lactate solution into the syringe containing the fat. The extracted fat in the syringe is then allowed to again separate into layers and the blood tinged infranatant fluid is eliminated.

There is also an oily supranatant layer, which is composed of broken fat cells and is not viable fat graft and is irritating to tissues when injected. Dealing with this may be as simple as not transferring it into the smaller syringes before definitive injection or by keeping the sy-

ringe in a near vertical orientation and not injecting the last 0.5 ml of material. The former is the easier method. Wicking methods are also sometimes employed to remove this oily supranatant component before injection (15). A portion of the harvested fat can be used immediately for augmentation. The rest is frozen in 10 ml syringes for future touch up sessions. A standard domestic freezer is sufficient for maintaining the fat in a constant frozen state. Most physicians feel comfortable storing the fat in the freezer for up to 6 months. Beyond this, it may discolor. Prolonged storage increases the risk of bacterial contamination.

Subsequent augmentations may or may not be necessary. Most fat and fluid resorption will occur over the first 3 to 4 weeks, in which time there is also some remodeling. Any further injections that may be required to fine tune or augment the original injection should be delayed until complete maturation of the fat graft has occurred after 4 to 6 weeks. The longevity of correction with fat varies with technique, injected area, and patient. There are a number of reports testifying to the long lasting correction attained by meticulous injection (16–19).

It is probably best to inject only to the level required for correction and to overcorrect no more than 10% as there will only be some limited resorption of fluid and nonviable fat (Fig. 21.7). When larger bolus fat injection was the preferred method, overcorrection by 30% to 40% was commonly employed. However, the smaller bolus fat transfer method with its smaller and better nourished aliquots of fat, runs a risk of long term overcorrection. Checking the patient at 6- to 12-month intervals will help determine if further correction is necessary (Fig. 21.8).

Fat transfer may be timed to coincide with resurfacing procedures or performed after the benefits of resurfacing are apparent (Fig. 21.9). If fat transfer is combined with resurfacing it should be performed immediately

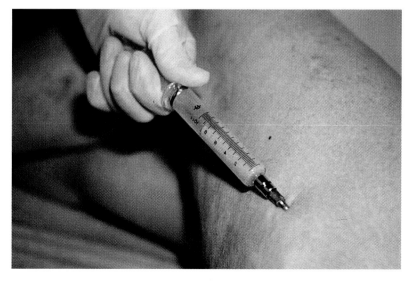

FIGURE 21.6
Harvesting bloodless fat using the tumescent technique and syringe suction.

FIGURE 21.7
The fat is injected only to the level required for correction.

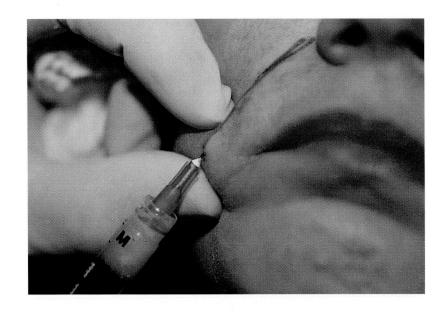

FIGURE 21.8
A, Appearance before fat transplantation of the central cheeks. B, Eight months after fat transplantation, the contours are significantly improved.

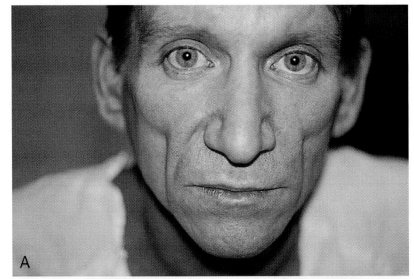

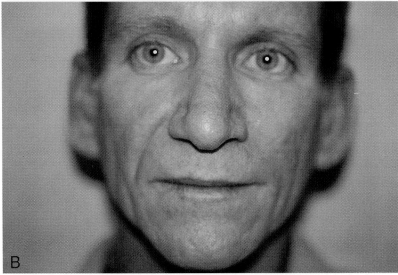

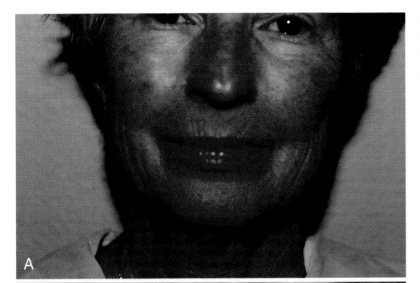

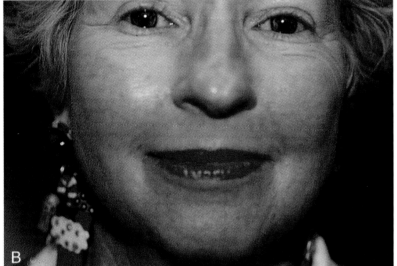

FIGURE 21.9
A, Appearance before laser resurfacing of the perioral area, followed by fat transplantation 3 weeks later to the cheeks and chin. B, Three months later the contours are nicely improved.

before the resurfacing is begun. The physician should outline the areas to be augmented while the patient is sitting or standing. If local anesthesia is employed either by direct infiltration or by tumescence, it should be delayed until after the fat transfer, or else the distortion induced by the anesthesia may interfere with the ability to accurately judge the necessary correction. If dermal grafts are employed as well, they should be implanted immediately before the fat is extracted from the donor site, usually while the tumescence is taking effect. Any focal subcutaneous incisionless undermining or subcision of scars may then be undertaken. After these initial steps, the resurfacing procedure can be performed in the normal manner.

Lam and Moy in 1992, identified several issues with the fat grafting technique (20). First, cells can be damaged on removal of the graft; second, reduced contact between graft and wound base could hamper the heal-

ing process; third, adipose tissue does not vascularize well; and fourth, when fat grafts are too large, nutrition can be inadequate. Most if not all these concerns can be dealt with by attention to atraumatic technique and implanting small parcels of fat carefully in multiple tunnels. This gives these small fat implants the best chance of being located within reach of the available blood supply and potential survival.

Postoperatively, the patient is advised to immobilize the augmented area. For facial fat transplantation, this usually involves no eating, smiling, and talking for 3 to 4 hours. Ice packs help to diminish bruising in both the recipient and donor sites. The small punctures are treated with an antibacterial ointment applied twice daily until they heal. Most patients have very little discomfort postoperatively and do not require analgesics. The donor area may remain tender (similar to muscle soreness) for 24 to 48 hours.

LIPOCYTIC DERMAL AUGMENTATION

Fournier first introduced the concept of dermal injection of fat for augmentation in 1985 (21). Zocchi and others have continued to investigate this approach (22). Fat does not survive well in the dermis. However, if reduced to a less viscous form that can be precisely placed into the dermis, it causes an inflammatory response resulting in the development of host collagen and thus long lasting soft tissue augmentation.

Although Fournier originally termed this technique "autologous collagen," there is evidence that very little collagen is present in human fat (23). The fat is processed by combining it with sterile distilled water. This emulsion is then frozen. On thawing two layers are discernable: a viscous supernate and a clear infranate. The infranate contains triglycerides and tissue fluid and is discarded (Fig. 21.10). This supernate is composed of ruptured fat cells. This material can be further broken down by centrifuging, ultrasound, and/or passing it back and forth between two syringes connected by a biluer lock adaptor.

The final product is a pale yellow material that passes through a 23- or 25-gauge needle. Using these smaller needles, the processed fat can be injected into the dermis of a depressed acne scar or wrinkle. The goal is to stimulate collagen production much like microdroplet silicone. The collagen is produced at the host site after augmentation with fat, thus the term "lipocytic dermal augmentation" (23).

Lipocytic dermal augmentation can be combined with microlipoinjection in a two layered approach. Microlipoinjection is performed in the subcutaneous tissue to elevate deep furrows. Some of the fat can be processed and used for dermal augmentation in the layer above (Fig. 21.11). This is similar to the bilevel technique of Zyderm I placed above Zyplast.

The chief advantage of lipocytic dermal augmentation is that the donor tissue is easily available and is not a foreign protein as is Zyderm collagen or Fibrel. The viscosity of the material however mandates the use of a larger needle which results in increased bruising and induration. If overcorrection is not employed however, most patients can return to work the day after the procedure.

DERMAL GRAFTING

Dermal grafts and derma-fat grafts have been used in many fields of surgery over the last 60 years (24). Until recently, dermal grafts have suffered from cyst formation and unpredictable resorption characteristics, but improvements in harvesting methods have recently provided an alternative soft tissue dermal augmentation method (25, 26). The strength of this technique lies in its autologous nature, its relative ease as a procedure, and its gratifying results.

The technique for this procedure begins with harvesting the graft from the donor site. Dermabrasion or laser resurfacing with either scanning or high-energy short-pulse carbon dioxide (CO_2) lasers may be used to prepare the retroauricular donor site. The donor site is marked to allow enough dermal material to be harvested but still permitting primary closure of the defect leaving an imperceptible line in the retroauricular sulcus (Fig. 21.12.A). The dermabrader or laser is used to remove the epidermis and the dermis to a level below the sebaceous glands as the depth of this preparation appears to make a difference in the incidence of epidermal cysts (27).

The next step depends on the shape of the defect. If the defect is a linear trough like a scar, a marionette line or a nasolabial furrow, then a strip of dermis is excised using a scalpel or cutting mode CO_2 laser (7 to 10 W). The strip is then trimmed with gradle or tenotomy scissors to match the defect (Fig. 21.12.B). It is better for the graft to be too small than too big to avoid tethering to entry or exit sites. It is permissible to leave fat on the base of the graft if the defect needs more bulk. The excess fat does not seem to influence graft survival or increase the incidence of cyst formation. If the defect to be

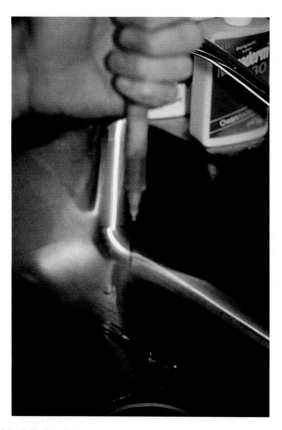

FIGURE 21.10

After freezing an emulsion of fat and distilled water and then thawing, two layers are discernable. The infranate contains triglycerides and tissue fluid and is discarded.

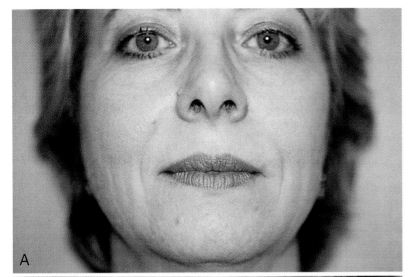

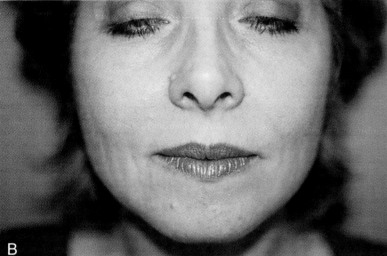

FIGURE 21.11
A, Appearance before lipocytic dermal augmentation
of the nasolabial furrows. B, Appearance 10 months
after augmentation and monthly superficial glycolic
acid peels.

corrected is circular, it is better to accurately measure the recipient site and harvest an appropriate size punch transplant of dermis.

Punch dermal grafts can be placed into pockets without guiding sutures, but linear grafts require attachment to a suture for their introduction into a pocket. Linear grafts may be tied with a 4-0 suture or similar suture on a straight needle. This suture will be guided into the recipient pocket using the plastic sleeve of a 14- or 16-gauge intravenous cannula (Fig. 21.12.C).

The cannula or a similar instrument is used to produce the pocket underlying the scar. Other instruments may be used for nonlinear pockets. Once the pocket is formed, the intravenous cannula is pushed through the skin at the distal end of the defect. The introducer is removed leaving the plastic sleeve in the recipient tunnel and exiting the wound at the proximal and distal ends. The suture is then passed into the distal end of the wound exiting proximally where the hub of the cannula is located. The suture is pulled through the

cannula until the dermal graft abuts the plastic sleeve (Fig. 21.12.D). The leading end of the dermal graft is passed into the beginning of the plastic sleeve and the sleeve and trailing dermal graft are eased into position with the assistant holding the other end of the graft with jewelers' forceps (Fig. 21.12.E). The suture is cut and either removed or left in situ. The cannula may be used for other dermal grafts. No attempt at further anchoring of the graft is necessary. The ends of the wound are stretched in either direction away from the recipient site to allow the graft to sit most comfortably in the bed and avoid any tethering of the graft to one edge. This can produce skin retraction. Trimming the graft to make it 2 to 3 mm shorter than the bed also helps in this regard.

Complications of this technique as described are few. It is important to de-epithelialize the graft completely and include removal of most of the papillary dermis to avoid cyst formation. Tethering of the graft is avoided by pulling the graft properly into the bed and not

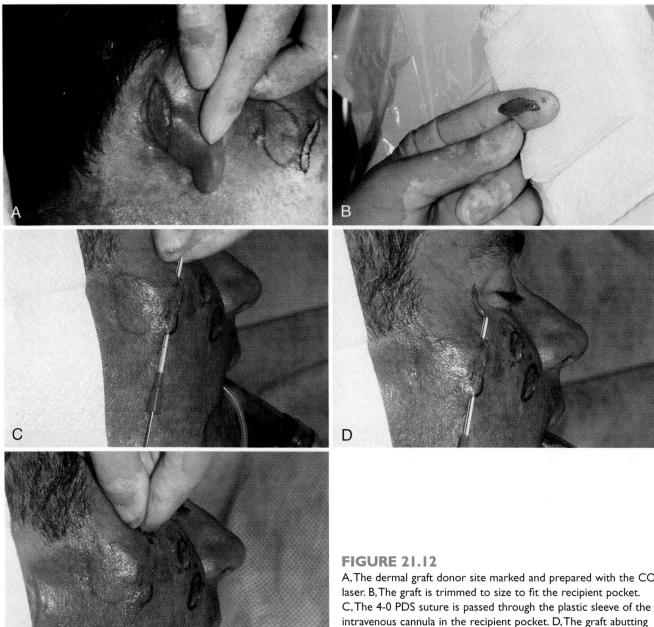

FIGURE 21.12

A, The dermal graft donor site marked and prepared with the CO_2 laser. B, The graft is trimmed to size to fit the recipient pocket. C, The 4-0 PDS suture is passed through the plastic sleeve of the intravenous cannula in the recipient pocket. D, The graft abutting the free end of the cannula ready to be drawn into the pocket. E, The graft in position just prior to severing the suture at either end of the recipient pocket.

allowing it to sit too close to entry or exit points. Examples of this technique may be seen in Figures 21.13, 21.14 and 21.15.

HYLAN GEL

Biomatrix Inc. (Ridgefield, NJ) began clinical trials in 1991 on an insoluble hyaluronic acid derivative (Hylan gel) (28). Hylan gel is low in antigenicity and pretreatment skin tests are not required. This material is injected in a similar fashion to Zyderm I. There is evidence that

Hylan gel correction is still partially maintained at 18 months. The patent for this material was recently licensed by the Collagen Corporation who will market it with their bovine collagen products. Popularity will depend on the longevity and ease of implantation.

GORE-TEX (SOFT FORM)

This material is a polytetrafluoroethylene material that was developed for vascular surgery (29). Gore-Tex is available in a suture form that is threaded through

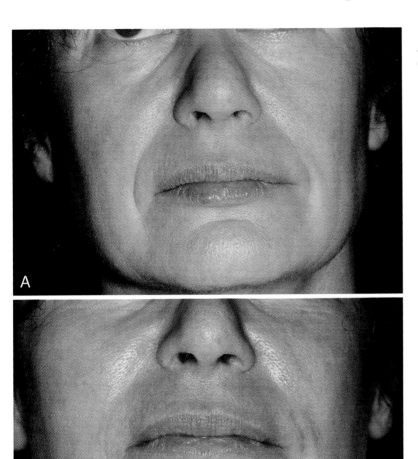

FIGURE 21.13
A, Preoperative nasolabial fold. B, Appearance 6 weeks after dermal grafting.

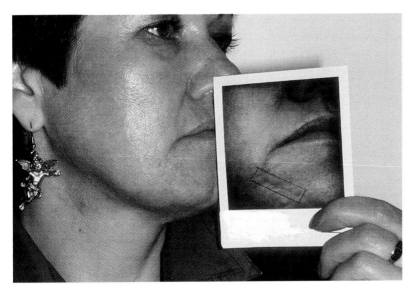

FIGURE 21.14
Appearance 1 month after dermal graft placement in the chin to correct scars.

FIGURE 21.15
A, Preoperative dermal grafting of a contour defect of the nasolabial folds. B, Postoperative results at 6 months. Note: the patient also had dermabrasion and laser to the cheeks 3 months before this, and fat transfer to the lateral cheeks at the time of the dermal grafting 6 months before this photograph.

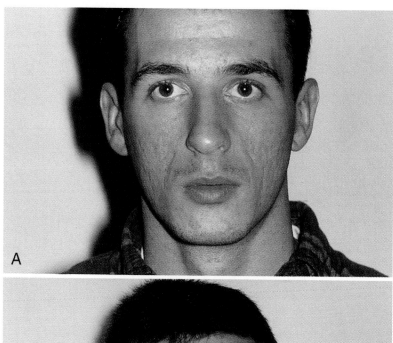

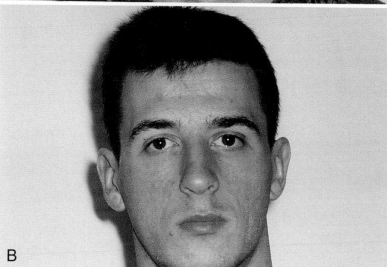

wrinkles using a guiding needle. This technique must be performed using local anesthesia. The number of threads implanted determines the degree of correction. After a sufficient number of threads are implanted, the ends are trimmed and the material pushed back through the punctures at either end of the furrow (Fig. 21.16). Since this material is implanted under the dermis, other soft tissue augmentation materials can be implanted over Gore-Tex. These would include Zyderm, Fibrel, or Hylan Gel.

The chief problem with Gore-Tex has been that this permanent material eventually "spits" in many patients. This dermal extrusion is annoying and the suture must be removed and be replaced when "spitting" occurs. Another problem is with movement of the material. This movement most often occurs at the vermillion border of the lips. The Gore-Tex suture creates a palpable ridge or roll above the intended area for augmentation. This ridge may be due to repeated muscle movement in this area.

Recently the Collagen Corporation acquired the right to market Gore-Tex as Soft Form®. Soft Form® is formed into a tube to allow growth of host collagen fibers through and into the implant. This collagen ingrowth presumably anchors the implant and decreases problems with extrusion. As this material is used more widely, it will become apparent how it compares to the currently available products.

AUTOLOGEN

Autologen is human autologous collagen that is produced by removing strips of skin which are then sent to Autogenesis Technologies, Inc. (Boston, MA) for preparation. The material is prepared much like bovine collagen into a form that can be reinjected back into the same patient from whom it was harvested (30). The cost of converting harvested skin into Autologen is expensive and there is inconvenience in mailing and receiving the specimen. Also, large amounts of skin must be harvested to obtain enough for significant correction of wrinkles or scars. Autologen probably is best suited for patients who have undergone face lifting, abdominoplasty, or breast reduction in whom large amounts of skin are removed. Theoretically, patients without the need for other surgery could have their skin harvested from an inconspicuous site such as the pubic area, but a significant scar would result.

The collagen concentration in the Autologen suspension is 50 to 100 mg/ml. There is no need for skin testing since the material is autologous. Longevity of correction has been reported to be 18 months. The final place of this product among other soft tissue augmentation products remains to be determined.

ARTECOLL

Artecoll (Rofil Medical, Breda, The Netherlands) is a long-term subdermal augmentation injection. It consists of fine polymethyl methacrylate (PMMA) microspheres suspended 1:3 in a 3.5% collagen solution. It is said that the microspheres are very smooth, homogenous and pure. The Artecoll can be injected via a 27-gauge needle with a tunneling technique, and because the material is viscous, it is injected deeply and requires no overcorrection. Artecoll is reinjected at 6 to 8 weeks if necessary. In this regard, Artecoll is similar to microdroplet silicone injections. Artecoll is mainly used for glabella frown lines, nasolabial and radial lip lines, marionette lines, philtrum augmentation, acne scars and other subdermal or deeper defects. PMMA seems to be an inert substance and has been used as bone cement for 30 years without immunological reaction (31). The collagen carrier, however, has the same reaction potential as bovine collagen and requires at least one skin test 4 to 8 weeks before definitive treatment. Side effects include redness, swelling and moderate pain and are reasonably common in the first 2 days. Type 4 allergy has not

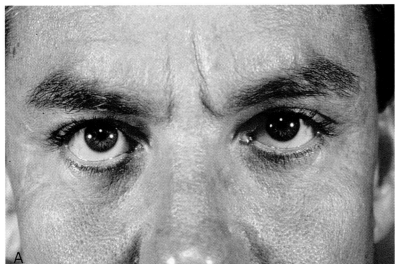
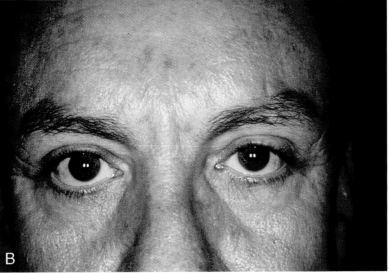

FIGURE 21.16
A, Glabellar folds preoperatively. B, After Gore-Tex augmentation, there is excellent improvement and contour. (Figure courtesy of Sue Ellen Cox, MD.)

been observed as yet, although an acute allergic reaction has been seen (31). Other side effects include itching, long lasting redness from too superficial injection technique, and hypertrophic scars on the lips of two patients. Migration has not been observed. Histologically, fibrosis ensues until the fourth month and usually a variable layer of new collagen fibers is noted.

SPECIFIC TREATMENT SCENARIOS

Nasolabial Furrows

Nasolabial furrows may vary from a superficial crease to a deep furrow. Skin resurfacing with deep chemical peeling, dermabrasion, or laser resurfacing may diminish the depths of these furrows. However, specific aggressive resurfacing into the furrow can risk scar formation. Anatomically, these furrows result from the movement of facial muscles and will recur to some extent after all forms of resurfacing. Full face resurfacing tightens the furrow from both the cheek and upper lip borders and achieves more improvement than resurfacing of the upper lip cosmetic unit only.

Patients with prominent nasolabial furrows will usually benefit from soft tissue augmentation as well as skin resurfacing (Figs. 21.9, 21.11, 21.13, 21.15). During the initial consultation, if the patient cannot schedule a prolonged recovery time as required with skin resurfacing, the physician can advise soft tissue augmentation of the furrows with Zyplast, Fibrel, Gore-Tex, or fat to temporarily improve contours. This can be repeated as the correction fades until the patient can undergo resurfacing. Once the resurfacing procedure has been completed, most patients will not see dramatic tightening of these furrows and often still require augmentation to achieve the best results. It is better to wait until the dermis has recovered sufficiently from the insult of the resurfacing procedure before dermal soft tissue augmentation is attempted. Thus, an interval of at least 3 months after laser, dermabrasion, or medium or deep chemical peeling is warranted before the use of Zyderm, Fibrel, or Hylan gel. Gore-Tex implantation should also wait at least 3 months. However, fat transplantation into the subcutaneous tissue is feasible approximately 2 weeks after resurfacing. The increased vascularization stimulated by the wound response to resurfacing may even enhance graft integration.

Perioral Lines

Many women over the age of 40 develop vertical lines of the upper or lower lips often with radiating rhytides at the lateral oral commissures. These rhytides are often dramatically improved after deep resurfacing whether abrasive, chemical or laser. Successful skin resurfacing may entirely eliminate these wrinkles. If only partial improvement is obtained however, soft tissue augmentation may be required to achieve the best

results (Fig. 21.9). Less viscous products such as Zyderm I or Hylan gel should probably be used in these lines. These products can be instilled into the superficial dermis. Many patients at the time of the consultation are not ready to undergo resurfacing immediately and may benefit from temporary augmentation with Zyderm I or Hylan gel until they can schedule the time for recovery.

Periorbital Lines

The dynamic effects of the orbicularis muscle often create crow's feet, even in patients in their early 20s. As the crow's feet become more severe, they are a cause of cosmetic distress. In many cases, aggressive resurfacing can entirely eliminate these lines. However, the lines recur to some degree with continued muscle movement. Botulinum toxin denervation using BOTOX (Allergan, Inc., Irvine, CA) before and after laser resurfacing helps to achieve continued improvement. Another alternative to correct crow's feet is soft tissue augmentation using Zyderm I or Hylan gel. These less viscous products can be instilled using a small gauge needle into these fine wrinkles. More viscous materials, such as Zyplast, fat, or Fibrel, often create beading and are not appropriate. As with other areas of the face, soft tissue augmentation may be performed as a delay tactic prior to resurfacing or subsequent to resurfacing as the rhytides reappear.

Glabellar Lines

These lines are the result of facial muscle movement especially with frowning. BOTOX denervation is the treatment of choice for this area. A more aggressive but permanent treatment involves forehead lifting with sectioning of the corrugator and procerus muscles. Even the more aggressive technique is often imperfect as the muscles may reform to some degree, sometimes resulting in a distorted frown line.

Augmentation with Zyderm II is an appealing temporary approach to smoothing out glabellar lines. More viscous materials such as Zyplast are occasionally associated with dermal necrosis most likely due to occlusion of small blood vessels (32). Sometimes Zyderm II augmentation is combined with BOTOX denervation. Zyderm II augmentation may also be used in conjunction with skin resurfacing in the glabellar area. Skin resurfacing alone however only temporarily improves these lines, and with continued muscle action they will recur. Consequently, BOTOX denervation should be at the heart of any treatment scheme for the lower forehead.

Another alternative to eliminate glabellar lines is fat transplantation, but rare cases of blindness have been noted after inadvertent intravascular injection of fat in this area (33). Blindness has also been noted after similar injection of Zyplast. Artecoll is advocated for this area, but given the above experience with fat and

Zyplast, caution is expressed regarding deep injection methods. Certainly, whatever agent is used should be injected on withdrawal of the syringe if implanted deeply in dermis or subcutis. Gore-Tex and SoftForm® augmentation avoids these problems (Fig. 21.16).

Horizontal Forehead Lines

Horizontal forehead lines occur due to movement of the underlying facial muscles (frontalis). Although skin resurfacing may temporarily improve these rhytides, they are likely to recur with continued muscle movement. BOTOX denervation is an excellent way to weaken the frontalis muscle and soften these lines. Further improvement may also be achieved with soft tissue augmentation using dermal fillers such as Zyderm II or Hylan gel (Fig. 21.5). A combination of BOTOX, soft tissue augmentation, and laser resurfacing may provide the best results. Forehead lifting, whether done conventionally or by endoscopic means, will also improvement these lines but requires much greater recovery and costs.

Marionette Lines

Patients developing aging changes in their lower face with resorption of the bony mandible and soft tissues such as the lower lip may develop quite marked hollowed areas below the lower lip, termed marionette lines. Fat and collagen are the most commonly used augmenting agents to treat these lines.

This is a difficult area to correct. Often the area is filled in a triangular fashion with special emphasis on lengthening the lower lip. Resurfacing alone has very little beneficial effect on this area.

Lip Augmentation

Soft tissue augmentation is an excellent way to enlarge the flattened lip, which often occurs with aging. Lips can be temporarily augmented using Zyplast at the mucocutaneous junction and Zyderm I injected directly into the vermillion. Alternatively, Gore-Tex may be threaded through the mucocutaneous junction. Fat transplantation also works well with injection directly into the body of the lips. Aggressive resurfacing causes enough skin tightening around the lips to pull the vermillion up to some extent. Often this results in the full lip the patient desired without the need for augmentation. Soft tissue augmentation may be deferred in patients who are contemplating skin resurfacing until after the resurfacing procedure.

Scars

Soft scars that are easily flattened by stretching the surrounding skin, usually respond well to tissue augmentation. An ice pick scar or deep fibrotic scar may require excision or punch grafting followed by skin resurfacing to obtain improvement. Resurfacing alone may suffi-

ciently improve soft pliable scars because of collagen tightening of the normal surrounding skin which stretches out the scars. In many cases, however, even aggressive resurfacing using dermabrasion or laser results in only partial improvement of deeper scars. Soft tissue augmentation with fat, Zyplast, Fibrel, or grafting with dermis often further improves the facial contours (Fig. 21.14). The augmentation should be deferred until skin resurfacing is complete unless the patient intends to delay resurfacing for at least 6 to 9 months. In these cases, temporary improvement of the scars can be accomplished using augmentation until the resurfacing is scheduled.

Depressed scars resulting from surgery or accidents often respond less favorably to soft tissue augmentation than post acne scars. Depressed scars are best treated by dermabrasion 6 weeks after the injury. If the patient consults the physician several months or years after the initial surgery or injury, scar excision and then abrasion 6 weeks postoperatively is appropriate to obtain the best results. Occasionally, additional benefits can be achieved using soft tissue implants, especially Zyplast or Fibrel after the results of the resurfacing are apparent.

SUMMARY

Skin resurfacing often results in partial improvement of deeper scars and wrinkles. Soft tissue augmentation is an excellent ancillary technique to further the benefits of skin resurfacing. Using a variety of modalities often achieves better results than aggressively employing skin resurfacing as a solo approach.

REFERENCES

1. Clark DP, Hanke CW, Swanson NA. Dermal implants: safety of products injected for soft tissue augmentation. J Am Acad Dermatol 1989;21:992.
2. Robinson JK, Hanke CW. Injectable collagen implant: histopathologic identification and longevity of correction. J Dermatol Surg Oncol 1985;11:124.
3. McPherson JM, Sawamura S, Armstrong R. An examination of the biological response to injectable, glutaraldehyde cross-linked collagen implants. J Biomed Mater Res 1986;20:93.
4. Coleman WP III. Assessment of a new device for injecting bovine collagen: the ADG needle. J Dermatol Surg 1996;22:175-176.
5. Delustro F, MacKinnon V, et al. Immunology of injectable collagen in human subjects. J Dermatol Surg Oncol 1978;17:49.
6. Elson ML. The role of skin testing in the use of collagen injectable materials. J Dermatol Surg Oncol 1989;15:301.
7. McPherson JM, Sawamura S, Conti A. Preparation of (3H) collagen for studies of the biological fate of zenogenic collagen implants in vivo. J Invest Dermatol 1985;86:673.
8. Spangler AS. New treatment for pitted scars. Arch Dermatol 1957;76:708.

9. Gottlieb S. GAP repair technique, poster exhibit. American Academy of Dermatology Annual Meeting. Dallas, TX December 1977.

10. Millikan LE. Long term safety and efficacy with Fibrel in the treatment of cutaneous scars–results of a multicenter study. J Dermatol Surg Oncol 1989;15:837.

11. Millikan L, Banks K, Purkait B, et al. A five year safety and efficacy evaluation with Fibrel in correction of cutaneous scars following one or two treatments. J Dermatol Surg Oncol 1991;17:223.

12. Neuber F. Fettransplantation. Chir Kongr Verhandl Dsch Gesellsch Chir 1893;22:66.

13. Illouz YG. The fat cell graft: a new technique to fill depressions. Plast Reconstr Surg 1986;78:122.

14. Lauber J, Abrams H, Coleman WP III. Application of the tumescent technique for hand augmentation. J Dermatol Surg 1990;16:369.

15. Carraway J, Mellow C. Syringe aspirations and fat concentration: a simple technique for autologous fat injection. Ann Plast Surg 1990;24:293.

16. Pinski KS, Roenigk HH. Autologous fat transplantation: long term follow up. J Dermatol Surg Oncol 1992;18:179.

17. Coleman SR. Long term survival of fat transplants: controlled demonstrations. Aesth Plast Surg 1995;19:421.

18. Moscona R, Ullman Y, Har-Shai Y, et al. Free fat injections for the correction of facial hemiatrophy. Plast Reconstr Surg 1989;84:501.

19. Niechajev I, Sevcuk O. Long term results of fat transplantation. Clinical and histologic studies. Plast Reconstr Surg 1994;94:496.

20. Lam A, Moy R. The potential for fat transplantation. J Dermatol Surg Oncol 1992;18:432.

21. Fournier P. Facial recontouring with fat grafting. Dermatol Clin 1989;8:523.

22. Zocchi M. Methode de production de collagene autologue par traitment du tissu graisseax. J de Medecine Esthetique et Chirurgie Dermatologique 1990;17:105.

23. Coleman WP III, Lawrence N, Sherman RN, et al. Autologous collagen lipocytic dermal augmentation: A histological study. J Dermatol Surg Oncol 1993;19:1032.

24. Peer LA, Paddock R. Histologic studies on the face of deeply implanted dermal grafts. Observation on sections of implants buried from one week to one year. Arch Surg 1937;34:268.

25. Swinehart JM. Pocket grafting with dermal grafts. Autologous collagen implants for permanent correction of cutaneous depressions. Am J Cosmet Surg 1995;12:321.

26. Abergel RP, Schlask CM, Garcia LE, et al. The Laser Dermal Implant: a new technique for preparation and implantation of autologous dermal grafts for the correction of depressed scars, lip augmentation, and nasolabial folds using Silk Touch laser technology. Am J Cosmet Surg 1996;13:15.

27. Goodman GJ. Laser assisted dermal grafting for the correction of cutaneous contour defects Dermatol Surg (in press).

28. Piacquadio D. Cross-linked hyaluronic acid (Hylan Gel) as a soft tissue augmentation material. A preliminary assessment. In: Elson ML, ed. Evaluation and Treatment of the Aging Face. New York: Springer-Verlag, 1995;340.

29. Camps-Fresneda A. The use of Gore-Tex combined with other fillers. In: Elson ML, ed. Evaluation and Treatment of the Aging Face. New York: Springer-Verlag, 1995;302.

30. Melton JL, Hanke CW. Soft tissue augmentation. In: Roenigk RK, Roenigk HHR, eds. Dermatologic Surgery. 2nd edition. New York: Marcel Dekker, 1996.

31. Lemperle G, Hazan-Gauthier, Lemperle M. PMMA microspheres (Artecoll) for skin and soft tissue augmentation. Part II: clinical Investigations. Plast Reconstr Surg 1995;96:627.

32. Hanke CW, Jolivette D, Stegman SJ, et al. Abscess formulation and local necrosis following treatment with Zyderm or Zyplast collagen implant. J Am Acad Dermatol 1991;25:319.

33. Driezen NG, Framm L. Sudden unilateral visual loss after autologous fat injection into the glabella area. Am J Ophthalmol 1989;107:85.

CHAPTER 22

Combining Botulinum Toxin Injection and Laser Resurfacing for Facial Rhytides

■ Jean Carruthers
Alastair Carruthers

Two powerful treatments for facial wrinkling have recently emerged—botulinum toxin injection (BOTOX, Allergan Inc., Irvine, CA) and carbon dioxide (CO_2) laser resurfacing. These approaches reduce wrinkles by different means. BOTOX denervates the underlying facial muscles that cause the wrinkles while CO_2 lasers vaporize photoaged epidermis and dermis, inducing formation of new epithelium, dermal collagen, and elastin. The onset of BOTOX muscle weakening occurs 24 to 72 hours after injection and the total response lasts 3 to 6 months. The healing process after laser resurfacing takes 3 to 6 months. Both methods treat static and dynamic facial rhytides, but each has a weighted effect, with BOTOX acting predominantly on the facial musculature and thus dynamic wrinkles, and the CO_2 laser acting primarily on altering the fabric of the skin at rest, or in other words, static wrinkles.

In this chapter, the use of the two modalities in combination will be explored since their combined effect can be greater than use of either method alone. In reality, most lines and wrinkles are due to both static and dynamic factors, and so the causes should not be considered in isolation. We propose that treatment with both BOTOX injection and laser resurfacing allows the newly-synthesized collagen that is laid down after laser ablation to be modeled in a less wrinkled pattern if the underlying musculature is inactive. Thus combined treatment in areas such as the crow's feet will produce better short and long-term results.

NEUROPHYSIOLOGY OF THE ACTION OF BOTOX

BOTOX prevents the release of acetylcholine at the neuromuscular junction (NMJ) of cholinergically innervated muscle, and thus causes reversible paralysis of affected striated muscle (1). This paralysis occurs through a four-step procedure, the first step being binding of the free end of the heavy chain to receptors on the presynaptic neurons. This binding process takes 32 to 64 minutes in an in vitro model (2). Secondly, the bound toxin is internalized to the presynaptic neuron, and thirdly, the toxin enters the neurocytoplasm. The fourth step is that the toxin inhibits acetylcholine packet release at the NMJ. The short chain of the BOTOX molecule is a zinc-dependent endoprotease that inactivates specific components of the neuroexocytic mechanism by enzymatic cleavage (3).

Histologically, human and experimental model vertebrate muscles behave similarly after BOTOX injection. Within 2 weeks, the muscles atrophy with some fibers being more atrophic than others. This atrophy stabilizes after 4 weeks. Acetylcholinesterase activity is seen over the whole sarcolemma and, after 4 to 5 months, returns to its pure NMJ location.

BOTOX accelerates the normal process of NMJ turnover and repair. Within 10 days, unmyelinated axonal sprouts develop at pre- and postsynaptic terminals and these create new NMJs that are less organized. One NMJ may have more than one axonal sprout and vice versa. Restoration and remodeling occur slowly and histological changes can be seen up to 3 years after exposure. This process has recently been reviewed (4).

IMMUNOLOGY, ALLERGY, AND CONTRAINDICATIONS TO BOTOX THERAPY

BOTOX is an immunogenic protein that can cause IgG antibody production. This is of clinical significance when larger doses of BOTOX (more than 100 units per session) are given. For example, in the treatment of cervical dystonia, antibody production may affect from 5% to 30% in treated individuals (5, 6). However, in one author's experience (J.C.), the development of secondary treatment resistance has not been seen in over 10,000 injection sessions of less than 100 units per session as would be expected if significant levels of blocking antibodies were present. Patients who develop this resistance problem may need treatment with another botulinum toxin such as botulinum toxin-B or botulinum toxin-F as there is no cross-reactivity between the toxins. The development of IgG antibodies is promoted by dosages greater than 100 units per treatment session and by booster injections within 4 weeks of the initial injection.

BOTOX therapy is extremely safe. The estimated human LD/50 is 40 units/kg, or 2500 to 3000 units for the average 70 kg patient (7–9). The dose range we use for cosmetic indications of 5 to 50 units is comfortably below the average and well within the therapeutic margin. Contraindications for BOTOX injection include pregnancy or lactation. Scott reported nine individuals inadvertently treated during pregnancy (10). Eight of the nine babies were completely normal at delivery, but the ninth was born prematurely, probably for reasons unrelated to the BOTOX. In addition, there is both experimental and clinical evidence that botulinum toxin does not cross the placenta in significant amounts. In spite of this, neither the manufacturers nor ourselves recommend the use of BOTOX during pregnancy.

Pretreatment evaluations should include inquiries about possible associated neurologic diseases. If a patient has a neuromuscular disease, such as amyotrophic lateral sclerosis, an opinion should be given by a neurologist as to the safety of treatment. BOTOX has however, recently become a staple in neurologists' treatment of spasticity, whether congenital, as in cerebral palsy, or acquired, as in post-strokes and multiple sclerosis. Most neurologists would probably recommend continued use of BOTOX in neurological conditions, but perhaps in a lower dose, especially in diseases affecting the neuromuscular junction, such as myasthenia gravis.

METHODS OF BOTOX TREATMENT

Crow's Feet

To denervate the muscle underlying crow's feet, BOTOX that has been kept frozen at −4°C is diluted using 1 ml of nonpreserved sterile saline and injected with a half-inch 30-gauge needle on a tuberculin syringe (11, 12). We inject 4 to 5 units in three sites (total 12 to 15 units per side), ensuring that the injection sites are outside the orbital margin (Fig. 22.1). Diplopia has been reported following treatment for crow's feet, which is presumably due to inappropriate placement of injections medial to the lateral orbital margin (13).

Garcia and Fulton recommend a more diluted toxin to treat patients using 10 ml of saline per vial and injecting approximately 4 units of BOTOX in the crow's feet area on each side (13). This is approximately one-third to one-quarter of the dose that we use in this area. In our judgement, the Fulton method does not produce as great an effect on wrinkles as does our method and does not appear to last as long.

Glabellar Frown Lines

For denervation of glabellar frown lines, we recommend injecting 15 to 20 units of BOTOX divided among the procerus, corrugator and medial orbicularis muscles (Fig. 22.2) (14–16). If fine vertical rhytides are seen temporally on forced frowning, or if the brow morphology

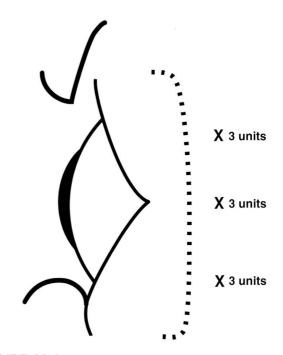

X 3 units

X 3 units

X 3 units

FIGURE 22.1

Injection sites and dosages for BOTOX treatment of crow's feet.

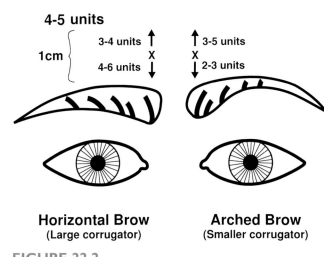

FIGURE 22.2
Injection sites and dosages for BOTOX treatment of the glabella.

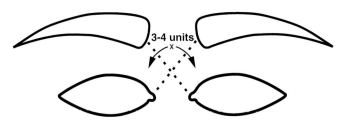

FIGURE 22.3
Injection sites and dosages for BOTOX treatment of procerus and depressor supercilii muscles.

is mainly horizontal instead of arched, an additional 3 to 4 units can be injected 1 cm above the bony orbital rim in the midpupillary line. Injection below this 1 cm gap can lead to lid ptosis. This injection treats the temporal orbicularis and possibly also the tail of the corrugator.

Five units of the diluted BOTOX solution should also be injected just above the intersection of the medial canthus and the opposite medial brow line to treat the procerus muscle (Fig. 22.3). Massage of this area directs the toxin toward the depressor supercilii muscle. We believe that part of the "angry" look seen in some patients is because of inferior movement of the medial brow due to the action of procerus and depressor supercilii muscles. In contrast, by relaxing these muscles and allowing unopposed action of the frontalis muscle, an "open-eyed" appearance is produced. The injection into the procerus muscle is the only injection in the central brow area that should be massaged.

Post-treatment Patient Instructions

Patients should not manipulate the injected areas for 4 hours after treatment. During that time, patients should remain vertical, (e.g., no naps) because the ptosis incidence for other BOTOX treated conditions

(blepharospasm and hemifacial spasm) shrinks from 11% to 2% with this simple change (15, 16). Recently, it has been shown that BOTOX binds preferentially to active muscles, so requesting patients to frown and smile for at least an hour after injection can enhance the overall degree of muscle paresis (17).

PATHOPHYSIOLOGY OF PULSED CO_2 LASER THERAPY ON HUMAN SKIN

The pulse of a CO_2 laser is designed to last less then 1 msec so that adequate thermal relaxation of the skin can occur. This short dwell time vaporizes the skin without leaving a residual underlying thermal burn to the dermis. The precision and flexibility of the various light application patterns of the computer pattern generator, and the density and power of the laser allows the surgeon to take into account the variability of skin thickness and clinical involvement between different facial areas (e.g., skin on the lower eyelid, which is very thin, versus skin on the brow, which is thicker) (18).

On each pass, the dermal collagen is heated to 55° to 60°C so that, although the collagen fibril will shrink, it will survive. In the 3- to 6-month period following the treatment, new collagen and elastin are formed in the dermis and collagen production may increase up to 600% in the Grenz zone. The dermal healing response to laser treatment is also seen when other resurfacing treatments, such as chemical peeling or dermabrasion, are used (19–29). The new collagen and elastin in the dermis and the new epithelium appear to correlate with the improved nonwrinkled clinical response (28).

COMBINING BOTOX AND CO_2 LASER TREATMENT

In a recent study by the authors, BOTOX and CO_2 laser resurfacing were combined on 9 patients. All patients had moderately severe to severe facial wrinkling with Glogau type III and IV skin with associated elastosis and dyschromia, and all had underlying Fitzpatrick skin type I to III. Patients were pretreated with 0.025% tretinoin cream, 10% glycolic acid, butylmethoxydibenzolmethane (Parsol 1789), titanium dioxide sunscreen, and 4% hydroquinone cream. Most patients routinely used tretinoin, glycolic acid, and Parsol 1789 in their ongoing skin care program and began use of the bleaching agent 2 weeks before laser therapy.

Four patients had BOTOX injected in their most involved side of crow's feet 1 week before either full-face or periocular laser resurfacing (Figs. 22.4, 22.5). Five patients underwent symmetrical bilateral BOTOX to the crow's feet area 1 week before laser therapy (Figs. 22.6, 22.7). Five units of BOTOX were injected into each site for a total of 15 units on each side.

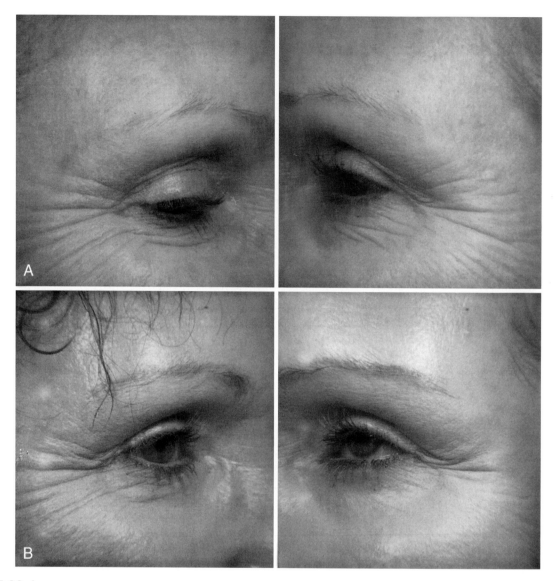

FIGURE 22.4
A, 43-year-old patient smiling before right-sided laser resurfacing and left-sided BOTOX injection with laser resurfacing. B, Same patient smiling 2 months postoperatively.

On the day of the procedure, patients began oral cephalexin (500 mg three times daily) and acyclovir (800 mg three times daily). After one patient developed facial herpes simplex vesicles on the sixth postoperative day while on acyclovir, subsequent patients were treated with oral famcyclovir (500 mg three times daily) because of its better gastrointestinal absorption. These medications were taken the day of the procedure and continued for 10 days postoperatively.

Before laser therapy, the face was cleansed with chlorhexidine and thoroughly rinsed with normal saline and dried. In patients receiving local anesthesia only, 1.5% lidocaine with 1:200,000 adrenaline was injected to block the supraorbital, infraorbital and mental nerves. Field blocks with the same medication were

continued so the entire face was blocked. Most patients who underwent full-face laser resurfacing had a general anesthetic with intravenous propofol and a laryngeal mask airway, monitored by an anesthesiologist.

The UltraPulse 5000 laser (Coherent Laser Corp., Palo Alto, CA) was used on all patients. In the glabella and crow's feet areas, the settings were density of 6-7, pattern three, spot size of seven, 225 to 300 mJ, with a 0.5 seconds repeat. Two laser passes were routinely used except on the pretarsal portion of the eye lids or where the patients were judged to have thin skin.

The generally accepted endpoint of "chamois" was not used because we believe that it may be more an indicator of thermal damage than of dermal depth. Thus, by some laser surgeons' parameters, our patients may

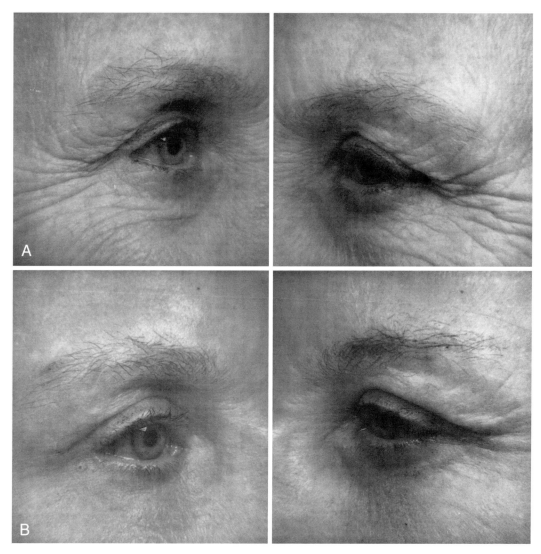

FIGURE 22. 5
A, 68-year-old patient smiling before right-sided BOTOX injection and bilateral whole face laser resurfacing. B, Same patient smiling at 10 weeks postoperatively.

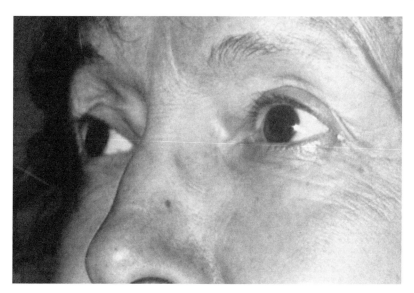

FIGURE 22.6
Semiprofile oblique view before bilateral laser blepharoplasties, bilateral BOTOX injection, and laser resurfacing.

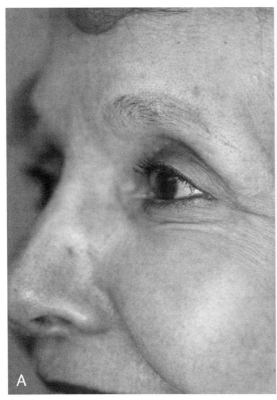

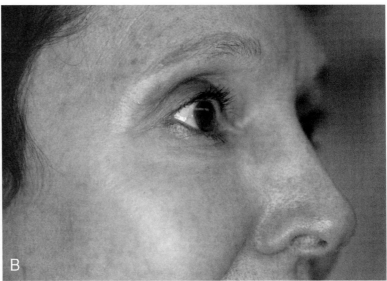

FIGURE 22.7

A and B, Oblique views of the same patient in Figure 22.6 after laser blepharoplasty, bilateral BOTOX injection and periocular laser resurfacing.

have been undertreated. We believe elective retreatment is a safer option than initial overtreatment.

Postoperative wound care included hourly soaking and debridement of the serous exudate and necrotic tissue with tap water containing one tablespoon of acetic acid (white vinegar), and maintaining a moist tissue surface. Continuous application of an ointment such as Vaseline (Chesebrough-Ponds Inc., Greenwich, CT), Crisco, or a plasticized base was used after the debridement. After re-epithelialization at 6 to 8 days, the soaks were discontinued and moisturizer or Vaseline continued for a further 7 to 8 days. In addition, make-up was used to cover postoperative erythema when patients went out in public. Pretreatment topical medications were restarted 2 weeks postoperatively for a minimum of 3 months (hydroquinone) to 6 months or more (tretinoin, alpha hydroxy acids, sunscreen).

At follow-up between 1 and 7 months (average 5 months), all patients were delighted with the relaxation of both static and dynamic periocular wrinkles. All of the patients, who had also undergone previous BOTOX injection procedures in the past, felt that the combined use of BOTOX injection and CO_2 laser resurfacing had given them a more relaxed, open and contented appearance than the use of either modality alone (Fig. 22.8). The four patients treated asymmetrically with BOTOX injections preferred the result on the side with combined therapy, over the side treated with laser resurfacing alone. One individual treated with BOTOX on one side only felt so strongly about the superior result on her BOTOX-treated side, that she underwent BOTOX injection on the other side 5 months after the laser therapy.

Complications included symmetrical areas of induration in the medial upper lids in one individual that were treated with intralesional 1 mg triamcinolone acetonide injections on each side and 1% hydrocortisone cream four times daily for a week. One patient (previously mentioned) developed herpes simplex virus infection despite taking acyclovir prophylaxis that settled completely without scarring on an increased dose of acyclovir to 800 mg five times daily. Another patient developed a *Staphylococcus aureus* infection around the mouth and responded to oral cloxicillin 500 mg three times daily and mupirocin ointment four times daily.

CONCLUSIONS

The wrinkle is symbolic of increasing public concern with facially visible aging. Studies of facial wrinkles of all types by light and scanning electron microscopy show that the wrinkles represent a configurational change rather than a specific structural change in the skin, except for elastic tissue network deterioration seen throughout the dermis (26–28). Laser vaporization of photoaged epidermis and dermis results in immediate clinical improvement due to collagen contraction and delayed clinical improvement due to increased collagen I deposition and collagen remodeling (22, 25).

BOTOX affects facial wrinkles by relaxing muscular action, further stimulating collagen remodeling and as a result facial wrinkles shorten, become shallower, or may disappear at rest after focal facial muscle paresis has been present for approximately a year (11).

Weakening the muscular control of the superficial musculo-aponeurotic system (SMAS) is a logical pretreatment adjunct to laser resurfacing. Dissections of the SMAS show that the system extends from the frontalis to the platysma muscle, including the temporal part of the orbicularis oculi (the crow's feet area) (30). Through its fibrous septal attachments to skin above and mimetic muscles below, the SMAS acts as a distributor of facial muscular contractions to the skin.

EVALUATING WRINKLE REDUCTION BY EACH MODALITY ON ITS OWN VERSUS IN COMBINATION

Fitzpatrick et al. demonstrated a 45% to 50% improvement in wrinkle scores when an UltraPulse CO_2 laser was used alone (18). We and others have shown similar improvement with BOTOX injections, but with the longest treatment response being about a year and the average, 4 to 6 months (10–13, 15). Study of BOTOX-treated facial wrinkles using casts showed a two-thirds improvement in wrinkle reduction that was still present 5 months after treatment (31).

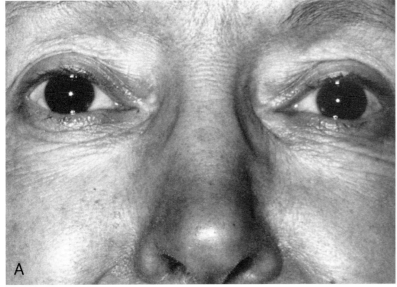
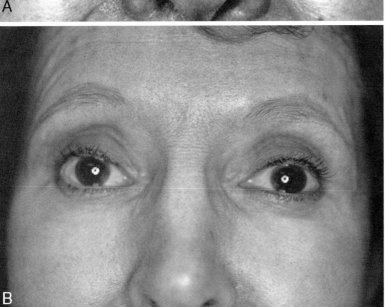

FIGURE 22.8
Front view of a 58-year-old patient before (A) and after (B) bilateral upper and lower lid laser blepharoplasty, bilateral prelaser BOTOX injection and periocular laser resurfacing.

Each modality allows new collagen to be laid down. By treating wrinkles in this fashion, new collagen formation does not reconfigure into the old wrinkle pattern. Timing the denervation of facial mimetic muscles before peak synthesis of new collagen at 3 to 12 weeks is important and may be more effective than waiting for months or years after laser treatment. In addition, the use of BOTOX to ameliorate a "dissolving" laser result may require several treatment sessions but may salvage a potentially discontented patient.

Combined therapy of BOTOX denervation and CO_2 laser resurfacing gives a dramatic improvement in wrinkling in the early (4 to 6 months) postresurfacing period. Based on the comparison of patients treated with only laser resurfacing, with laser resurfacing on both sides and BOTOX on one side, and with laser resurfacing and BOTOX on both sides, the combination consistently enhances the short-term result.

Unanswered questions concerning BOTOX injections include whether the injections will affect the long-term result of CO_2 laser resurfacing. Theory indicates that BOTOX injections should have a positive effect and our own results give initial positive indications on this theory as does the experience of others who have used BOTOX preresurfacing for up to a year (R. Fitzpatrick, presentation at the American Academy of Cosmetic Surgery Meeting, Rancho Mirage, CA 1997). However, proof will require a long-term within-patient comparison. Such studies are under way but there is difficulty persuading individuals to continue with one-sided BOTOX treatment because the short-term result is so obviously superior.

REFERENCES

1. Simpson LL. Peripheral actions of the botulinum toxin. In: Simpson LL, ed. Botulinum neurotoxin and tetanus toxin. New York: Academic Press, 1989:153-178.
2. Simpson LL. Kinetic studies on the interaction between botulinum type A and the cholinergic neuromuscular junction. J Pharmacol Exp Ther 1980;212:16-21.
3. Schiavo G, Rossetto O, Benefati F, et al. Tetanus and botulinum neurotoxins are zinc-dependent proteases specific for components of the neuroexocytosis apparatus. Ann NY Acad Sci 1994;710:65-75.
4. Carruthers A, Kiene K, Carruthers J. Botulinum exotoxin use in clinical dermatology. J Am Acad Dermatol 1996;34: 788-797.
5. Borodic GE, Joseph M, Fay L, et al. Botulinum A toxin for the treatment of spasmodic torticollis: dysphagia and regional toxin spread. Head Neck 1990;12:398-399.
6. Tsui JK, Wong NLM, Wong E, et al. Production of circulating antibodies to botulinum toxin A in patients receiving repeated injections for dystonia (abstract). Ann Neurol 1988;23:181.
7. Scott AB, Suzuki D. Systemic toxicity of botulinum toxin by intramuscular injection in the monkey. Mov Disord 1988;3:333-335.
8. Meyer KF, Eddie B. Perspectives concerning botulism. Z Hyg Infect Krankheiten 1951;133:255-263.
9. Lamanna C, Hillowalla RA, Alling CC. Buccal exposure to botulinum toxin. J Infect Dis 1967;117:327-331.
10. Scott AB. Clostridial toxins as therapeutic agents. In: Simpson LL, ed. Botulinum neurotoxin and tetanus toxin. New York: Academic Press, 1989;399-412.
11. Carruthers A, Carruthers JDA. Botulinum toxin in the treatment of glabellar frown lines and other facial wrinkles. In: Jankovic J, Hallet M, eds. Therapy with botulinum toxin. New York: Marcel Dekker, 1994;577-595.
12. Carruthers A, Carruthers JDA. The use of botulinum toxin to treat glabellar frown lines and other facial wrinkles. Cosmet Dermatol 1994;7:11-15.
13. Garcia A, Fulton JE. Cosmetic denervation of the muscles of facial expression with botulinum toxin. Dermatol Surg 1996;22:39-43.
14. Carruthers A, Carruthers JDA. Cosmetic uses of botulinum toxin. In: Coleman WP, Hanke W, Alt TH, eds. Cosmetic surgery of the skin. New York: Mosby, 1997;231-235.
15. Carruthers JDA, Carruthers JA, Bagaric D. Can ptosis incidence be reduced after lid injections for blepharospasm and hemifacial spasm? Can J Ophthalmol 1995;30:147.
16. Carruthers A, Carruthers JDA. Cosmetic uses of botulinum A exotoxin. Advances in dermatology. Volume 12. New York: Mosby Yearbook, 1997;325-348.
17. Deutschl G, Glocker SX. Evidence for differential uptake-mechanisms in hypercontracting muscle fibres. Mov Disord 1995;10:366.
18. Fitzpatrick RE, Topa WD, Goldman MP, Saturn NM. Pulsed carbon dioxide laser, trichloracetic acid, Baker-Gordon phenol and dermabrasion: a comparative clinical and histologic study of cutaneous resurfacing in a porcine model. Arch Dermatol 1996;132:469-471.
19. Nelson BR, Fader DJ, Gillard M, et al. Pilot, histologic and ultrastructural studies of the effect of medium depth chemical facial peels in dermal collagen of patients with actinically damaged skin. J Am Acad Dermatol 1995;132:470-480.
20. Kligman AM, Baker TJ, Gordon HL. Long-term histologic follow-up from phenol facial peels. Plast Reconstr Surg 1985;75:652-659.
21. Spira M, Dahl C, Freeman R, et al. Chemosurgery: a histologic study. Plast Reconstr Surg 1970;45:247-253.
22. Baker TJ, Gordon HL, Moczienko P, et al. Long-term histological study of skin after chemical face peeling. Plast Reconstr Surg 1974;53:522-525.
23. Pollack SV. Wound healing: A review: The biology of wound healing. J Derm Surg Oncol 1979;5:389-393.
24. Nelson BR, Majmudar G, Griffiths EM, et al. Clinical improvement following dermabrasion of photoaged skin correlates with synthesis of collagen I. Acta Dermatol 1994;130:1136-1142.
25. Benedetto AV, Griffin TD, Benedetto EA, et al. Dermabrasion therapy and prophylaxis of the photoaged face. J Am Acad Dermatol 1992;27:439-442.
26. Winton GR, Salasche SJ. Dermabrasion of the scalp as a treatment for actinic damage. J Am Acad Dermatol 1986;14:661-668.
27. Fitzpatrick RE, Goldman MP, Saturn NM, Tobe WD. Pulsed carbon dioxide laser resurfacing of photoaged facial skin. Arch Dermatol 1996;132:395-407.

28. Stegman SJ. A comparative histologic study of the effects of three peeling agents and dermabrasion on normal and sun-damaged skin. Aesth Plast Surg 1982;6:123-135.

29. Nelson BR, Met RD, Mashmundar G, et al. A comparison of wire brush and diamond fraise superfacial dermabrasion for photoaged skin: a clinical, immunohistologic and biochemical study. J Am Acad Dermatol 1996;34:235-243.

30. Mitz V, Peyronie M. The superficial muskuloeponeurotic system (SMAS) in the parotid and cheek area. Plast Reconstr Surg 1976;58:80-88.

31. Ascher B, Klap P, Marion MH, et al. La toxine botulinique dans la traitement des rides fronto-glabellaires de la région orbitaire. An Clin Plast Esthet 1995;40:67-76.

CHAPTER 23

Combining Laser Resurfacing and Blepharoplasty

■ Greg Goodman

"There are three things needed for beauty: harmony, wholeness and radiance." — *Aquinas*
"I know only one thing and that is that I know nothing." — *Socrates*

The baby boomers born after World War II spent the better part of the 1950s and 1960s in the sun ruining their skin. When they weren't sun-baking their periorbital skin, they were either squinting to avoid the sun's rays or smoking. As a consequence they are now middle-aged, demanding patients with more than their fair share of periorbital sun damage and rhytides. The periorbital region of these patients often illustrates a number of different aging changes that are best dealt with at a similar time in the patients lives. Specifically, patients may require resurfacing of the periorbital skin together with the correction of the hooded upper eyelid or the removal of lower eyelid herniated fat pads.

There are a number of other periorbital lesions that may be treated by periorbital resurfacing such as appendageal or cutaneous tumors. At this time, patients may often consider simultaneous blepharoplasty as they are already contemplating a procedure (laser resurfacing) with considerable recovery time that is commensurate with or longer than that of laser blepharoplasty.

With appropriate safety precautions, it is now possible to treat the entire periorbital zone with laser resurfacing. However, it is not always appropriate to do so at the time of blepharoplasty surgery. Whether or not it is appropriate at the same time, laser treatment is often still a useful adjunct to blepharoplasty.

METHODS OF TREATING PERIORBITAL SKIN

Skin resurfacing is a technique that can be used to correct abnormalities in the epidermis or superficial dermis. There are a number of methods to evenly wound these layers to produce a new epidermis (from surrounding intact epidermis and the appendageal structures) and a regenerated dermis (1-6). These methods include chemical peeling, dermabrasion and, more recently, carbon dioxide (CO_2) laser resurfacing.

Chemical peeling is a valuable technique for all grades of sundamage and wrinkling, however, it does tend to have a certain unpredictability of depth of penetration. This is especially so of the deeper peels. Phenol peels impair melanocyte function and may result in some degree of permanent hypopigmentation (5, 6). Also, peels tend to not totally eradicate wrinkling in this area. They are useful as a spot treatment for xanthelasmas in the form of strong trichloroacetic acid (TCA) or 88% phenol, but generally peeling agents are not very useful for treatment of appendageal tumors. TCA or 88% phenol are useful for treating the periorbital region in the absence of CO_2 laser technology, however, they rarely efface all wrinkles.

Brody has stated that it may be relatively safe to perform chemical peels at the same time as transconjunctival blepharoplasty, but medium and deep chemical peels should be delayed at least 1 to 3 months and possibly up to 6 months after transcutaneous lower eyelid blepharoplasty (7). Ectropion has occurred from peeling earlier. Lower eyelid peeling is less of a risk if only upper eyelid blepharoplasty is being performed (8).

Morrow is more confident of the simultaneous use of chemical peels and CO_2 laser upper and transconjunctival lower eyelid blepharoplasty. He refrains from using phenol as a peeling agent in this case and treats the infrabrow area with 35% TCA down to, but not including the incision line. The lower eyelids were treated with 35% to 50% TCA (9).

Dermabrasion has never been a realistic option in the periorbital region because of the delicate eyelid skin and the proximity of the orbital structures. In dermabrasions which are carried into the lower eyelid skin or those of the crow's feet area, it has been my experience that wrinkles are not particularly effaced with this technique.

Periorbital wrinkling particularly of the crow's feet area is well treated by collagen injections (Collagen Biomedical Corporation, Palo Alto, CA) but is limited. First, it is a temporary solution which patients may not prefer. Secondly, it is difficult to inject the infraorbital wrinkles without edema of this area interfering with vision. Third, the tendency for collagen to "bead" in the fine wrinkles of this area is a difficulty. This technique requires considerable expertise to perform well and attention should be paid to not overfilling the injected lines (10, 11). Fine wire diathermy (electrosurgery) is a reasonable technique for some small eyelid lesions such as milia, syringomas, sebaceous hyperplasia, acrochor-

dons and pedunculated warts, however, it is less effective than laser at treating widespread lesions and is of no use in the treatment of periorbital rhytides.

THE ADVENT OF MODERN CO_2 LASER RESURFACING

Since the first cases of laser resurfacing reported by David in 1985 and then David and Lask in 1989, there have major advances in CO_2 lasers for treating the surface of the skin (12, 13). Technology has reduced operator dependence, improving reproducibility of results. Two distinct approaches have been used to achieve char-free tissue ablation that appears to be so vital in reducing the complication rate associated with laser use (14–16).

High Energy, Short Pulsed Defocused CO_2 Lasers

The first approach involves very high energy, short pulsed CO_2 lasers, such as the UltraPulse CO_2 laser system (Coherent Laser Corp, Palo Alto, CA). This laser can deliver peak pulse powers of 500 W, with an energy density of 5 J/cm^2 to a 3 mm defocused spot size (17, 18). The pulse is very short, well under 1 ms. This vaporizes tissue so rapidly and completely that little heated tissue is left to transmit heat to nontargeted tissues (Fig. 23.1). Similar results are attainable with the SurgiPulse XJ-150 (Sharplan Lasers, Inc., Allendale, NJ), which produces energies up to 400 mJ by closely pairing two 200 mJ pulses.

The second characteristic of a high energy, short pulsed CO_2 laser system is that the power applied to the skin is determined solely by the number of pulses per second which can be varied. With this system, each pulse is an individual event that applies a certain amount of energy to the skin; the energy density per

FIGURE 23.1
Short pulse CO_2 laser systems deliver char-free ablation.

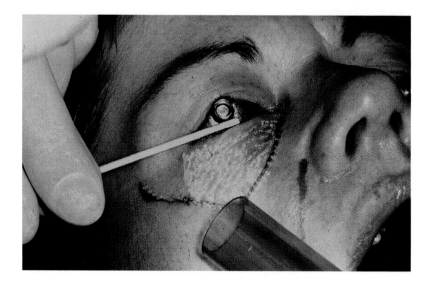

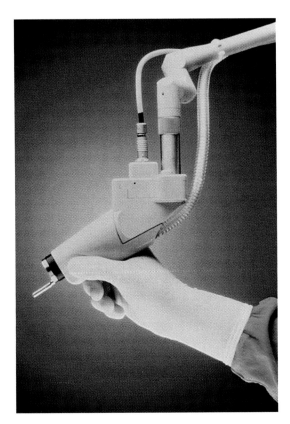

FIGURE 23.2
Scanners, such as the computer pattern generator, improve reproducibility of periorbital resurfacing.

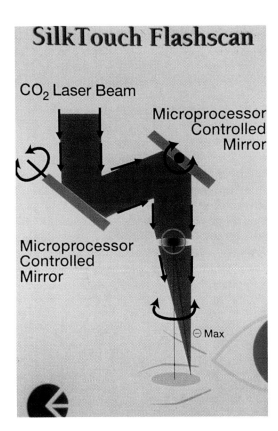

FIGURE 23.3
Scanning short-dwell-time focused CO_2 lasers also deliver reproducibility of results.

unit area (fluence) determines the effect on tissue. The laser is passed over the skin at a speed that allows each area to be treated by a single pulse. Further passes may be necessary to achieve the desired depth of tissue ablation. For maximum surgical control, (e.g., when removing small lesions) minimum power or number of pulses per second is employed. However, for treatment of large areas, a higher pulse rate is used commensurate with the ability of the operator to keep these pulses separate or only slightly overlapping.

A major advance in laser resurfacing is the 'collimated' hand piece, a lens which keeps the beam always defocused, that allows the distance from the target tissue to vary without varying the spot size or power density. This ensures even vaporization of tissue.

Scanning devices, such as the computerized pattern generator, have now become available and has reduced the need for hand speed variation (19). Pulses are placed in patterns of different sizes, shapes and area of overlap, enabling uniform application of laser energy to the skin and precise reproducibility between operators (Fig. 23.2). These devices also collimate the beam, enabling the operator to work at a distance from the skin. It is with these devices that most treatment is now given as it produces results of uniform quality if correctly used and the patients are correctly assessed.

The TruPulse laser system (Tissue Technologies, Albuquerque, NM) produces extremely short pulses of 90 msec duration but with a high energy pulse of 250 to 500 mJ. This induces less thermal transmission than other major CO_2 laser systems with only approximately 20% of patients still demonstrating postoperative erythema at 4 weeks. This laser may be useful in periorbital resurfacing where significant thermal injury may not be required for clinical effect.

Short Dwell Time Scanning CO_2 Lasers

The SilkTouch flash-scanning system (Sharplan, Allendale, NJ) is an example of a short dwell time scanning CO_2 laser. This produces char-free ablation by sharply focusing the beam, allowing high energies to be applied from a comparatively low energy laser system. The scanner rapidly moves a continuous beam in a spiral, keeping the dwell time at any particular point below 1 ms (20, 21). Recently, Sharplan further decreased the dwell time of the laser on tissue with the production of their "Feather-touch" adaptation (Fig. 23.3). Short dwell time scanning CO_2 lasers may have application especially in the periorbital regions where more delicate treatment is often desirable.

Both the high energy, short pulsed lasers and lower energy focused scanning lasers achieve superficial ablation by delivering their energy within the thermal relaxation time of skin (less than 1 ms). This achieves selective photothermolysis. The characteristic brown char caused by earlier CO_2 lasers, which correlates with a slow boiling of tissue and indicates heat transmission outside the intended target is largely absent with these laser systems when used correctly and results in faster healing with less complications.

The Erbium:YAG Laser

Erbium:YAG lasers, with a relatively near infrared wavelength (2,940 nm) when compared to CO_2 laser wavelength, has been recently suggested for resurfacing. Erbium:YAG lasers do not provide hemostasis comparable to CO_2 lasers and induce skin bleeding. These lasers induce rapid healing and its results are readily repeatable and again may have a future role in eyelid resurfacing.

LASER RESURFACING OF THE PERIORBITAL REGION

It is not always necessary or desirable to isolate part or all of the periorbital region since it is part of the full face procedure (Fig. 23.4). However, quite often the periorbital region is the only zone that needs resurfacing. When this circumstance arises, merging or feathering the new fresh periorbital skin into unresurfaced skin is important.

In general, when resurfacing the periorbital area the first rule that should be adhered to is to resurface the entire zone (Fig. 23.5). This probably exempts cases when only a few lesions are being treated, however, there are several reasons to treat the entire cosmetic unit if possible. Treating multiple lesions, such as syringomas in the midst of a sea of wrinkles, may cause disruption of these wrinkles and an unnatural appearance may result. In most circumstances, however, the main reason for

FIGURE 23.4

A, It is often unnecessary nor desirable to isolate the periorbital area. This patient is seen here before full face laser resurfacing incorporating periorbital resurfacing. B, Patient 2 months after full facial resurfacing.

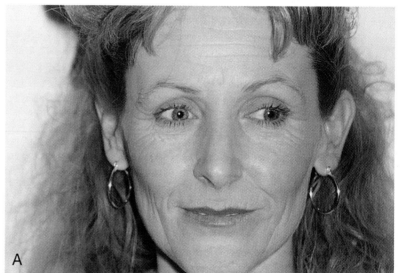

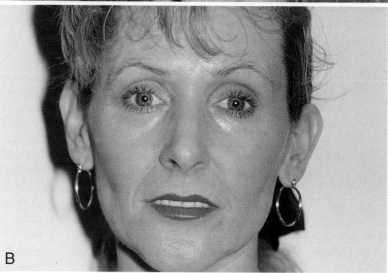

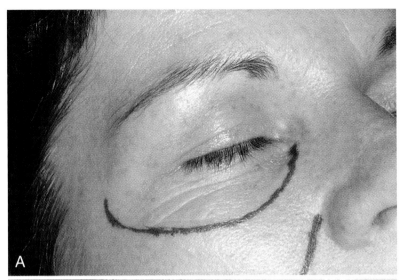

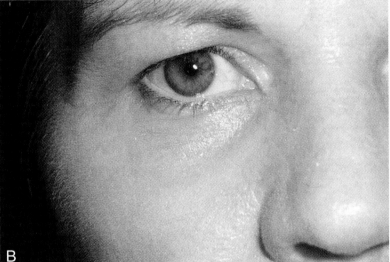

FIGURE 23.5
A, Preoperative view of a patient in whom the lower eyelid area is being resurfaced as a regional procedure. B, Postoperative view of the patient after eyelid resurfacing. (Reprinted with permission from Goodman GJ, Bekhor PI, Richards S. Advances in laser therapy—the importance of selective photothermolysis. Med J Aust 1996:164(11):681-686.)

periorbital resurfacing is the eradication of sundamage and periorbital wrinkling. For this indication, the complete periorbital cosmetic unit should be resurfaced when possible.

Despite this purist's view, treatment of only the periorbital cosmetic unit is regularly transgressed by treating well into the temple region to take in the lateral periorbital rhytides (crow's feet). A concept of a "greater cosmetic unit" has to be embraced. Due to this "transgression" it is even more important that attention be paid to blurring the edges of this treatment zone.

Generally, the entire periorbital zone is treated, however, the lower eyelid area or upper eyelid may be similarly resurfaced in isolation. In combination with blepharoplasty a number of combinations are performed. These are:

1. Lower eyelid transconjunctival blepharoplasty with simultaneous infraorbital, periorbital or full face laser resurfacing.

2. Lower eyelid transcutaneous blepharoplasty with delayed infraorbital, periorbital or full face laser resurfacing.

3. Upper eyelid blepharoplasty with simultaneous infraorbital laser resurfacing but with delayed upper eyelid resurfacing if required.

The lower eyelid area is treated from the malar ridge inferiorly, follows the line of the zygomatic arch laterally and to the eyelid margin superiorly. The eyes are protected with metal corneal shields or a Jaeger bone plate. The lower eyelid lashes are moved superiorly to protect these from the laser beam using the wooden end of a cotton swab (Fig. 23.6). The upper eyelid is treated from the eyelashes or the superior margin of the tarsal plate inferiorly up to the eyebrow superiorly and following the line of the orbital ridge laterally. Laterally, the periorbital perimeter may shift depending on where the crow's feet lead. It is important to realize that laser resurfacing only addresses fully crow's feet that are present at rest and only softens dynamic or hyperkinetic wrinkles in this area. A useful partnership in the treatment of this area is the use of laser for those wrinkles visible at rest and botulinum toxin for the hyperkinetic lines.

Merging periorbital resurfacing with unresurfaced facial skin requires increased skill and includes lighter power settings, less passes and angled beams at the perimeter of the treatment zone. Some experts peel the unresurfaced skin with light peeling agents or use manual dermabrasion to blend the skin.

THE COMBINATION OF LASER RESURFACING AND BLEPHAROPLASTY (TABLE 23.1)

Indications for Combined Blepharoplasty and Resurfacing

The major indication for combining laser resurfacing and blepharoplasty is the concurrence of epidermal or dermal disease in association with protuberant lower eyelid fat pads or redundant upper eyelid skin. The skin disease may include:

1. Rhytides and other aspects of sundamage, such as dyschromia, solar keratoses and elastosis (Fig. 23.7).
2. "Pseudo-laxity'" of the lower eyelid skin even including some festoons. If the eyelid tone is adequate, laser resurfacing may be the only therapy required.
3. Multiple periorbital benign tumors such as seborrheic keratoses, milia, syringomas, trichoepitheliomas and xanthelasma (Fig. 23.8).
4. Unsatisfactory scars from previous surgery on upper or lower eyelids including those of blepharoplasty surgery.

Why Combine These Procedures?

The major reason to combine laser resurfacing and blepharoplasty is that the result is better in these patients than if only one or other procedure is performed. In the circumstance of lower eyelid resurfacing and simultaneous lower eyelid transconjunctival blepharoplasty, it allows replacement of an operation with a problematic complication rate, namely transcutaneous lower eyelid blepharoplasty with skin excision, with a superior and safer technique (22).

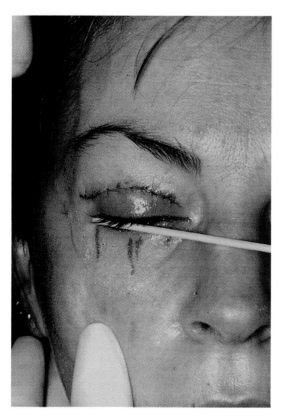

FIGURE 23.6
The lower lid lashes are moved superiorly with a moistened wooden end of a cotton swab to protect them from the laser beam.

FIGURE 23.7
Patient with marked solar damage and rhytides who would benefit by a combined blepharoplasty and resurfacing.

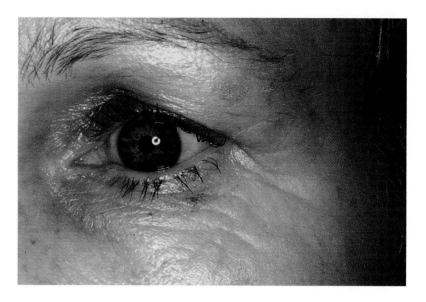

TABLE 23.1

TABLE 23.1

GOLDEN RULES OF LASER PERIORBITAL RESURFACING AND BLEPHAROPLASTY (MOST USEFUL IN BOLD)

A. Lower Lid Laser Blepharoplasty

1. Procedure
   Transconjunctival
   Unless another reason
   If Transcutaneous
   - Do not take skin
   - Unnecessary
   - Quality or contour, not quantity
   - Risk of scleral show, round eye, ectropion, "done" look
2. Local Anesthetic
   - Protect globe
   - Retract lower eyelid
   - 30-gauge needle
   - Aim to orbital rim
   - One injection
   - 1 ml
   - Between vascular arcades
   - **Wait and ice**
3. Laser Safety
   - Nonreflective instruments
   - Aluminum foil or wet cloth
   - No O_2 unless metal taped
   - Glasses, warning signs, etc.
   - **Globe and skin protection (e.g., Trelles or Cox eye shields, Jaeger or Sutcliffe plates)**
4. The Incision
   - Tilt head back
   - Incise 4 to 5 mm below lower tarsal border
   - Gentle pressure globe
   - Aim to orbital rim/bulge
   - Incise punctum to end tarsal plate
   - **If no fat, move Desmarres and think that it may be anterior to where you're looking**
5. Laser Use
   - 0.2 mm continuous wave focused 6 to 7 Watts to incise
   - Check posterior aspect fat pads, especially nasal for blood vessels, other structures
   - Drape fat against nonreflective surface
   - **Defocus before cutting fat pads**
6. Fat Pads
   - Plan, look & photograph
   - Only take what comes
   - Drape over cotton tip or aim at Jaeger plates, not eye
   - Redrape, come out & compare sides
   - Compare fat
   - **Take the lateral pad first**

Tips in Periorbital Resurfacing
7. Realize the limitations
   Excellent
   - Static & infraorbital Rhytides
   - Sun Damage
   Good
   - Scars
   - **Crow's feet - softening only**
   Variable
   - Benign skin tumours
   - Dyschromia "dark circles"

8. Follow the "Vertical Landmarks"
   Epidermis
   - Bubbling
   - Color loss when wiped
   Superficial Dermis
   - **Contraction and transient blanching tissue**
   - **Effacement of fine wrinkles**
   - Transient blanching blood vessels
   Deeper Dermis - not necessary
   - Greying of tissue
   - Chamois change
   - Bleeding
9. Periorbital Resurfacing - Upper Lids
   - Rhytides, appendage tumours on upper lid
   - Useful if mild to moderate upper lid redundancy
   - **Light or no resurfacing to pretarsal skin**
   - Use low settings and/or single pass
   - Dress open
10. Periorbital regional resurfacing
    Lower lid
    - Malar rim inferiorly
    - Lower lashes superiorly
    - Laterally end crow's feet or orbital rim
    Upper lid
    - Into eyebrows superiorly
    - Upper lid crease or lashes
    - Laterally orbital rim
11. Resurfacing combined with blepharoplasty
    - Upper lid blepharoplasty and immediate lower lid resurfacing
    - Upper lid blepharoplasty and delayed upper lid resurfacing
    - Lower lid transconjunctival blepharoplasty and immediate periorbital or lower eyelid resurfacing
    - Lower lid transcutaneous blepharoplasty and delayed lower lid resurfacing
12. Upper Lid Blepharoplasty - Think & Plan
    - Think Brow
    - **Think Symmetry**
    - Think quality vs quantity skin
    - If early and skin only, think resurfacing
13. Upper Lid Blepharoplasty - Local Anaesthetic
    - **Place local anesthetic injection inside marking**
    - Place just under skin, between vessels
    - 2 ml lidocaine/epinephrine laterally & milked
    - 1 ml medially
    - Pressure & ice
14. Upper Lid Blepharoplasty - Incision
    - **Don't dwell, steady hand movement**
    - Start excision laterally, skin only till over orbital rim, then skin and orbicularis
    - Nonreflective back stop
    - Move skin not laser
15. Upper Lid Blepharoplasty - Underdo excision
    - **If full orbit and aggressive debulking of tissue is main thrust do not take maximum skin excision**
    - Mark maximum then decrease this by 2 to 5 mm
    - Think Brow
    - Laser resurfacing if redundant skin especially medial canthus

FIGURE 23.8
A, Patient with syringomas who underwent both laser resurfacing and simultaneous lower lid blepharoplasty. Preoperative view. B, Postoperative view at 2 weeks.

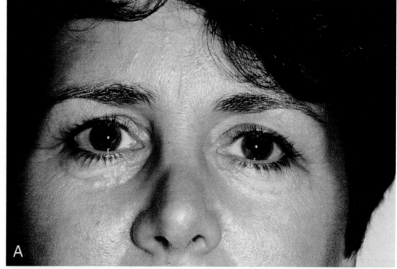

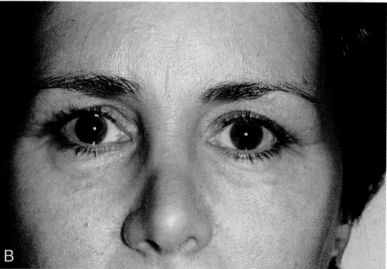

In the upper eyelid, resurfacing after blepharoplasty may replace the need for surgically revising postoperative irregularities and scars. Also, it is often better to combine procedures in a single operation for convenience to the patient. Otherwise the patient is subjected to two anesthetics, two operations and two recovery times.

Lower Eyelid Nuances

Transconjunctival Versus Transcutaneous Lower Eyelid Blepharoplasty and the Issue of Skin Quality Versus Skin Quantity

Although transconjunctival blepharoplasty was described as early as 1924, many surgeons continue to use the transcutaneous procedure in the misguided belief that skin resection in the lower eyelid region is necessary (23).

If a patient seeks treatment for chronic sun exposure and wrinkles of the lower eyelids, and possesses other-

wise normal eyelid structure with no undesirable fat bulges or shadows, excision of a portion of this skin will not only fail to solve the problem, but will probably result in lower eyelid retraction to some degree. This common error is caused by a failure to recognize that wrinkles represent dermal elastosis and alterations in other dermal elements. If the skin problem is quality and not quantity, then no skin should be removed. One would not excise an area of lip to remove upper lip wrinkles and the same concept is true for the periorbital region. It is difficult to understand how the removal of eyelid skin and attempting to virtually hang the weight of the cheeks on an unsupported lower eyelid can do other than produce downward pull of the eyelid. A patient who demonstrates their desired change during the preoperative interview by pulling the lower eyelid skin to the sides and up must be told that surgery cannot be expected to produce that change. Given the high incidence of resultant complications after traditional lower transcutaneous lower eyelid blepharoplasty (such as scleral show, ectropion and dry, irritable eyes), it is difficult to justify cutting lower eyelid skin for any reasons other than for lateral canthotomy or tumor removal (24–27).

David and Goodman have stated that lower eyelid blepharoplasty must be considered a "contouring" procedure (meaning surgery that designs a bed or platform to support skin) and not a skin procedure (28). The skin is then able to conform to the bed on which it lies and normally does not need to be excised. Lower eyelid blepharoplasty rarely leaves any appreciable excess skin. However, it does leave behind wrinkles that are addressed by resurfacing techniques devised to improve the quality of the skin surface layers. The rise in popularity of the transconjunctival approach has been further fueled because of the ability to provide a simultaneous solution to the dual problems of contour from the herniated infraorbital fat pads and the skin quality from the ravages of time and environmental insults.

Upper Eyelid Blepharoplasty Nuances

Whether one uses laser, scalpel or any other instrument for the blepharoplasty is largely irrelevant. There are some cogent arguments for separating the upper eyelid blepharoplasty from laser resurfacing of the upper eyelid. Performing the two procedures at the same operative session but with the blepharoplasty performed first presents some difficulties. The presence of the wound and sutures would make resurfacing of this zone technically difficult. More importantly, the additional shrinkage attained with laser resurfacing is considerable. If certain skin resections occur before resurfacing is commenced, problematic lagophthalmos could ensue.

There are also theoretical advantages in waiting several weeks after the first procedure to perform a second one. Resurfacing at 4 to 8 weeks after dermabrasion often yields an improved scar (29). There is every reason

to be optimistic that this is also the case with CO_2 lasers. From Katz's paper, it appears that resurfacing with dermabrasion 8 weeks after the scar infliction is the optimum scar revision interval (30). Harmon et al. have shown that dermabrasion alters the events of primary scar formation by modifying cell to cell and cell to matrix interactions within the epidermis and dermis and between these tissue compartments (31). These main findings were an upregulation of tenascin expression throughout the papillary dermis, an increase in collagen bundle density with a tendency towards unidirectional orientation parallel to the epidermal surface and expression of alpha 6/B-4 integrin subunit throughout the stratum spinosum. In essence, this translates into an ability to ablate scars if dermabrasion is performed at an appropriate interval after the scar invoking procedure (4 to 8 weeks). These results need to be repeated with laser resurfacing to see if the same scenario of scar ablation is possible with laser resurfacing. Most often the scar on the upper lid is imperceptible even without further treatment, but if the scar is unacceptable, then delayed resurfacing remains an attractive option.

Other reasons to offer resurfacing after upper eyelid blepharoplasty include refining results from the initial operation. Occasionally, the medial canthus can be problematic and various attempts to deal with skin redundancy in this area have been entertained. A number of techniques including the use of M plasties, storiform incisions and burrow's triangles have been suggested (32). Another tool for this difficult area is the CO_2 laser if the medial canthal redundancy still exists (Fig. 23.9). The tightening effect of the laser-induced tissue shrinkage is sufficient to obviate this problem. Similarly, the laser can be used in other areas of skin redundancy of the upper eyelid that may ensue from a less than totally satisfactory blepharoplasty. Unlike the scar scenario where it is best to resurface within 4 to 8 weeks of the

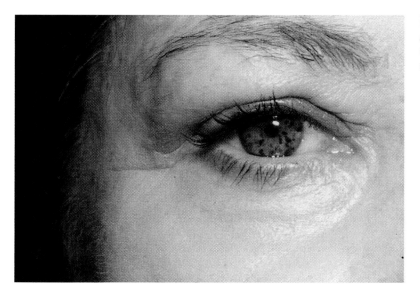

FIGURE 23.9
Appearance after blepharoplasty of a patient who may benefit from future laser resurfacing to the upper lid.

FIGURE 23.10

A, Patient who has had previous blepharoplasty elsewhere with some residual upper eyelid skin redundancy. B, 6 weeks after upper eyelid laser resurfacing showing improvement in redundant upper eyelid skin without blepharoplasty.

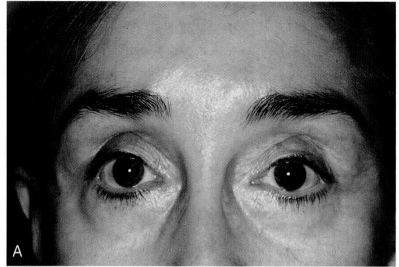

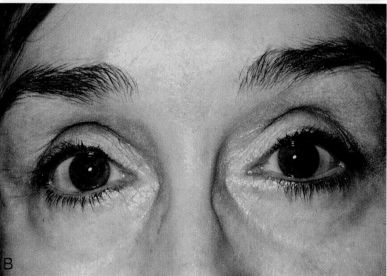

initial procedure, there is no particular time frame operative for the treatment of these irregularities.

When combining upper eyelid blepharoplasty with lower eyelid resurfacing, it is important to be conservative with both techniques. The skin shrinkage of a heavily treated lower eyelid resurfacing added to a tight upper eyelid blepharoplasty may be a recipe for disaster with lagophthalmos and dry eye, with resultant corneal disease a real possibility.

Occasionally a patient with mild skin redundancy alone may be helped purely by resurfacing the upper eyelids without skin excision (Fig. 23.10).

An interesting approach has recently been advocated by Fulton in which the forehead, infrabrow and upper eyelid zones are resurfaced first (33). After appreciating the shrinkage, which is usually considerable, the remaining blepharoplasty excision is marked directly on the resurfaced skin and the skin and deep structures are removed as required. A trans-blepharoplasty brow suspension is added to hold the brow in position.

PATIENT SELECTION, PREOPERATIVE EVALUATION, AND THE INAPPROPRIATE PATIENT

Blepharoplasty Selection Criteria

Appropriate patient selection (or omission) along with careful preoperative planning are the most important aspects in assuring a successful outcome to this technique. The two main aspects to be considered in patient selection are the patients' psychological well being and the structures to be modified.

The Patient's Psychological Well Being

As with any cosmetic procedure the enemy of the surgeon is unrealistic expectations sometimes held by the patient. The psychologically troubled patient with minimal objective disturbance should be avoided. This procedure, like any other cosmetic procedure, is not going to change the patient's relationships with spouses, friends, or make him or her more popular. It is just going to fix their eyelids. Eliminating these patients is essential, as a surgeon's reputation is made as much by those patients he or she declines to operate on as on those that he or she does.

What Structures Should be Modified?

To determine what structure should be modified, the following questions should be answered.

A. For lower eyelids: Does the patient require skin resurfacing or fat removal or both?

As indicated above, there is seldom any indication for skin removal in any patient. Is an eyelid tightening procedure required? (Fig. 23.11).

B. For upper eyelids: Does the patient just have mild excess skin or appendageal tumors that can be treated with resurfacing or does the patient need blepharoplasty as well? Does the patient need a brow lift, ptosis repair or other supplemental procedure? (Fig. 23.12).

If a patient has a ptotic eyebrow, it may need correction or else the patient may end up with a subop-

timal result consisting of a sunken eye appearance, and in the extreme case, may have the appearance of the eyebrow sewn to the eyelid.

Blepharoptosis is not corrected by skin resection and requires shortening of the levator aponeurosis or Muller's muscle (34–36). The easiest preoperative screening method is to lift the brows to the normal position and note the position of the upper eyelid margin which should lie 1 to 2 mm below the upper limbus. If this margin is lower, blepharoptosis is probably present. Other signs include high or absent upper eyelid crease but with good levator excursion, thinning of the eyelid above the tarsus, compensatory brow hike, eyelash prolapse, and in some cases, a palpable defect in the aponeurosis (34).

Eyelid excursion should also be checked. This is done with the brow in its correct position and the patient directed to close the eyelids. If they cannot close their eyes fully blepharoplasty should not be performed. Supratarsal fixation may be required in female blepharoplasty and is certainly required in

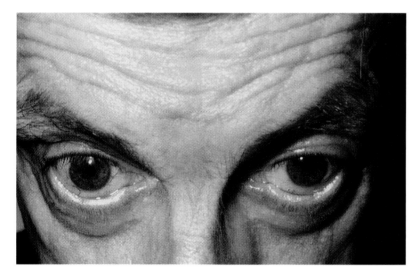

FIGURE 23.11
Patient with lax lower lid tone for whom lid shortening would be advantageous.

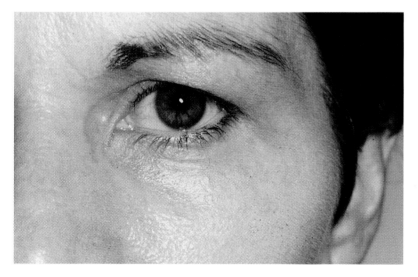

FIGURE 23.12
Patient with brow ptosis for whom browpexy would be advantageous.

FIGURE 23.13
Patient with prominent, well-positioned brow and deeply set eyes who would benefit from supratarsal fixation.

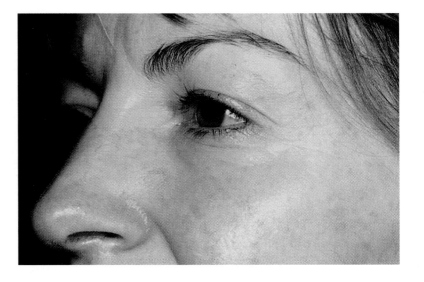

the Asian blepharoplasty, but it is avoided in people with prominent globes. It is very useful in patients with deeply set eyes and prominent supraorbital rims (Fig. 23.13).

C. Does the patient suffer from thyroid disease, seventh nerve palsy, myasthenia gravis, sicca syndrome, past trauma or other general medical causes of eyelid or eye pathology that require consideration before surgery?

   Studying photos of the patient at various stages in the life of the individual is useful in determining if the patient's problem is congenital, acute (suggestive of a medical cause), or if the problem is the more common involutional or gravitational cause (35).

D. Does the patient suffer from general medical conditions that may preclude the procedure or require attention before the operation such as diabetes, hypertension, or bleeding dyscrasias? Routine complete blood counts and coagulation profile should be undertaken on all patients.

E. Is the patient on medications that will interfere with the procedure?

   Remember in particular that aspirin is a very common and not always known ingredient in many diverse medications such as antacid preparations, headache and cold remedies. Aspirin use should be halted at least 2 weeks before the procedure occurs. Other nonsteroidal anti-inflammatory drugs, alcohol, and Vitamin E are also best avoided for a week before the procedure.

   Has the patient normal visual acuity, and corneal integrity before the operation? This should be specifically tested. In some cases referral for specialist ophthalmologic examination would seem prudent.

Preoperative Assessment and Planning for Periorbital Resurfacing

A successful outcome to periorbital resurfacing begins with the preoperative assessment and the planning. The deceptive ease of periorbital resurfacing may lull the inexperienced surgeon into feeling that this procedure is not worthy of more than a superficial glance. The trap is that, as in transcutaneous blepharoplasty, the lateral canthus is poorly supported by the lateral canthal tendon in comparison to its medial counterpart and tends not to cope well with any stress imposed by surgery in this region. The same tests that are undertaken for transcutaneous blepharoplasty are required in assessing the patient for periorbital resurfacing.

One of these tests is the snap test. The snap test is performed with the patient staring straight ahead. The lower eyelid is grasped and retracted away from the globe and then released. The time taken for the eyelid to revert back to its normal position is about 1 second. If this takes longer, then it is an indication of poor eyelid support. Another test is the distraction test which involves pulling the lower eyelid out from the globe as far as is comfortable and measuring. This measurement from the globe should not exceed 7 mm. If the patient fails either or both of these tests then they are at risk of postoperative ectropion.

One should beware of patients who have had previous eyelid surgery as these patients are at increased risk of postoperative problems. It is wise to remember that the potential problem of eyelid closure is being altered both superiorly through upper eyelid blepharoplasty or upper eyelid resurfacing, and inferiorly through lower eyelid resurfacing-induced tightening.

Protuberance of the globe should also be assessed, whether being due to true exophthalmos or shallow orbits and hypoplastic malar eminences. These conditions tend to lift the lower eyelid anteriorly and superiorly out of the supporting plane and produce an increased tendency for postoperative retraction (37).

Lagophthalmos should be assessed with the eyebrows in their normal position and the patient should lightly close their eyes. If the eyelids do not totally close, then any lower eyelid retraction or ectropion may not be tolerated by the cornea. Any history of corneal compromise or dry eyes should also be ascertained.

The Dark Circles

Dark circles under the eyes are multifactorial. Contributions appear to be made in some patients by fine wrinkling. In others, the problem is shadowing from prominent infraorbital prolapsed fat pads and in others appears to be a true dermal melanocytosis. For many patients, dark circles are caused by a combination of some or all of these factors (Fig. 23.14).

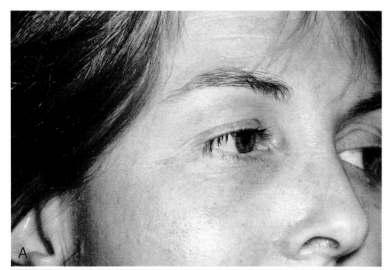
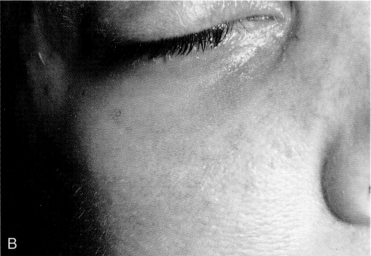
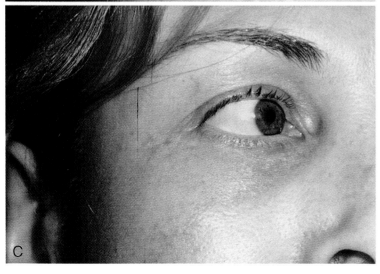

FIGURE 23.14

A, Patient with dark circles especially medially. B, Same patient undergoing laser resurfacing showing dark circles still present after first pass of laser resurfacing. C, Patient after healing from resurfacing. This patient may benefit from Q-switched laser therapy.

Treatment of dermal melanocytosis with the Q-switched ruby laser has been suggested (38). If herniated fat pads are evident in some patients, a combined lower eyelid blepharoplasty and lower eyelid resurfacing is worthwhile and appears to adequately treat the dark circles. If, however, there is no obvious herniation or fine wrinkling, then Q-switched ruby laser treatment may be very useful instead of CO_2 laser resurfacing or blepharoplasty. A teardrop deformity may also cause shadowing and may require fat augmentation to correct this cause of dark circles.

Dynamic Versus Static Wrinkling

There is a difference between the dynamic wrinkling associated with hyperkinetic activity of orbicularis oculi and the static wrinkling of older, sun ravaged periorbital skin. However, there is some overlap with these two conditions. Under the influence of the sun and other environmental insults, such as smoking, the skin tends to thicken and become less pliable. The evanescent wrinkling of youth seen with facial expressions, such as smiling, grimacing and squinting, is replaced by more permanent lines etched into the face. These static lines are those removed with resurfacing using the CO_2 lasers. More severe wrinkling appears when the patient animates as the skin is quite coarse and folds more like cardboard than skin. These wrinkles produced with movement are softened by laser therapy but are not removed. This "dynamic wrinkling" is best addressed by other methods, such as botulinum toxin injection (Fig. 23.15) (39, 40). Botulinum toxin injections are best delayed until the resurfacing has healed and the final result appreciated or performed in advance of laser resurfacing. These two procedures make excellent companions and are commonly required in the same patient.

LASER SAFETY ASPECTS

In this chapter we will only deal with safety issues as pertaining to laser resurfacing of the periorbital area

FIGURE 23.15
A, Patient with active periorbital wrinkling after resurfacing but before botulinum toxin injection.
B, Patient 1 month after botulinum toxin injection.

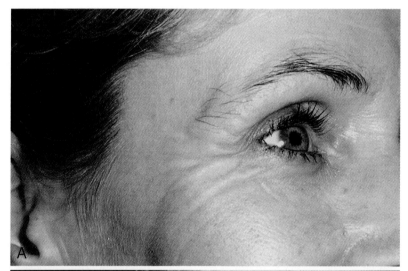
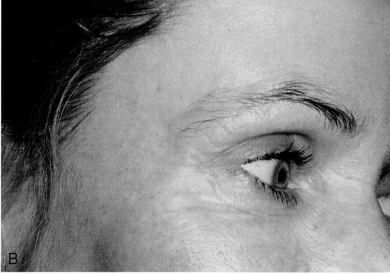

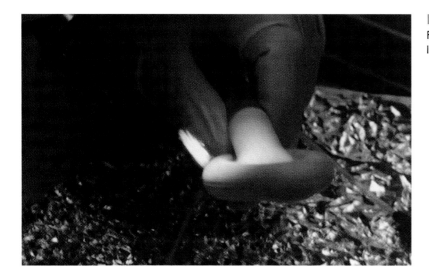

FIGURE 23.16
Flammability test of a laryngeal mask aflame after laser beam interaction.

and blepharoplasty. Fire is one of the most feared aspects of laser therapy (Fig. 23.16). Personal injury to surgeon, staff or patient and operating room fires are possible and it behooves anyone who uses lasers to acquaint themselves with the necessary safety that must be applied when using this powerful tool.

Staff must wear appropriate protective eyewear and laser plume masks at all times when the laser is being used. Movement in the operating room should be minimized. No staff should enter the operating room without warning and distractions to the surgeon should be minimized. The laser should be placed in standby mode whenever it is not in use during a procedure.

There are common operating room practices and anesthesia techniques that must be modified for CO_2 laser therapy. The first is the common use of supplemental oxygen. Oxygen should not be used at all when the laser is active. Generally laser resurfacing and blepharoplasty do not require full general anesthesia. Local anesthesia or intravenous sedation is usually all that is required. If supplemental oxygen is temporarily required, laser resurfacing should be stopped and the laser placed on standby until the need is passed. If oxygen is deemed necessary throughout the case, then laser resistant airways and equipment should be employed. Flammable skin cleansing agents should be replaced by aqueous ones and acetone should not be used when laser use is planned.

Collimation of the laser beam has added to the predictability and reproducibility of laser resurfacing, but it also has added to its risks. The laser, if it misses its mark, can shoot a collimated beam quite a distance with relatively little diminution in its ability to ignite flammable materials. The focused beam of the scanning lasers will also still reach quite a distance before the divergent beam loses sufficient power density not to be a health hazard. It is good policy to always provide a non reflective back drop for the laser beam and to keep the scan size small

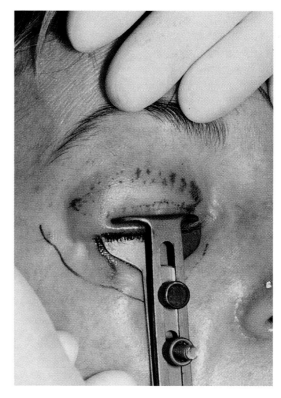

FIGURE 23.17
David-Baker clamp in situ to protect the eye during upper lid blepharoplasty.

enough and the frequency of scan slow enough that one knows where the beam is going at all times. If drapes are used, they should be wet, however, open field technique without drapes provides better safety.

The patient's eyes must be protected at all times. During the upper eyelid blepharoplasty the best instrument to use is the David-Baker clamp (Byron Inc, Tuscon, AZ), but well fitting eye shields or a Jaeger plate are also useful (Fig. 23.17). During lower eyelid blepharoplasty the lower eyelid is best protected with a Jaeger plate or metal eye shields (Fig. 23.18). Plastic eye shields are not laser safe and should not be used. For lower eyelid resurfacing, the Jaeger plate is an excellent instrument, but for upper or periorbital resurfacing, metal eye shields are preferable (Fig. 23.19). Two common varieties are the Trelles eye shield (Byron Inc., Tucson, AZ) (Fig. 23.19), which has a central dimple that is

attached to a removable rod, and the Cox eye shield (Oculo Plastik, Montreal, Quebec), which is metal and is easily placed and removed with a rubber suction holder. Both instruments are available in different sizes, the larger size applicable for most men and the smaller sizes for most women. They are appropriately buffed to reduce scattering of the CO_2 laser beam and are safe for patient, staff and surgeon. When inserting any of the eyeshields, appropriate use of local anesthetic drops and lubricating ointments is advised. However, too much ointment should be avoided as it may smudge operative markings and will be a barrier to resurfacing and could theoretically become a fire safety risk. Wet gauze is useful to cover the eyes when treating other areas of the face, but is not sufficient protection when treating the immediate periorbital area and does not permit complete resurfacing of all infraorbital wrinkling.

Laser plume requires several considerations for staff and surgeon safety. Laser safety masks are designed to filter plume down to 0.1 μm and should be worn (Fig. 23.20). Smoke evacuation with filters able to extract down to 0.1 μm should also be used and should be within 2 cm of the laser head to achieve best performance. Laser plume has some inherent microbial risks and operating staff should be protected (41).

TECHNIQUE

Formal preoperative photography should include frontal shots of upward, downward, and neutral gazes, as well as oblique and lateral views. Instant photos of the patient are also useful for reference during the procedure.

Skin Marking–Upper Eyelid

Upper eyelid incision lines should be marked with a fine-tip sterile marking pen and the eyes gently closed.

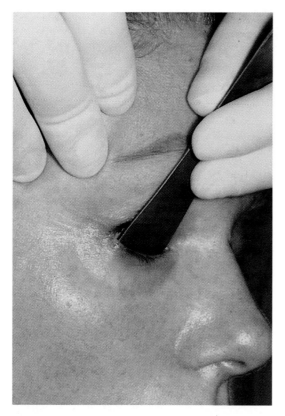

FIGURE 23.18
Jaeger plate in position during lower lid procedure.

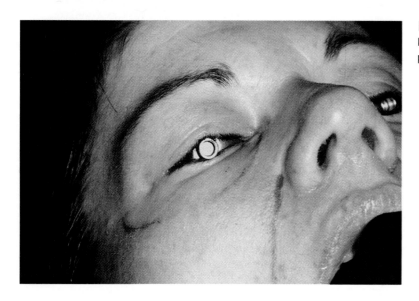

FIGURE 23.19
Metal eye shields suitable for laser periorbital procedures.

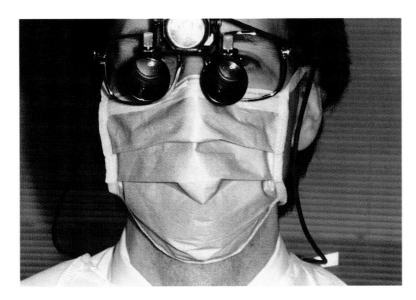

FIGURE 23.20
Appropriate protective masks should be worn during laser procedures.

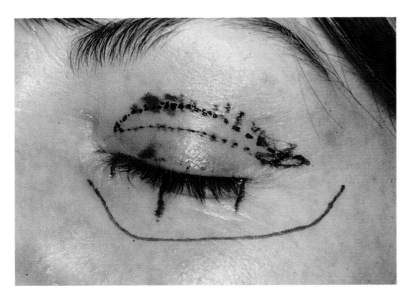

FIGURE 23.21
Three marks are useful for aiding symmetrical marking of the upper lid marking the upper lid punctum, the pupil on distant gaze and the lateral canthal angle.

The most important marking is the inferior upper eyelid crease which preferably follows the top of the tarsal plate or the patient's natural supratarsal fold. If this crease is not visible or is unsatisfactorily low for the patient, it will be necessary to create a new crease, but this should be no higher than one third the distance from lash to brow. The natural upper eyelid crease ranges between 6 to 12 mm from the ciliary margin at the mid pupillary line. In females, the location of this crease depends on the postoperative appearance that the patient desires. Placing the lower incision higher from the ciliary fold (10 to 12 mm) produces a more wide eyed, feminine appearance. This may be desired by patients who wish a large platform for accentuation of their eyes with eye shadow. Males should have a lower eyelid crease of 6 to 8 mm at the mid pupillary line as otherwise a feminine appearance is produced.

The line should not be drawn medially past the punctum as excisions into the area of the medial canthus are prone to postoperative webbing or banding. Laterally, however, it is important to carry the incision line out far enough to avoid webbing and hide it in a skin crease in the crow's feet area with an upward turn to the end of this line. In younger patients, this lateral extension should be minimized. The incision should leave at least 4 mm clearance between the lateral canthus and the incision line to allow lymphatic drainage and avoid a long term or permanent swelling of the upper eyelid.

Three vertical marks placed on the eyelid are helpful in determining the level of the upper eyelid crease. These are placed in line with the upper eyelid punctum, the pupil at distant gaze, and the lateral canthal angle. This helps in comparing the two sides when marking the patient (Fig. 23.21).

A number of techniques for marking the superior incision line have been described. One technique is, with the patient seated, to grasp the skin with fine-toothed or Green forceps and use an overlapping or pinch technique to estimate the redundant skin laid over the lower line and determine the amount of skin to be removed (42, 43). This estimation of skin removal can be made when the eyelids are gently closed in a natural position, when they are just opening, or when there is 1 to 2 mm of eyelid opening (35, 37, 44).

An interesting and simple technique is described by Hawtof (45). This involves marking a lower line at the tarsal plate with the eyelids closed and the brow suspended until the eyelids are just opening. The pen is held still at a number of points along this line and in each instance the eyelid is gently pulled downwards. The skin is then moved beneath a stationary pen.

Others excise on clinical grounds (46–49). Weber cautions that the upper eyelid blepharoplasty markings should follow the patient's natural creases whenever possible and to leave at least 10 mm between the lowermost eyebrow hairs and the incision line (32). He also stresses using fine dot points 2 mm apart to avoid smudging the line. In patients with a full orbit, when deeper contents such as fat and orbicularis are to be debulked aggressively, one should place the superior line 2 to 5 mm below the maximum skin markings to allow the skin to drape into its new bed.

The most important thing to remember about marking for upper eyelid surgery is to ensure that symmetry is maintained. Postoperative asymmetry will not be tolerated by the patient even if the patient was asymmetric preoperatively. It will forever mar an otherwise perfect surgical result. Asymmetry is the most common complication of upper eyelid blepharoplasty and the most common cause for re-operation. If there appears to be too much laxity at the medial end of the incision, a Burrow's triangle may be taken base down, but the incision should end at the medial punctum. This area may be helped by laser resurfacing. In the central section of the incision line, remember that the apex of the curve is in the mid pupillary line when the patient is gazing at a distant object. This is especially important when one is fashioning a new crease and not following the natural superior border of the tarsal plate. On the lateral aspect of the incision line it is best to try to keep the thin eyelid skin in this area and not move the heavier eyebrow skin inferiorly into this region. Bulging seen in this region is most likely the lacrimal gland and not fat.

Skin Marking–Lower Eyelid

The skin markings on the lower eyelid outline the fat pads visible on clinical examination. These are delineated by asking the patient to bow their head and then look up at you from that position, and thus medially and laterally illustrate any herniated fat pads (Fig. 23.22). Light pressure on the globe with the eyes closed accentuates the prolapsed fat. It is useful to mark the outer limits of this prolapsed fat. The laser resurfac-

ing marks are drawn to illustrate the cosmetic unit of lower eyelid or periorbital zone and further instant photography may be useful at this stage.

The technique of combining laser lower eyelid transconjunctival blepharoplasty and laser upper eyelid blepharoplasty with periorbital laser resurfacing is described later in this chapter. For descriptions on transcutaneous lower eyelid blepharoplasty and non-laser upper eyelid blepharoplasty, readers should consult other notable references (27, 35, 50–54).

Anesthesia

Although the procedure may be performed completely under local anesthesia, some intravenous sedation delivered by an anesthesiologist is preferred, especially when upper eyelid resurfacing is performed and during the initial stages of blepharoplasty surgery.

After induction with an agent, such as midazolam, further intravenous sedation may be added with popular agents such as ketamine and propofol. An airway or laryngeal mask can be used and an intravenous line established to maximize patient safety (Fig. 23.23). Oxygen is not used unless required and patients should be monitored with a pulse oximeter. While the anesthesiologist administers intravenous sedation, the surgeon should instil a drop of 0.5% ophthalmic proparcaine into each eye. Local infiltration of 1% lidocaine containing epinephrine 1:100,000 is then performed by the dermatologic laser surgeon.

A thumb or finger should be used to pull the lower eyelid down as far as possible and an assistant should place the Jaeger plate under the lower eyelid from above to protect the globe. After assessing the position of the orbital rim with a pair of forceps (Fig. 23.24), insert a 30-gauge needle through the conjunctiva until the point contacts the bony orbital rim (Fig. 23.25). Choose a relatively blood vessel-free area of conjunctiva overlying the fat bulge for the injection, or at least an area between larger vessels. Back the needle out about 1 mm and then inject 1 ml of local anesthetic. As the tip of the needle is withdrawn to lie just under the conjunctiva, slowly inject a small additional quantity (about 0.1 to 0.3 ml) of local anesthetic. To minimize trauma, it is important to not move the needle around or side-to-side while it is in the tissue. Wait at least 5 minutes for the anesthetic to distribute throughout the lower eyelid. No additional agents or further anesthetic agents are usually required. A 2.5 ml syringe is probably a good shape and size syringe to perform this local infiltration.

If the upper eyelids are also being treated, immediately infiltrate with a single puncture of the 30-gauge needle inside the planned incision at the lateral and upper extent of the predetermined excision area. This permits delivery of 2 ml of local anesthetic just under the skin, creating a large weal. The needle itself should not

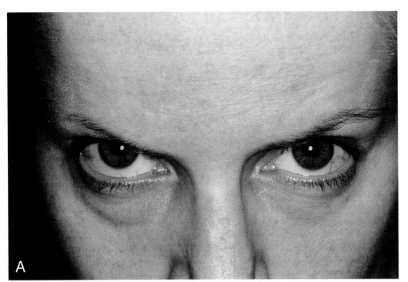

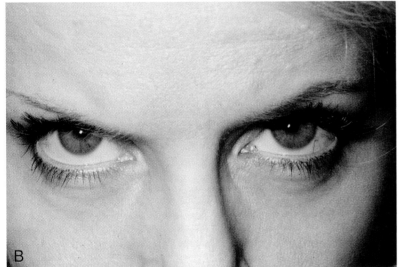

FIGURE 23.22
A, Prolapsed fat of the lower lid is more evident with the patient looking up at the observer. Preoperative view before lower lid blepharoplasty and full face laser resurfacing. B, Postoperative view of a patient after lower lid blepharoplasty and full face laser resurfacing.

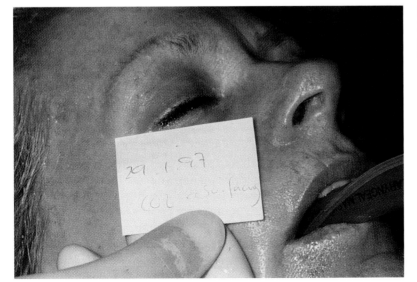

FIGURE 23.23
Patient with previous upper lid blepharoplasty undergoing full face laser resurfacing with a laryngeal mask in situ. This is a useful airway in laser procedures.

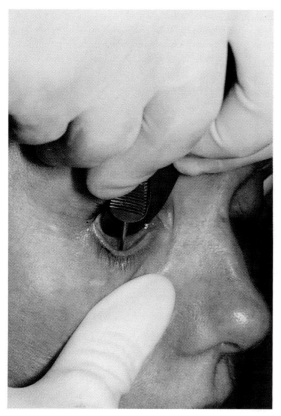

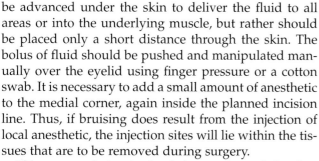

FIGURE 23.24
The lower eyelid is distracted inferiorly as far as possible with the Jaeger plate in situ. A pair of fine forceps is used to locate the infraorbital rim.

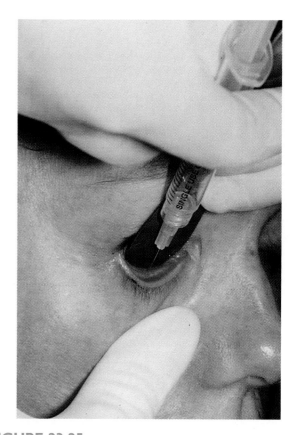

FIGURE 23.25
Local anesthetic is injected carefully in the direction of the infraorbital rim.

be advanced under the skin to deliver the fluid to all areas or into the underlying muscle, but rather should be placed only a short distance through the skin. The bolus of fluid should be pushed and manipulated manually over the eyelid using finger pressure or a cotton swab. It is necessary to add a small amount of anesthetic to the medial corner, again inside the planned incision line. Thus, if bruising does result from the injection of local anesthetic, the injection sites will lie within the tissues that are to be removed during surgery.

If laser resurfacing is also being performed, local or field block infiltration may be used if the patient is to be treated while awake. However, it is useful to supplement this anesthesia with a topical anesthetic cream (e.g., EMLA, Astra Pharmaceuticals, Westborough, MA). In most cases I use continuous intravenous sedation when performing periorbital resurfacing or blepharoplasty and concurrent resurfacing.

Lower Eyelid Incision

When performing lower eyelid incisions, apply light pressure to the globe using a metal Jaeger plate. This forces the fat to bulge under and distend the conjunctiva. Use a CO_2 laser (5 W in the focused mode, 0.2 mm

spot size, 3 W if 0.08 mm handpiece), to make an incision through the conjunctiva (Fig. 23.26). The incision is made approximately 4 to 5 mm below the lower tarsal border and over the protruding bulge. The length of this incision will vary between the punctum and the end of the tarsus, following the arching contour of the globe, and depends on the exposure necessary to remove the various amounts of fat.

One of the most common problems faced by beginning laser blepharoplasty surgeons is the inability to consistently find the lower eyelid fat through the transconjunctival approach. The landmark of importance is the lower orbital rim. By placing a forceps in the incision and feeling for the orbital rim, the incision can be deepened with the laser aiming for the rim through the level of retractors and the capsulopalpebral fascia until the fat compartments are seen. If the fat is not immediately apparent as a bulge when pushing gently on the globe, the wound can be teased open posteriorly with forceps and the bulge may become more apparent.

To excise the fat pad, insert a non-reflective eyelid retractor inside the incision and, using forceps, gently elevate the fat without tugging. Pulling with too much effort may cause bleeding and resultant bruising. Applying gentle finger pressure on the globe causes excess fat to bulge into the incision. Drape the fat over a dripping wet cotton-tip applicator and excise the unwanted fat with the laser. The exact amount of fat to be taken is largely a matter of experience and is that amount which protrudes outside of the orbital rim when the patient is sitting (Fig. 23.27). The instant photos taken preoperatively, with the patient gazing upward, define the intraoperative procedure.

It is technically easier to remove the lateral fat pad first, and subsequently remove the middle and nasal pads. If no visible bulge is present preoperatively in an area, it is best not to remove fat in that area just because it is found intraoperatively. It is wise to remember that a normal amount of fat is what gives a youthful appearance and removing too much fat produces a gaunt appearance or a focal hollowed area that will not make for a happy patient.

After the fat has been removed, reapproximate the incision edges by pulling both the anterior lower eyelid skin and the posterior lamella (posterior edge of the wound) superiorly and laterally. Check for additional fat bulging by applying gentle pressure on the globe. If indicated, go back and remove more fat. It is important to ensure that the globe is protected whenever additional laser use is required. After completion, check that

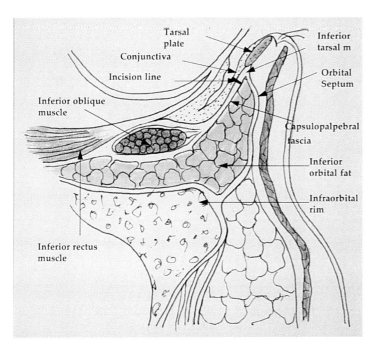

FIGURE 23.26

Diagram showing sagittal section view showing orbital fat bounded by orbital septum anteriorly which is not transgressed. The incision is through the conjunctiva and the capsulopalpebral fascia and the inferior retractors which are bounding the orbital fat posteriorly. (Redrawn and adapted from Zarem HA, Resnick JI. Expanded applications for transconjunctival lower lid blepharoplasty. Plast Reconstr Surg 1991;88(2): 215-221.)

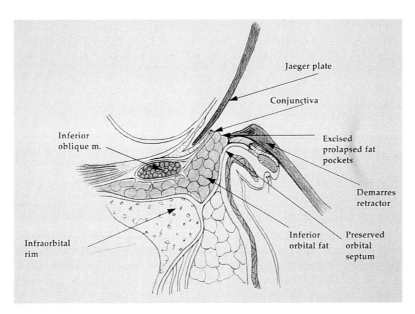

FIGURE 23.27

The postoperative view showing the transected orbital fat. (Redrawn and adapted from Zarem HA, Resnick JI. Expanded applications for transconjunctival lower lid blepharoplasty. Plast Reconstr Surg 1991;88(2):215-221.)

FIGURE 23.28
Extracted fat kept for side to side comparison.

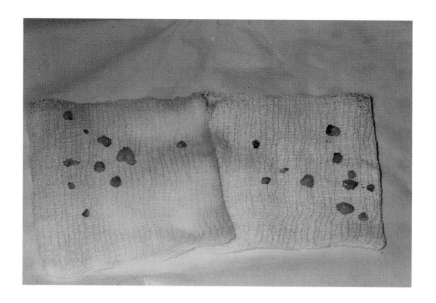

hemostasis is complete. The excised fat should be retained for side-to-side comparison (Fig. 23.28). No suturing of the lower eyelid incision is needed as healing is usually painless and rapid, and it may also be safer not to suture this wound in case of any postoperative bleeding.

Upper Eyelid

Although the Jaeger eyelid plate has customarily been used during the upper eyelid blepharoplasty to protect the cornea and globe, and for placing tension on eyelid skin during laser blepharoplasty, the more recently designed David-Baker eyelid retractor has several advantages over the Jaeger plate (28, 55, 56).

After lubricating both sides of the David-Baker retractor, it should be positioned under the upper eyelid and in contact with the conjunctiva to protect the cornea and globe. The retractor also places tension on the skin of the upper eyelid. A sharp incision through the skin and muscle should be made holding the laser perpendicular to the skin and maintaining a uniform hand speed. The lateral corner of the skin and muscle is then grasped with forceps and undercut using the laser. Laterally, past the orbital rim, only skin should be taken, but as one crosses the orbital rim the incision should be deepened to include the orbicularis oculi. For men, a residual of thin muscle tissue is frequently left, but for women, complete removal of orbicularis muscle along with skin is recommended (Fig. 23.29). Use of sterile saline-soaked dental rolls or gauze or a non-reflective Jaeger plate is recommended to protect adjacent skin from inadvertent overshoot. If bleeding occurs, it is often in the lateral incision and defocusing the laser is usually sufficient to induce hemostasis. Gentle pressure on the globe makes the fat pads bulge against the septum at which point the underlying septum should be in-

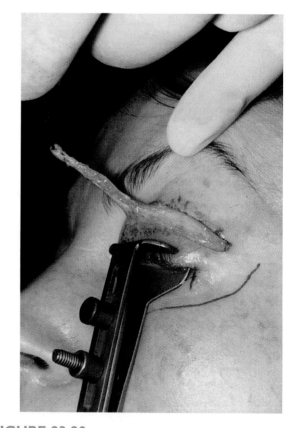

FIGURE 23.29
Skin and orbicularis being excised. Note the hemostasis associated with laser excision.

cised, again using the laser. The septum is then divided transversely.

The fat should then be elevated using forceps and the excess draped over wet cotton-tipped applicators, similar to the lower eyelid procedure, and excised. It should be noted that each non-laser maneuver may add to bleeding and subsequent postoperative bruising and swelling. Care must be taken not to pull too vigorously on the fat. The amount to be removed will elevate easily. The transection of the fat is accomplished with a straight, clean incision using the laser in cutting mode.

Upper eyelid incisions may be closed in a variety of ways, including continuous or interrupted suturing, taping, and gluing, all of which are acceptable (Fig. 23.30). Antimicrobial ointment should be applied to the suture line if sutures are used. Ice, slush, or a cold compress may be begun immediately after surgery and continued for 24 hours with the head elevated for the first 48 hours. No dressings are needed. Strenuous activity should be avoided for at least a week and contact lenses should not be worn for 2 weeks.

Periorbital Resurfacing

It is better treatment to treat the whole face than to treat the periorbital area alone. However, in many cases this area may be the only site of disease or at least is significantly out of step with other areas of the patient's face and it is the only area the patient wishes to have treated. As discussed above, resurfacing the periorbital area is usually performed immediately after transconjunctival lower eyelid blepharoplasty. Similarly, infraorbital resurfacing is performed on completion of either upper or lower eyelid blepharoplasty or both. Upper eyelid resurfacing is often not performed at the same time as upper eyelid blepharoplasty, but may be performed as a delayed procedure.

Technically, periorbital resurfacing requires less laser energy and passes than the rest of the facial skin. Typically, resurfacing is accomplished with an UltraPulse laser (Coherent Laser Corp., Palo Alto, CA) with a computer pattern generator (CPG) square pattern (No. 3), a small pattern size (4 or 5) and a 10% to 20% overlap. The power is usually set at 60 to 100 W at 300 mJ/pulse with a 2.25 mm spot size. A single complete pass that encompasses the entire cosmetic unit is executed.

Depending on the pathology being treated, the next pass varies. For widespread dermal tumors such as syringomas, trichoepitheliomas, or xanthelasmas, the next pass may be a focal spot directed at the center of the tumor and can be delivered by the CPG on a single spot setting (No. 1). Alternatively changing handpieces may be required to use a smaller spot size and hence higher focal power density (such as the 1 mm handpiece). This focal treatment is usually followed by a light general second pass. The Erbuim:YAG laser is particularly efficient in dealing with benign eyelid lesions because, when set on repeat pulse and directed at a papular target, the laser almost acts like a drill repeatedly removing small wafers of tissue until the lesion is flattened. It does not tend to run out of steam on these papular lesions like a CO_2 laser might. However, for the far more common problems of rhytides and sun damage, observing the state of the wrinkles after the first pass is the best guide whether more therapy is needed.

Usually, a second pass is performed similar to the first but avoids the delicate skin of the lower eyelid pretarsal area and especially the skin in the region of the poorly supported lateral canthal angle. When treating the lower eyelid or upper cheek, keep an eye on what is happening at the lateral canthal angle as even treatment at quite a distance from this site can exert downward pressure on this delicate area. This is especially so in the poorly supported eyelid as seen after previous lower eyelid surgery. Ectropion, scleral show and round eye are complications of the skin muscle resection of the transcutaneous lower eyelid blepharoplasty. The same complications can be produced by over exuberant

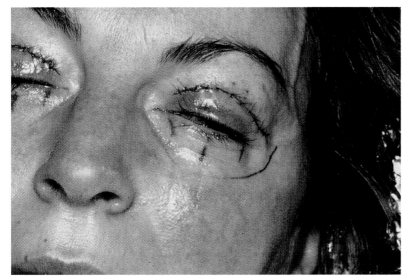

FIGURE 23.30
Dissolvable sutures in place after upper lid blepharoplasty. Cox eye shields are in place for the impending lower lid resurfacing.

FIGURE 23.31
Patient with incipient lower eyelid pull down after resurfacing.

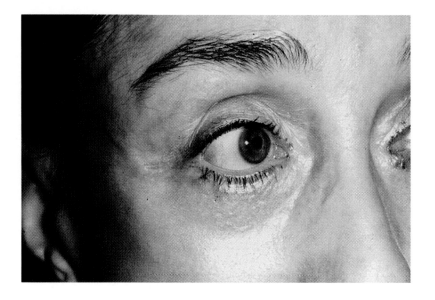

resurfacing (Fig. 23.31). It is extremely rare for eyelids to require a third pass.

With the SilkTouch flash scanning system (Sharplan Lasers Inc., Allendale, NJ), a small spot size (3 mm) is used with 6 to 7 W and a 125 mm handpiece. The focused scan is completed in 0.2 seconds. Except when treating appendageal tumors, a second pass is not required because of the increased depth of penetration of this laser compared to the UltraPulse laser. If rhytides are severe, a scattered second pass is useful on the more severe areas. Again this pass should avoid the delicate pretarsal and lateral canthal angle skin zones.

The newer FeatherTouch laser from Sharplan Laser Inc. dwells on tissue for a much shorter time than the SilkTouch laser and appears more gentle to the delicate periorbital zone. The FeatherTouch unit is usually set at 30 to 36 W with the 200 mm handpiece and a 5 to 7 mm square pattern, with one pass being typically adequate.

The Tru-Pulse laser system (Tissue Technologies Inc., Albuquerque, NM), with an extremely short pulse of 90 msec has been delivered successfully with a 250 to 500 mJ pulse with 1 to 4 passes being necessary (58). The long term outcome of this technology and that of the Erbium:YAG laser will demonstrate whether safety of periorbital resurfacing can be further improved without sacrificing efficacy.

COMPLICATIONS OF LASER RESURFACING

It should be stressed that complications of laser resurfacing appear to be fewer than for other resurfacing procedures such as phenol face peeling or dermabrasion. It is useful to differentiate the expected clinical course and outcome from complications.

Normal Morbidity of CO_2 Laser Healing

Edema

Postoperative edema occurs 24 to 72 hours after laser procedures. This phase may be altered by intraoperative parenteral corticosteroids and/or postoperative oral steroids. However, some edema, in a more subtle form, is seen for up to 6 weeks after the procedure (Fig. 23.32). It is important to explain this phase of the postoperative period to the patient before the operation as clinical appearances at this time are not totally predictive of the final outcome.

Erythema

A much criticized aspect of laser resurfacing is the postoperative erythema it induces. To some extent, the erythema is determined by the number of passes, the type of CO_2 laser used, the production of char, and the peculiarities of individual patients. However, some erythema is part of the normal wound healing and may persist for over 2 months after the procedure (Fig. 23.33). Erythema seems to persist longer in olive skin patients and should probably not be considered abnormal unless it appears focal in nature where it may be a premonitory sign of scarring. If generalized, erythema probably does not require treatment, but topical steroids such as mometasone furoate, methylprednisolone aceponate, or silicon gel have been advocated. Whether these patients make up a group that is more prone to longer term hypopigmentation deserves further study.

Hyperpigmentation

In any patient who has Fitzpatrick type III skin and above, temporary hyperpigmentation should be anticipated (Fig. 23.34). This hyperpigmentation is not a complication, but a natural part of wound healing. It may be that this phase prevents the melanocytes

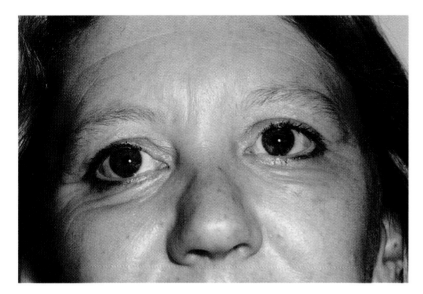

FIGURE 23.32
Patient 3 weeks after resurfacing with unusually significant edema of the lower eyelid zone.

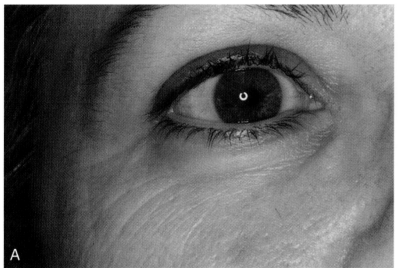

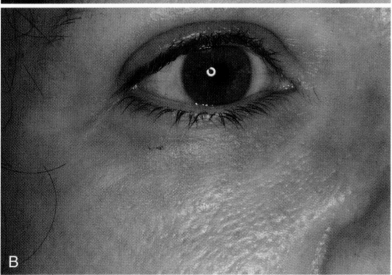

FIGURE 23.33
A, Patient before resurfacing showing lower eyelid rhytides. B, Patient 3 weeks after resurfacing displaying "normal" postoperative erythema.

FIGURE 23.34
Patient with "normal" hyperpigmentation postoperatively.

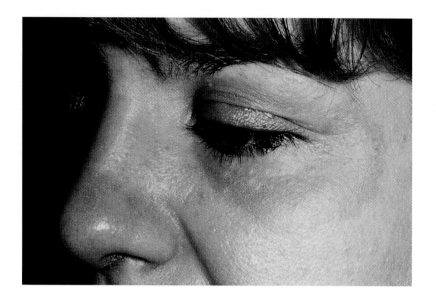

from the shoulders of appendageal structures from populating the lining epidermis and suppling the network or keratinocytes with melanosomes. Normal regulatory mechanisms occur evening pigmentation in the intermediate to long term postoperative period. The phase of hyperpigmentation usually occurs at about 3 weeks and continues until about 6 to 8 weeks postoperatively. It is possible to reduce the effect of the more active melanocytes by using hydroquinone or kojic acid beginning at 2 weeks after the resurfacing procedure.

Increased Sensitivity to Topical Agents
This should be anticipated in the first few weeks after the procedure. It is uncertain why this resurfacing procedure suffers this fate compared to dermabrasion, for example. Even inert substances such as white soft paraffin appear to produce an irritant contact dermatitis. This is manifest by symptoms of itch and signs of edema, vesiculation and small pustules. Lowe et al. have advocated Crisco as being relatively free of these problems (58). However, I have used bio-occlusive dressings alone, such as Flexan (Dow B. Hickson Inc., Sugarland, TX) or Duoderm (Convatec, Princeton, NJ), and have found these the best for facial and lower eyelid resurfacing. If a topical agent is to be used, a non-comedogenic light moisturizer is best. Greasy ointments including antibiotic ointments are best avoided in the early stages of re-epithelialization although they are permissible and useful for the upper eyelid areas where dressings are not practical.

Scarring
Scarring is unusual after periorbital CO_2 laser resurfacing. Contributing events can be divided into patient factors and operative factors.

Patient Factors
Past Isotretinoin. Our experience with dermabrasion and chemical peeling during or soon after isotretinoin therapy should make us cautious with any skin wounding for at least 6 months after isotretinoin is completed (59–61). Opinions vary as to how long one must wait before resurfacing after completion of this agent, with 6 to 24 months commonly being the range (62). To my knowledge, no reports of abnormal healing after CO_2 laser resurfacing have been described attributable to the use of this agent.

Past Disease Producing Appendageal Depletion. Any disease or surgery sufficient to substantially decrease appendageal structures may risk abnormal healing in the postoperative period. Examples of these diseases may include:

Radiotherapy sufficient to diminish appendages
Grafts–either split skin or full thickness, unless quite small
Scarring skin diseases, such as discoid lupus erythematosus or scleroderma

Infection. The only facial infection that is likely to lead to scarring is herpes simplex (Fig. 23.35). Any patient who personally has ever had herpes simplex infection should be protected with antiviral agents beginning at least 24 hours before the procedure and given until re-epithelialization is complete. If a resident family member contracts and develops a herpetiform lesion during the time of re-epithelialization then the patient should also be protected with prophylactic antiviral agents. Examples of acceptable agents include acyclovir, valcyclovir and famcyclovir. Rarely, candidiasis or bacterial infections may be seen.

Trauma. Patients should be instructed to not attempt their own debridement of scabs or pick at healing wounds. Patients who have previously suffered from excoriated acne are particularly at risk.

Operative Factors

The reason that the modern CO_2 laser systems are able to result in low scarring potential is because they avoid char. Char represents a heat sink and a central superheated point from which conduction of that heat may impact unwanted targets. The adage "char means scar" should be borne in mind by all laser resurfacing practitioners.

Eyelids require very little treatment and the number of passes and the power used should be the minimum to achieve the desired results.

Treatment of Scarring

Scarring may be averted by early recognition. Active treatment of herpes simplex is essential. Treatment of any focal erythema needs to be aggressive. Topical steroids, such as mometasone furoate or methylprednisolone aceponate should be used once or twice daily. If unsuccessful after 1 to 2 weeks, intralesional triamcinolone or a vascular laser may be required.

Pigmentary Abnormalities

It appears that laser resurfacing is comparatively safe for all skin types. Hyperpigmentation appears to be a temporary concern. However, hypopigmentation is a relatively late sign with other resurfacing techniques and is a definite complication of CO_2 resurfacing. Since the advent of scanning technology, it appears to be a less likely event.

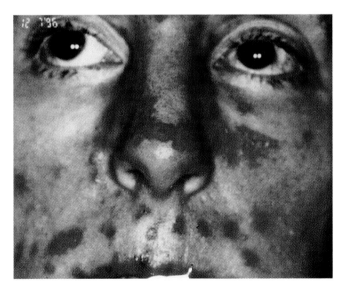

FIGURE 23.35

Patient with Herpes Simplex viral infection after laser resurfacing.

Ectropion

Ectropion should, in most circumstances, be avoidable. The ability of the CO_2 laser to "tighten" the dermis is visible whenever this layer is treated, but in the periorbital region it is exaggerated. Some patients require special care in this region. Among those are patients with atonic lower eyelids as assessed by snap and retraction tests. Patients with previous transcutaneous blepharoplasty and those with any symptoms of dry eyes need to be treated cautiously, if at all. David et al. has suggested that eyelids require very little in the way of treatment using a −10% setting on the CPG and performing only one pass (63). If one considers the eyelid zone of a patient to be at any risk, these guidelines are best heeded.

The end point of treatment for lower eyelid rhytides is disappearance of wrinkles, remembering that the lower border of the lower eyelid tarsal plate is not a wrinkle. The skin overlying the lower tarsal plate never needs more than one light pass. It is prudent in any person with less than optimal lower eyelid tone to under treat this area and accept an improvement rather than eradication of these wrinkles. Attention should be paid to prevention of char in this area. Also, attention should be paid to patients whose skin tightens excessively and adjustment made for this during the procedure.

Pulling down of the lower eyelids is usually temporary, improving over the first 2 to 3 weeks. If this is noted during the operation, two remedial steps may be taken. The first involves always using a bio-occlusive dressing up to the lashes and the second is to use this dressing to suspend the lateral canthus upwards towards the temple (Fig. 23.36).

Bizarre, Poorly Merged or Uneven Appearance

Bizarre, poorly merged, or uneven appearance may just be a temporary phenomenon due to patchy pigmentation or delayed erythema in certain areas. However, it may represent inadequate attention to detail by the operator. If a single pass of laser treatment is being performed, careful attention must be made to keeping the treatment coverage even and complete. Untreated areas are obvious among treated areas. In general, square, hexagonal or rectangular patterns fit together better than circular patterns. Adequate attention to feathering the edges of the resurfaced zone and performing full face or regional resurfacing will hide demarcation lines.

Dressing and Cream-Induced Complications

Dressing and cream-induced complications include irritant contact dermatitis that can be treated by ceasing agent use and applying appropriate cool compresses (e.g., Burrow's solution dilute 1:20 with water and topical steroid cream). Acneiform eruptions are common and avoiding occlusive ointment and use of noncomedogenic moisturizers is important. All pustules are not acne and cultures to rule out staph and Candida infections should be carried out. Pustules can also occur with Pityrosporon infections.

Dressings keep patients from traumatizing the skin. They also limit cream-related reactions. Leaving these dressings intact for 2 days usually gives excellent results but changing them daily is also reasonable, although unnecessary. Occasionally, imprints of the newer high adhesive Flexan dressing (Flexipore in Australia) may leave imprints on the skin but this has not been seen in the periorbital area The dressings are removed in the shower on the second postoperative day and a film dressing applied or the use of simple ointments, such as emulsifying ointment or silicon containing moisturizers, is a safe and reasonable alternative.

Incomplete Satisfaction

The low complication rate of laser resurfacing combined with a high satisfaction rate will ensure a strong future for CO_2 laser use in the armamentarium of the cosmetic surgeon. In a recent as yet unpublished study of 100 patients who had laser resurfacing, 78.8% of patient outcomes were classed as good to excellent, 68.9% of patient outcomes met patient expectations, 78% of patients would have the procedure done again if required, and 84% would recommend the procedure to others (64).

COMPLICATIONS OF BLEPHAROPLASTY

Successful blepharoplasty does not end on the operating table. The after care period is important. To reduce the incidence of nausea, anesthesia that has a high rate of associated nausea should be avoided. Postoperatively, patients should not strain after the operation, avoid constipation, bending over, sneezing and cough-

ing as feasible. Nonsteroidal anti-inflammatory drugs should also be avoided and activities minimized. Ice is very useful for the first 12 to 24 hours to reduce swelling. Artificial tears and lubricants are useful in this period. Women should avoid make up until suture lines have healed.

Mild perioperative problems usually resolve with time and support. These include edema, mild pain, bruising and mild lower eyelid conjunctival irritation. Others complications, such as diplopia, blepharoptosis and lagophthalmos, may settle expectantly but may need further surgical intervention. Asymmetry, persistent fat bulges, and residual excess skin may be corrected electively at a later date. However, the major complications of this procedure, such as enophthalmos, retrobulbar hemorrhage and blindness, corneal injuries and ectropion, obviously need to be avoided (65, 66).

Retrobulbar hemorrhage is a true emergency with about an hour and a half to save the eye. An ophthalmologist should be immediately called for assistance, the wound immediately opened, and any hematoma evacuated and the eye massaged. Any bleeding points that can be identified should be cauterized. If this fails to resolve the problem, medical management consisting of 1 gm/kg mannitol and 500 mg Diamox (Lederle, Wyeth, Baulkham Hills) intravenously to reduce intraocular pressure should be undertaken. The next step is lateral cantholysis or even orbital decompression. Certainly, ophthalmological help is necessary at this point.

Enophthalmos and focal areas of hollowing from overly aggressive fat removal should be avoided by only taking fat that is easily presented at the operation with no overt tugging and pulling at fat pockets to get every morsel of retro-orbital fat attainable.

The incidence of dry eye, round eye, scleral show and ectropion (Fig. 23.36) should decline as the transcu-

FIGURE 23.36
Dressings in situ after laser resurfacing. They offer coverage, enhancement of wound healing and support.

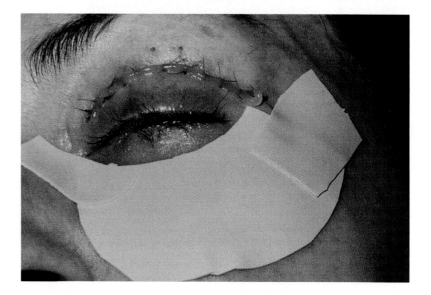

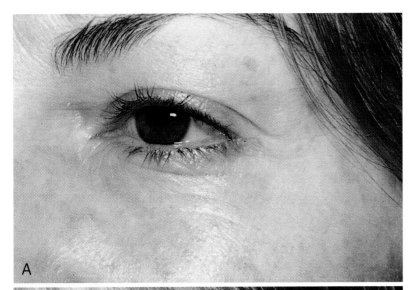

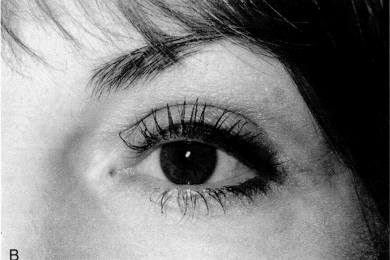

FIGURE 23.37
A, Preoperative view of a patient who underwent upper lid blepharoplasty and lower lid resurfacing. B, Postoperative view at 4 weeks showing effacement of fine rhytides. Patient is wearing mascara and eye shadow that can now be used to advantage on an expanded upper eyelid platform.

taneous blepharoplasty is performed less often (24–26, 33, 67–72). In a large multicenter clinical survey by Glassberg, Babapour and Lask involving 16 responding practitioners and 4,269 cases of laser blepharoplasty there were no serious complications attributable to the laser component of the blepharoplasty technique (73).

SUMMARY

The commonest indication for blepharoplasty is redundant skin and deeper structures of the upper eyelid and herniated fat pads and a "pseudoredundancy" of skin on the lower eyelid. In the past, we have had no good method of addressing the quality of the eyelid skin affected by wrinkling or dermal and epidermal tumors at the same time as addressing the true redundancy of tissues (Fig. 23.37). This has led to the less satisfactory solutions, such as skin muscle flaps and chemical peels, being used in the past. With the rise of new laser systems has come the ability to reliably resurface the peri-

orbital area safely and effectively. In certain situations it is permissible to perform the resurfacing at the time of the blepharoplasty, in other circumstances it allows us the ability to tidy up and improve the results of the blepharoplasty at a later date. As with every new technique, there are nuances to learn and in this circumstance, new technologies to tackle.

REFERENCES

1. Stegman S. A study of dermabrasion and chemical peels in an animal model. J Dermatol Surg Oncol 1980;6:6.
2. Hill T. Cutaneous wound healing following dermabrasion. J Dermatol Surg Oncol 1980;6:6.
3. Winton GB, Salasche SJ. Dermabrasion of the scalp as a treatment for actinic damage. J Am Acad Dermatol 1986; 14:661-668.
4. Alt TA, Goodman GJ, Coleman WP III, et al. Dermabrasion. In: Coleman WP III, Hanke CW, Alt TA, Asken S, eds. Cosmetic surgery of the skin: principles and techniques. 2nd ed. Mosby: St. Louis 1997:131-151.

5. Rubin MG. Trichloroacetic acid and other non phenol peels. Clin Plast Surg 1992;19(2):525-536.
6. Kligman AM, Baker TJ, Gordon HL. Long term histologic follow up of phenol face peels. Plast Reconstr Surg 1985; 75:652-659.
7. Brody HJ. Chemical peeling. St. Louis: Mosby Yearbook, 1992:129.
8. Litton C, Trinidad G. Chemosurgery of the eyelids. In: Aston ST, ed. Third International symposium of plastic and reconstructive surgery. Baltimore: Williams and Wilkins, 1982:341-345.
9. Morrow DM. Chemical peeling of eyelids and periorbital area. J Dermatol Surg Oncol 1992;18(2):102-110.
10. Hanke CW, Coleman WP. Collagen filler substances. In: Coleman WP III, Hanke CW, Alt TA, Asken S, eds. Cosmetic surgery of the skin: principles and techniques. 2nd ed St. Louis: Mosby Yearbook, 1997:217-230.
11. Yarborough JM, Millikan LE. Gelatin matrix implant and collagen. In: Parish LC, Lask GP, eds. Aesthetic dermatology. New York: McGraw-Hill, 1991.
12. David L. Laser vermilion ablation for actinic cheilitis. J Dermatol Surg Oncol 1985;11:605-608.
13. David L, Lask GP. Laser abrasion for cosmetic and medical treatment of facial actinic damage. Cutis 1989;43: 583-587.
14. Goldman MP, Fitzpatrick RE. CO_2 laser surgery. In: Goldman MP, Fitzpatrick RE, eds. Cutaneous laser surgery: The art and science of selective photothermolysis. St Louis: Mosby Yearbook, 1994:198-258.
15. Anderson RR, Parrish RR. Selective photothermolysis: precise microsurgery by selective absorption of pulsed radiation. Science 1983;220:524-527.
16. Anderson RR. Laser tissue interactions. In: Goldman MP, Fitzpatrick RE, eds. Cutaneous laser surgery. The art and science of selective photothermolysis. St Louis: Mosby Yearbook, 1994:1-18.
17. Lowe NJ, Lask G, Griffin ME, et al. Skin resurfacing with the ultrapulse carbon dioxide laser: observations on 100 patients. Dermatol Surg 1995;21:1025-1029.
18. Goodman GJ. Facial resurfacing using a high energy short pulse carbon dioxide laser. Aust J Dermatol 1996;37: 125-132.
19. David LM, Sarne AJ, Unger WP. Rapid laser scanning for facial resurfacing. Dermatol Surg 1995;21:1031-1033.
20. Lask G, Keller G, Lowe N, et al. Laser skin resurfacing with the Silk Touch flashscanner for facial rhytides. Dermatol Surg 1995;21:1021-1024.
21. Goodman GJ, Bekhor PS, Richards SW. Advances in laser therapy–the importance of selective photothermolysis. Med J Aust 1996;164:681-686.
22. Weinstein C. Ultrapulse carbon dioxide laser removal of periocular wrinkles in association with laser blepharoplasty. J Clin Med Surg 1994;12(4):205-209.
23. Bourget. Les hernies graisseuses de l'orbite: notre traitment ethirugical. Bull Acad Med (Paris) 1924;92:1270.
24. Weinberg DA, Baylis HI. Transconjunctival lower eyelid blepharoplasty. Dermatol Surg 1995;21(5):407-410.
25. Perkins SW, Dyer WK II, Simo F. Transconjunctival approach to lower eyelid blepharoplasty. Experience, indications, and technique in 300 patients. Arch Otolaryngol Head Neck Surg 1994;120(2):172-177.
26. Asken S. The preseptal and the retroseptal approaches in transconjunctival blepharoplasty. J Dermatol Surg Oncol 1992;18(12):1110-1116.
27. Neuhaus RW. Lower eyelid blepharoplasty. J Dermatol Surg Oncol 1992;18(12):1100-1109.
28. David LM, Goodman G. Blepharoplasty for the laser dermatologic surgeon. Clin Dermatol 1995;13:49-53.
29. Yarborough JN. Scar revision by dermabrasion. In: Roenigk RK, Roenigk HH, eds. Dermatologic surgery. New York: Marcel Dekker 1989:909-933.
30. Katz BE, Oca AG. A controlled study of the effectiveness of spot dermabrasion ('scarabrasion') on the appearance of surgical scars. J Am Acad Dermatol 1991;24(3):462-466.
31. Harmon CB, Zellickson BD, Roenigk RK, et al. Dermabrasive scar revision: immunohistochemical and ultrastructural evaluation. Dermatol Surg 1995;21:503-508.
32. Weber PJ. Nuances in ophthalmic plastic surgery. A dermatologic surgeon's perspective. J Dermatol Surg Oncol 1992;18:1117-1121.
33. Fulton JE. World Congress of Cosmetic Surgery. Manila, Philippines, February 6-9, 1997.
34. Baker SS. Carbon dioxide laser ptosis surgery combined with blepharoplasty. Dermatol Surg 1995;21:1065-1070.
35. Perman KI. Upper eyelid blepharoplasty. J Dermatol Surg Oncol 1992;18:1096-1099.
36. Wilkins RB, Papita M. The recognition of acquired ptosis in patients considered for upper eyelid blepharoplasty. Plast Reconstr Surg 1982;70:431-434.
37. Shorr N, Enzer YR. Considerations in aesthetic eyelid surgery. J Derm Surg Oncol 1992;18:1081-1095.
38. Lowe NJ et al. Infraorbital pigmented skin. Preliminary observations of laser therapy. Dermatol Surg 1995;21:767-770.
39. Carruthers A, Carruthers JD. Botulinum toxin in the treatment of glabella frown lines and other facial wrinkles. In: Jankovic J, Hallett M, eds. Therapy with botulinum toxin. New York: Marcel Dekker 1994:577.
40. Garcia A, Fulton JE. Cosmetic denervation of the muscles of facial expression with botulinum toxin. A dose response study. Dermatol Surg 1996;22:39-43.
41. Garden JM. Papillomavirus in the vapour of carbon dioxide treated verrucae. JAMA 1988;259:8.
42. Rees TD. Blepharoplasty. In: Rees TD, Wood-Smith D, eds. Cosmetic facial surgery. Philadelphia: W.B. Saunders, 1973:61.
43. Spira M. Blepharoplasty. Clin Plast Surg 1978;1:58.
44. Asken S. The preseptal and the retroseptal approaches in transconjunctival blepharoplasty. J Dermatol Surg Oncol 1992;18(12):1110-1116.
45. Hawtof DB. Marking the upper lid blepharoplasty [letter]. Plast Reconstr Surg 1987;80(3):469.
46. Castanares S. Blepharoplasty for herniated infraorbital fat. Plast Reconstr Surg 1951;8:46.
47. Flowers RS. Zigzag blepharoplasty for upper eyelids. Plast Reconstr Surg 1971;47:557.
48. Lewis JR II. The Z blepharoplasty. Plast Reconstr Surg 1969;44:331.
49. Baker TJ, Gordon HL, Mosienko P. Upper lid blepharoplasty. Plast Reconstr Surg 1977;60:692.
50. Alt TH. Blepharoplasty. Dermatol Clin 1995;13(2):389-430.
51. Dingman DL. Transcoronal blepharoplasty. Plast Reconstr Surg 1992;90(5):815-820.

52. Becker BB, Berry FD. Eyelid level after lower lid blepharoplasty with skin excision. The relationship of intraoperative and postoperative lid levels. Arch Otolaryngol Head Neck Surg 1992;118(9):959-962.

53. Kamer FM, Mikaelian AJ. Preexcision blepharoplasty. Arch Otolaryngol Head Neck Surg 1991;117(9):995-1000.

54. Asken S. Cosmetic eyelid surgery–blepharoplasty. In: Coleman WP III, Hanke CW, Alt TH, Asken S, eds. Cosmetic surgery of the skin: principles and techniques. Philadelphia: BC Decker 1991:267-291.

55. Baker SS. Carbon dioxide laser upper lid blepharoplasty. Am J Cos Surg 1992;9:141-145.

56. David LM, Baker SS. David-Baker eyelid retractor. Am J Cosmet Surg 1992;2:147-148.

57. Bell T, Schachter D, Harris D, et al. Tru-Pulse CO_2 laser resurfacing of the lower eyelids: dosimetry and erythema. Internet: Tissue Technologies home page (http:/kumo.swcp.com/-trupulse/bell2-ab.htm). Technical papers summary of BiOS Lasers in Dermatology, Plastic and Tissue repair (8000,8004).

58. Lowe NJ, Lask G, Griffin ME. Laser skin resurfacing. Pre and post treatment guidelines. Dermatol Surg 1995;21:1017-1019.

59. Rubenstein R, Roenigk HH, Stegman SJ, et al. Atypical keloids after dermabrasion of patients taking Isotretinoin. J Am Acad Dermatol 1986;15:280.

60. Roenigk HH Jr, Pinski JB, Robinson JK, et al. Acne, retinoids, and dermabrasion. J Dermatol Surg Oncol 1985;11:396.

61. Zachariae H. Delayed bound healing and keloid formation following argon laser treatment or dermabrasion during Isotretinoin treatment Br J Dermatol 1988;118:703.

62. Alt TH, Goodman G, Hanke CW, et al. Dermabrasion. In: Coleman WP III, Hanke CW, Alt TA, et al., eds. Cosmetic surgery of the skin: Principles and techniques. 2nd ed. St Louis: Mosby, 1997:112-151.

63. David LM, Sarne AJ, Unger WP. Rapid laser scanning for facial resurfacing. Dermatol Surg 1995;21:1031-1033.

64. Goodman GJ. CO_2 laser resurfacing: Preliminary observations on short term followup. A subjective study of 100 patient's attitudes and outcomes. Dermatol Surg (in press).

65. Mahaffey PJ, Wallace AF. Blindness following cosmetic blepharoplasty: a review. Br J Plast Surg 1986;39(2):213-221.

66. Callahan MA. Prevention of blindness after blepharoplasty. Ophthalmology 1983;90:1047-1051.

67. McCord CD Jr, Ellis DS. The correction of lower lid malposition following lower lid blepharoplasty. Plast Reconstr Surg 1993;92(6):1068-1072.

68. Baylis HI, Nelson ER, Goldberg RA. Lower eyelid retraction following blepharoplasty. Ophthal Plast Reconstr Surg 1992;8(3):170-175.

69. McGraw BL, Adamson PA. Postblepharoplasty ectropion. Prevention and management. Arch Otolaryngol Head Neck Surg 1991;117(8):852-856.

70. Zarem HA, Resnick JI. Expanded applications for transconjunctival lower lid blepharoplasty. Plast Reconstr Surg 1991;88(2):215-221.

71. Carraway JH, Mellow CG. The prevention and treatment of lower lid ectropion following blepharoplasty. Plast Reconstr Surg 1990;85(6):971-981

72. Jordan DR, Anderson RL. The tarsal tuck procedure: avoiding eyelid retraction after lower blepharoplasty. Plast Reconstr Surg 1990;85(1):22-28.

73. Glassberg E, Babapour R, Lask G. Current trends in laser blepharoplasty. Results of a survey. Dermatol Surg 1995;21:1060-1063.

CHAPTER 24

Laser Assisted Endoscopic Forehead Lifting Combined with CO$_2$ Laser Resurfacing

■ Cynthia Weinstein

Upper facial rejuvenation is a popular cosmetic procedure. In the past, aesthetic procedures to correct upper facial aging produced significant morbidity, often with an exaggerated and unnatural appearance. With advances in medical technology, it is possible to achieve excellent results using minimal incisions, with lower morbidity and a more natural look. These new techniques require extensive training and a willingness to climb the steep learning curve in order to obtain the best results. Consumer acceptance of the newer endoscopic and laser techniques has been universally positive, yet acceptance among physicians has been slower and greeted by significant scepticism. Dermatologists have led the way in the development of many laser procedures, and can readily incorporate the more invasive endoscopic techniques into their armamentarium.

MECHANISMS OF UPPER FACIAL AGING

The three major components of upper face aging are gravity, muscle activity, and sun damage.

1. Gravity (Table 24.1)
   A. Brow ptosis. Gravity produces descent of the eyebrows, leading to "crowding" of the eye area and apparent redundancy of upper eyelid skin. It is particularly marked in the lateral eyebrow area.
   B. Looseness of eyelid skin.

C. Herniation of preseptal fat pads. These fat pads produce "puffiness" of upper eyelids and "bags" under lower eyelids.
   D. Ptosis of the temperomalar region.
2. Muscle Activity (Figure 24.1)
   The muscles of facial expression contribute to permanent folds and creases and also control brow position.
   A. Frown muscles. Although there is much controversy about which muscles produce glabella frown lines, it is likely that both the depressor supercilii portion of the orbicularis oculi muscle and the corrugator muscle contribute to the vertical glabella frown lines. Frown muscles also produce descent of the medial eyebrow. The procerus muscle produces horizontal wrinkles at the nasal root and leads to descent of the medial eyebrow.
   B. Smile lines. The lateral portion of the orbicularis oculi muscle produces "smile" lines at the outer aspect of the eyelid. Hyperactivity of this portion of the orbicularis muscle also leads to descent of the lateral eyebrow.
   C. Horizontal forehead creases. Although the frontalis muscle contributes to horizontal forehead lines, it is the *only* muscle which elevates the eyebrow. Interference with this muscle will lead to some degree of brow ptosis. Hyperactivity of this muscle and consequent horizontal forehead lines often occurs secondary to brow ptosis or redundant upper eyelid skin as a compensatory action

FIGURE 24.1
Surgical Anatomy of the Forehead Region.
(Reprinted with permission from Seckel, Brooke R.
Facial Danger Zones: Avoiding Nerve Injury in Fa-
cial Plastic Surgery. Quality Medical Publishing,
1994.)

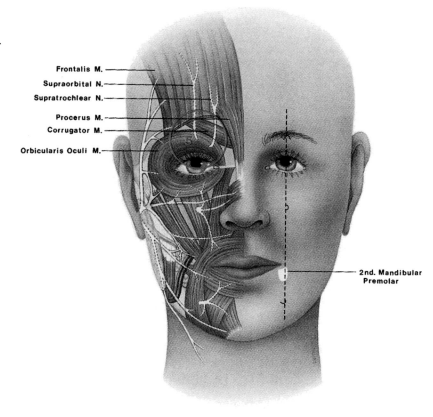

Frontalis M.
Supraorbital N.
Supratrochlear N.
Procerus M.
Corrugator M.
Orbicularis Oculi M.
2nd. Mandibular Premolar

TABLE 24.1

CAUSES OF AGING UPPER FACE

1. **Gravity**
   Brow ptosis
   Loose eyelid skin
   Herniation eyelid preseptal fat pads - Puffy eyes
   Ptosis of temperomalar region
2. **Muscular Activity**
   Glabella frown lines
   Smile lines
   Horizontal forehead lines (dynamic)
3. **Photoaging (Sundamage)**
   Sallow skin
   Pigmented lentigenes
   Dyschromia
   Horizontal forehead lines (static)
   Crow's feet
   Periocular wrinkles
   "Loose" upper and lower eyelid skin

TABLE 24.2

OPEN FOREHEAD LIFTING: DISADVANTAGES

1. Long incision, scar
2. Risk of permanent hair loss
3. Risk of numbness and hyperaesthesia
4. Elevation of the hairline (coronal approach)
5. Increase in eyebrow to hairline distance

which leads to permanent horizontal forehead wrinkles, fine periocular wrinkles and deep crow's feet.

TRADITIONAL METHODS OF UPPER FACIAL REJUVENATION

Traditional methods of upper facial rejuvenation include:

1. Open coronal and hairline brow lifting with resection
   of the corrugator and procerus muscles under direct
   vision. The forehead wrinkles are stretched, and "excess" skin resected. The frontalis muscle may also be
   scored, in order to weaken its activity (1, 2).
2. Upper and lower eyelid blepharoplasty with resection of "excess" skin on upper and lower eyelids.

Open Forehead Lifting (Table 24.2)
The open approach to forehead lifting (coronal or hairline) although effective, has significant morbidity and

to try to lift the eyebrow back to its normal position (pseudoptosis).
3. Sun Damage (Photoaging)
Chronic sun exposure leads to disruption of collagen
fibers (solar elastosis) with consequent loss of skin
elasticity. Repeated movement leads to wrinkles and
creases being permanently printed onto the skin

often poor patient acceptance. Furthermore, this method is rarely suitable for men or women with receding or thinning hairlines. Undesirable side effects of the open approach to brow lifting include:

1. Long incision.
2. Risk of visible scar.
3. Risk of permanent and visible hair loss.
4. Itching scalp.
5. Altered sensation.
6. Elevation of the hairline (coronal approach).
7. Exaggeration of brow elevation in order to "pull out" forehead wrinkles, creating a surprised expression.
8. Difficulty in achieving differential eyebrow lifting especially of the lateral aspect.
9. Occasional difficulty in eyelid closure.

Traditional Blepharoplasty

Traditional transcutaneous blepharoplasty is a popular procedure. However, significant disadvantages with the standard approach can lead to a level of dissatisfaction including:

A. Excess upper eyelid skin resection may lead to further brow ptosis and "crowding" of the periorbital region.
B. Excision of "loose" skin on the lower eyelid, may cause distortion of eye shape and even frank ectropion.
C. Periorbital wrinkles are unchanged by the traditional approach to blepharoplasty.
D. The scalpel approach to blepharoplasty often leads to significant bleeding, bruising and swelling.

IDEAL APPROACH TO UPPER FACIAL REJUVENATION (TABLE 24.3, FIGURE 24.2)

If fashion magazines are a realistic guide to ideal beauty, we should aim to achieve the following parameters in rejuvenating the upper face:

1. The eyebrow in women should be just above the orbital rim laterally, and at the orbital rim medially. The "ideal" brow should be 2.5 cm above the mid pupil and 5 cm from the anterior hairline. In men the "ideal" brow should be at the orbital rim.

TABLE 24.3

"IDEAL" UPPER FACIAL REJUVENATION

1. Eyebrow above orbital rim laterally, at the orbital rim medially
2. Reduce glabella frown lines
3. Remove redundant skin and prolapsed fat on upper eyelid to produce a "crease"
4. Reduce wrinkles of the forehead, crow's feet and periorbital regions
5. Maintain an eyebrow to hairline distance of approximately 5 cm

2. Reduce glabella frown lines by diminishing the activity of the corrugator and or depressor supercilii portion of the orbicularis oculi muscles.
3. Remove wrinkle lines and sun damage from the forehead skin.
4. Resect redundant skin on the upper eyelid and prolapsed fat pad to produce a well defined upper eyelid crease.
5. Remove prolapsed fat from lower eyelid, without distorting eye shape.
6. Smooth wrinkles and reduce "loose" skin on lower eyelid, without causing round eyes or ectropion.
7. Reduce the appearance of crow's feet.

RATIONALE FOR ENDOSCOPIC MINIMAL INCISION BROW LIFT

Eyebrow position is determined by the balance between the muscles of eyebrow elevation and eyebrow depressors. If the eyebrow depressors can be weakened or inactivated, the eyebrow elevators will pull the eyebrows superiorly (3-14). The muscles responsible for elevating or depressing the eyebrow are listed below.

1. Elevators of eyebrow
   Frontalis muscle (joined to occipitalis)

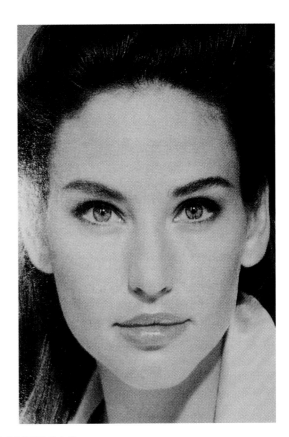

FIGURE 24.2
Ideal upper facial proportion (magazine model). (Reprinted with permission from ITA Magazine.)

2. Depressors of the eyebrow
   Orbicularis oculi (lateral)
   Orbicularis oculi-depressor supercilii portion (medial)
   Corrugator muscle (medial)
   Procerus muscle (medial)

If the eyebrow depressors can be weakened, and the periosteum is released at the orbital rim, the frontalis will produce elevation of the eyebrow due to its "unopposed" action.

VARIETIES OF MINIMAL INCISION ENDOSCOPIC FOREHEAD LIFTING (TABLE 24.4)

There are a variety of approaches to minimal incision endoscopic forehead lifting, which include:

1. Subperiosteal - dissection.
2. Subgaleal.
3. Combined subperiosteal and subgaleal approach.
4. Combined transblepharoplasty resection of corrugator and depressor supercilia muscle with subperiosteal brow lift (15-17).

The majority of surgeons now favor the subperiosteal approach with varying methods of corrugator resection. I prefer the transblepharoplasty approach combined with subperiosteal endoscopic dissection.

RATIONALE FOR LASER RESURFACING THE FOREHEAD (TABLE 24.5)

Carbon dioxide (CO_2) laser resurfacing has enjoyed great popularity due to its ability to improve skin quality, remove wrinkles due to sun damage and produce skin tightening. Laser resurfacing can readily improve horizontal forehead lines while simultaneously producing skin contraction, and thus prevent excessive elevation of the frontal hairline and an increase in the brow to hairline distance.

RATIONALE FOR COMBINING MINIMAL INCISION FOREHEAD LIFT WITH CARBON DIOXIDE LASER RESURFACING

By combining endoscopic minimal incision forehead lift with CO_2 laser resurfacing, the different components of upper facial aging can be addressed. Endoscopic minimal incision browlift elevates the brow and weakens the depressors of the eyebrow (especially medial depressors) and decreases frowning (corrugator and the depressors supercilia portion of the orbicularis oculi muscles), while CO_2 laser resurfacing will reduce wrinkle lines, producing smooth, contracted skin (9).

TABLE 24.4

TYPES OF MINIMAL INCISION FOREHEAD LIFTING

1. Subperiosteal lift
2. Subgaleal lift
3. Combined subperiosteal and subgaleal lift
4. Combined transblepharoplasty resection of the corrugator and depressor supercilli muscle with subperiosteal browlift

TABLE 24.5

RATIONALE FOR LASER RESURFACING THE FOREHEAD

1. Remove actinic damage, dyschromia, sallow skin
2. Remove static wrinkle lines, horizontal forehead lines, crow's feet and periocular wrinkles
3. "Shrink" forehead skin
4. Prevent excessive elevation of hairline

TABLE 24.6

RATIONALE FOR COMBINED TRANSBLEPHAROPLASTY WITH ENDOSCOPIC MINIMAL INCISION BROW LIFT

1. Rejuvenate forehead and eyelid complex
2. Correct proportion of eyelid resection versus eyebrow lift
3. Avoid exaggeration of browlift
4. Frown muscles resected under direct vision
5. Small scalp incisions
6. Resection of preseptal fat pads

RATIONALE FOR TRANSBLEPHAROPLASTY RESECTION OF FROWN MUSCLES COMBINED WITH ENDOSCOPIC MINIMAL INCISION FOREHEAD LIFT (TABLE 24.6)

There are a number of advantages in combining CO_2 laser blepharoplasty with endoscopic minimal incision forehead lift including (15-17):

1. It is possible to rejuvenate the whole upper face, including the eyelids.
2. It is possible to obtain the most aesthetic proportion of eyebrow to eyelid lifting without exaggerating either, thereby avoiding unnatural eyebrow elevation.
3. It is easy to resect the depressors of the eyebrow (i.e., resect the corrugator and the depressor supercilia portion of the orbicularis oculi under direct vision).
4. It is often desirable to resect the preseptal fat pads on the upper eyelid to create a definite eyelid crease.
5. It is possible to make smaller scalp incisions.

INDICATIONS FOR MINIMAL INCISION FOREHEAD LIFT WITH CO_2 LASER RESURFACING (TABLE 24.7)

Because endoscopic forehead lifting combined with transblepharoplasty resection of frown muscles is minimally invasive with few incisions, the indications for forehead lifting have broadened somewhat, especially to men with thinning hair, and younger patients. Indications include:

1. Brow ptosis especially lateral brow.
2. Deep glabella frown lines.
3. Horizontal forehead lines associated with brow ptosis.

4. Men with thinning front temporal hair and brow ptosis.
5. Young patients with brow ptosis.
6. Patients with a combination of brow ptosis plus loose, upper eyelid skin.
7. Patients with puffy eyelids and brow ptosis.

PREOPERATIVE ASSESSMENT (TABLE 24.8, FIGURES 24.3, 24.4)

Very few patients understand that some of the heaviness and looseness of upper eyelid skin is caused by descent of the eyebrows. Many who request a blepharoplasty are surprised when a brow lift is suggested as an alternative. It is useful to show the patient, preferably on a computer imaging system, that part of their eyelid

TABLE 24.7

INDICATIONS FOR MINIMAL INCISION FOREHEAD LIFT COMBINED WITH CO_2 LASER RESURFACING

1. Brow ptosis
2. Glabella frown lines
3. Horizontal forehead lines with brow ptosis
4. Male patients with thinning hair, brow ptosis and horizontal forehead lines
5. Combination brow ptosis and "excess" upper eyelid skin
6. "Heavy" eyelids

TABLE 24.8

PREOPERATIVE ASSESSMENT

1. Forehead height (ideal 5 cm)
2. Eyebrow position (relation to orbital rim)
3. Thickness of hair in the frontotemporal region
4. Skin type - Laser resurfacing
5. Glabella frown lines
6. Wrinkling root nose - Procerus muscle activity

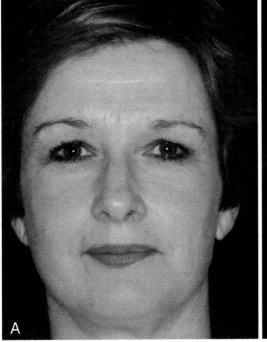 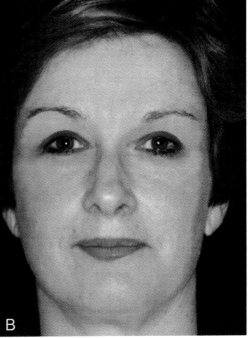

FIGURE 24.3
Computer imaging is a useful tool in assessing the amount of eyebrow versus eyelid surgery that will provide maximal rejuvenation of the upper face. A, Appearance before computer imaging. B, Appearance after computer imaging, brow lift, upper eyelid blepharoplasty, corrugator resection, and forehead resurfacing.

FIGURE 24.4
Manual assessment of the degree of eyebrow versus eyelid rejuvenation. A, 10 mm manual brow lift. B, Brow lift and upper eyelid blepharoplasty manual technique to mimic the desired result.

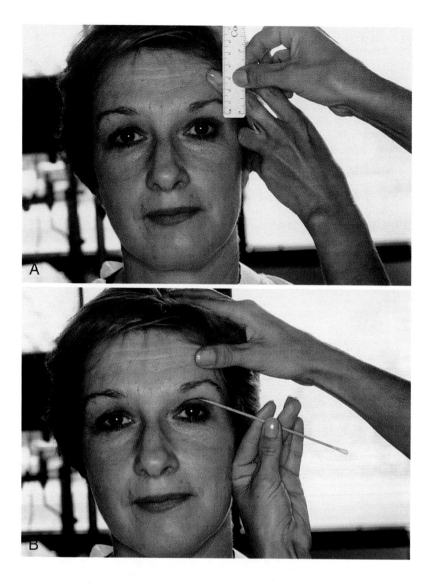

problem is in fact due to brow ptosis. Using the imaging system, one can demonstrate what can be accomplished with a blepharoplasty, a browlift, and a combination of the two procedures. The results of laser resurfacing can also be demonstrated. This allows the patient to actively participate in the decision as to their proposed future surgery. If computer imaging is unavailable, a mirror may be used to demonstrate the above changes. It is also important to assess:

1. Forehead height. The distance from the superior border of the eyebrow to the anterior hairline. If the forehead height is already greater than 5 cm or the frontal hairline is receding, it may be desirable to perform a more conservative forehead lift, or an anterior hairline incision.
2. If patients have thin hair in the frontal or temporal region, it is best to keep incisions as small and as few as possible.
3. Skin type is important when considering laser resurfacing. Resurfacing the forehead alone may produce

a cosmetically obvious difference in the quality of the skin in the resurfaced region compared to their normal skin. If possible, consideration to full face resurfacing should be given to those patients with significant sun damage.
4. The degree of wrinkling on the nasal root will be indicative of procerus activity. If the wrinkling is pronounced, proper attention to procerus ablation is advised.

PATIENT COUNSELING

Preoperative patient counseling is probably the most important step that ensures that the patient remains confident during the early postoperative "healing" phase. Many patients have the belief that the laser resurfacing is a minor procedure and are unprepared for the normal morbidity associated with it. Regional versus full face resurfacing should always be discussed, pointing out all the possible problems of regional erythema, change of skin texture and possible hypopigmentation in the long term. Patients who undergo fore-head lifting need to be informed about the possibility of considerable swelling for the first 2 to 3 days postoper-atively, especially in the periorbital region. Also, the placement of fixation screws in the hairline need to be discussed with the patient.

Preoperative counseling should occur at least 10 days before the procedure so the patient may ask questions and have consent forms fully explained. Preoperative photographs can be taken at the time of counseling.

THE DAY OF PROCEDURE

1. Marking the Patient (Figure 24.5)
   The patient is marked in the sitting position to cor-rectly establish the amount of eyebrow lifting and

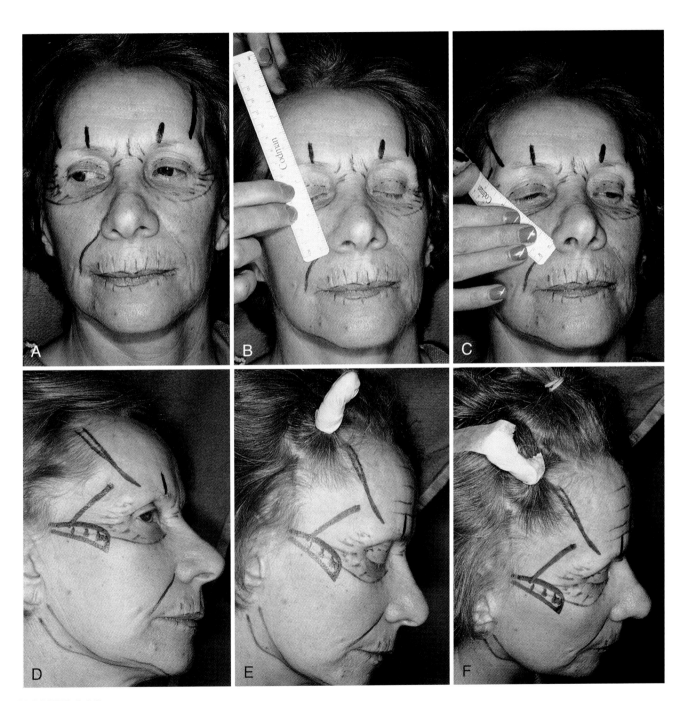

FIGURE 24.5

Marking the patient. Important landmarks. A, Supraorbital nerve, and temporal crest. B, Temporal crest, zygomatic arch, path of temporal branch of facial nerve. C, Extension of line from nasal alar through mid pupil to create paramedian scalp incision. D, Extension line from nasal alar through lateral orbital rim to create T-shaped temporal incision. E and F, Hair parted to create scalp incisions.

eyelid skin resection. The pupil to brow distance is measured and the amount of brow elevation is determined. The following marks should be made:

A. Eyelid crease. This is marked for the transblepharoplasty corrugator resection and lateral orbital rim release.

B. Supraorbital notch. This is marked to identify the position of the supraorbital neurovascular bundle which must be preserved.

C. Paramedial scalp incision. This mark denotes a 1 cm incision behind the hairline at an oblique angle. The position of this incision is in line with the alae of the nose and mid pupil.

D. Temporal incision. A T-shaped incision is marked posterior to the hairline in the temporal region. This mark is made along the line of the nasal alae and lateral orbital rim.

E. Temporal crest. The attachment of the temporal fascia to forehead periosteum is at the temporal crest. This marks the transition from the plane between superficial and deep temporalis fascia to the subperiosteal plane of the central forehead.

F. Malar arch. The malar arch marks the inferior limit of the dissection for the endoscopic forehead lift.

G. Frontal branch of the facial nerve. This nerve must be preserved as it passes between the lateral orbital rim and the temporal hairline in the superficial temporal fascia. It is helpful to mark its pathway.

2. Preparing the Scalp Incisions

In order to accomplish the endoscopic forehead lift, 4 or 5 scalp incisions are made. To avoid hair protruding into the incisions it is best to tie the hair into small ponytails and wrap each one in a rubber finger glove. This clears the incision sites and avoids the need to shave the hair.

3. Anesthesia

In most cases, intravenous sedation is used combined with local anaesthetic. A combination of intra- venous propofol, midazolam, and fentanyl are used. Alternatively, general anaesthesia may be employed. The local anaesthetic is prepared fresh on the day of the procedure (0.2% lidocaine, 1 : 200000 epinephrine and 0.5% Marcaine are combined).

The following sites are injected:

A. Supraorbital nerve block. A long needle is used to ensure that the local anaesthetic is injected subperiosteally along the superior margin of the eyebrows.

B. Eyelid. The crease of the eyelid is injected using a short 30-gauge needle superficially to avoid muscle hematoma.

C. Scalp incisions. Local anaesthesia is injected deeply to reach the subperiosteal plane in the central forehead and the deep temporalis fascia in the temple region.

D. Malar arch. Local anaesthetic is injected along the arch, and extended to the post auricular region.

E. Other nerve blocks may be used if laser resurfacing of other facial regions is performed at the same time.

4. Equipment

A CO_2 laser is used for the eyelid incision, the transblepharoplasty corrugator resection, and release of the periosteum at the orbital rim. A rigid 4 mm endoscope is used for the scalp dissection and periosteal elevators are used to lift the periosteum. Both regular and special endoscopic elevators are used. I use Ramirez elevators (Snowden Pencer, Tucker, GA). Snowden Pencer sand blasted metal eye shields are also used as are Baker-David clamps (Byron Medical, Phoenix, AZ).

5. Procedure (Figures 24.6–24.10)

In most cases, a combined transblepharoplasty and endoscopic forehead lift procedure is used. First, eyelid incisions are performed using a continuous wave CO_2 laser at 3 to 5 W, and the incision is carried down

FIGURE 24.6

Transblepharoplasty incision and dissection into the forehead. Note sand blasted Baker-David clamp in situ. Note supraorbital nerve (A) visualized posterior to corrugator muscle (B) (medial pocket). Dissection into subperiosteal plane.

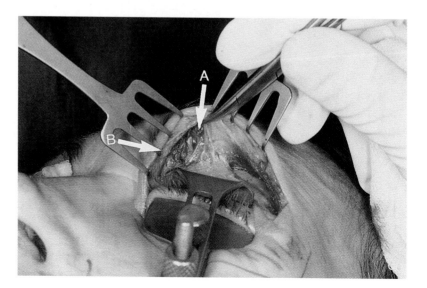

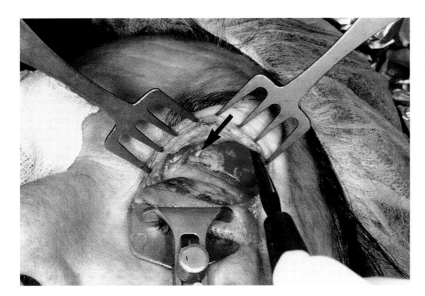

FIGURE 24.7
Periosteal elevator dissection from eyelid to scalp in the subperiosteal plane. Note the presence of the supraorbital nerve, readily visualized (*arrow*).

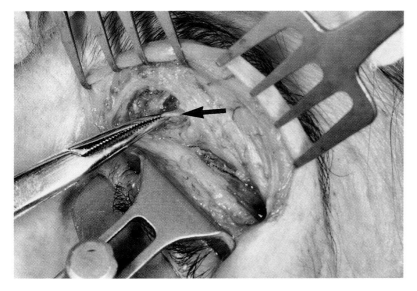

FIGURE 24.8
Fibers of the supratrocheal nerve seen coursing through the corrugator muscle (*arrow*).

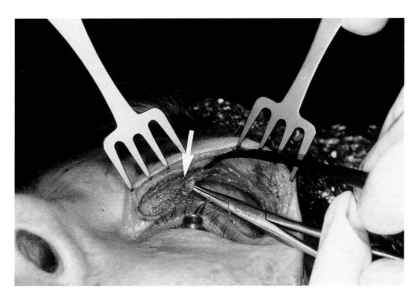

FIGURE 24.9
The supraorbital nerve is seen when the periosteum has been released (*arrow*).

FIGURE 24.10
After release of periosteum degree of eyebrow elevation shown on right.

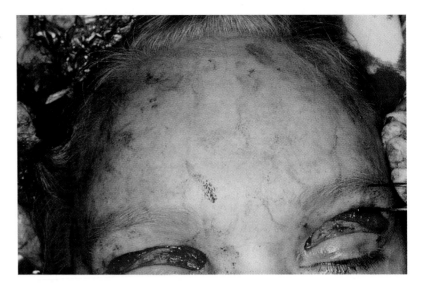

to the orbital septum. The septum is then incised across its whole length using a sand blasted teaser. The fat pads are identified, released and excised. An incision is made in the infrabrow subcutaneous tissue aiming for the superior orbital rim. This bloodless dissection is possible due to the coagulation properties of the CO_2 laser. The focusing hand piece and 5 to 7 W continuous wave is used. The first important structure identified is the depressor supercilii portion of the orbicularis oculi muscle, which is medial and superficial to the supraorbital nerve. This muscle is coagulated and/or excised using the CO_2 laser.

Deep to the orbicularis muscle is the corrugator muscle. The corrugator muscle is much redder, more vascular, and more friable compared to the orbicularis muscle, which is paler and more fibrous. Running through the corrugator muscle are branches of the supratrochlear nerve. Usually 3 or 4 branches are readily visualized. The corrugator muscle can be coagulated, excised or incised. I favor coagulation of the muscle to prevent recurrence of frowning. The whole muscle is treated, preserving some supratrochlear nerve branches. Behind and lateral to the corrugator muscle are the supraorbital nerve and vessels which can be visualized once the periosteum is incised.

The periosteum is then incised and lifted. A periosteal elevator is used to lift up the periosteum from the orbital rim to the hairline, avoiding injury to the supraorbital nerve. The complete central forehead should be lifted up to the temporal crest. It is advisable to leave the dissection at the temporal crest and not go beyond, as it is possible to reach the wrong plane in the temporal region and risk injury to the frontal branch of the facial nerve. It is best to dissect the temporal pocket from the temporal scalp incision to ensure that the correct plane is maintained.

6. Scalp Incisions

A T-shaped incision is made using a scalpel in the temporal hair posterior to the hair line with the top of the T parallel to the hair line. I prefer to not use the laser for this incision, as some loss of hair follicles may lead to localized permanent hair loss.

The dissection is made into the plane between the superficial and deep temporalis fascia. At this stage it is best to introduce the endoscope to ensure the correct plane is maintained. The loose areolar tissue will appear as "angel hair." Superficial to the plane between the superficial and deep temporalis fascia, the frontal branch of the facial nerve runs within the superficial temporal fascia. A periosteal elevator (e.g., Ramirez No. 4) is used to dissect this plane towards the lateral orbital rim and the malar arch. The pocket is also dissected posteriorly towards the vertex and inferiorly to the post auricular zone.

The dissection is then carried superiorly to the temporal crest. The attachment of the fascias is broken so that the temporal pocket will connect with the central forehead subperiosteal plane. There are usually veins present along the orbital rim (sentinel veins). These may be left intact, or carefully coagulated under endoscopic vision.

The paramedian scalp incision is then made with a scalpel and the incision carried down to bone incising the periosteum. A periosteal elevator is introduced and dissection proceeds in the subperiosteal plane inferiorly to connect with the pocket created by the subperiosteal dissection from the blepharoplasty approach. Posteriorly the scalp is dissected subperiosteally to the vertex.

The procerus muscle, which is a brow depressor and situated at the root of the nose, may be incised or coagulated which releases the most medial aspect of the brow and decreases the tendency for horizontal creases at the base of the nose.

7. Fixation of the Forehead

Once the periosteum has been released and the brow depressors coagulated, incised or excised, the brow is lifted to the desired position. Fixation screws are used to hold this position. A drill is introduced via the paramedian incision and a shallow hole is made into the bone. A drill with a stopper should be used to ensure that the hole is not made too deeply.

Titanium screws are used and skin staples are placed behind the titanium screw to lift the brows into the desired position. The screws are placed in line with the arch of the eyebrow as this should be the highest point of the eyebrow. If one wishes to obtain further medial eyebrow elevation, a second titanium screw may be placed through a more medial incision. In the author's experience, placement of a second screw is rarely needed and could lead to exaggeration of the brow lift.

The temporal incision is then sutured, initially using 4-0 PDS suture, beginning inferiorly in the subcutaneous tissue and suturing this to the temporalis fascia superiorly, thus lifting the temporal region of the upper face. The skin is then closed with skin staples. A small minivac drain is placed through a separate incision in the scalp and forwarded within the subperiosteal plane.

LASER RESURFACING

As the forehead has thick skin with an excellent blood supply, it is possible to perform simultaneously both the endoscopic forehead lift and laser resurfacing. Once the forehead is fixed into position, laser resurfacing is performed to remove wrinkles of the forehead (static lines) and produce skin shrinkage (18, 19). In contrast to the eyelid incision, a pulsed laser system preferably with a computerized pattern generator is used. Using the Coherent 5000 laser (Coherent Laser Corp, Palo Alto, CA) at a setting of 300 mJ, 100 W, pattern 3, 9, 6 or 3, 9, 7, one complete pass is made, gently wiped and a second pass at 3, 9, 6 is made.

If deeper wrinkles exist, a smaller pattern and 1 further pass can be made on the forehead. It is important to use two laser passes as 1 pass may "print" the square pattern on the skin. With the second pass, the square pattern should be oriented at a different angle to the first pass.

Using the Sharplan 40c laser system (Sharplan Laser, Inc., Allendale, NJ), deeper wrinkles are treated using the SilkTouch mode using a 260 mm handpiece, a 12.0 mm square pattern and 28 to 30 W. After one pass, the ablated tissue is gently wiped and a second pass using 24 to 28 W is made, changing the pattern or orientation. No more than two passes are made.

For patients with superficial wrinkles, the FeatherTouch mode is used with a 200H handpiece and an 11 mm square pattern. The time that the laser is in contact with the skin when the FeatherTouch mode is used is one-third that of the SilkTouch mode, with the depth of resurfacing being correspondingly less. The first pass is made using 34 to 40 W, and the second pass using 30 to 36 W. After CO₂ laser resurfacing, further eyebrow elevation occurs due to tissue shrinkage.

CLOSURE OF EYELID INCISION

The eyelid incision is closed as the final step of the operation. Once the eyebrows have been elevated to the desired position, it is then possible to estimate the amount of upper eyelid skin resection that is needed. This is performed using a focused handpiece of the CO₂ laser in continuous wave mode. Following this step, the upper eyelid incision is closed using 6-0 mild chromic or 6-0 nylon interrupted sutures.

ADDITIONAL PROCEDURES

Additional procedures can also be done with the CO₂ laser and include:

1. CO₂ Laser Resurfacing Other Regions.

Performing full-face CO₂ laser resurfacing at the same time as the forehead lift avoids demarcation zones, or mismatch between sun damaged skin and the resurfaced skin.

2. Neck Liposuction and Submentoplasty.

In the author's practice, neck liposuction and submentoplasty is commonly performed with endoscopic forehead lift and full face laser resurfacing. This combination is ideal for the younger patient, who does not have significant loose neck skin. An excellent facial rejuvenation is possible with this particular combination.

POSTOPERATIVE CARE (FIGURE 24.11)

Most patients are able to go home several hours after the procedure.

1. A minivac drain is placed in the subperiosteal space of the forehead and left in for 24 hours. A light (noncompression) dressing is also used for 24 hours.

2. A semi-permeable dressing, such as Silon (BioMedical Sciences, PA) or Opsite (Smith-Nephew Inc, Key Largo, FL), is used on resurfaced areas and changed after 24 hours. A fresh dressing is then left in place for 7 days if possible.

3. The patient is instructed to use ice packs on his or her eyes and forehead for 24 to 48 hours. We suggest 20 minutes on, 5 minutes off.

4. The patient is instructed to sleep on 4 pillows at night to prop the head up and minimize eyelid swelling.
5. Broad spectrum oral antibiotics, such as 1 g cephalosporin daily, are prescribed for 10 days postoperatively.
6. Oral steroids are useful to minimize edema. A medrol dose pack may be used.
7. Oral valacyclovir or famcyclovir 500 mg daily should be administered to patients who have undergone laser resurfacing of any region.
8. Skin staples, sutures and the titanium screws are removed at 7 days postoperatively.
9. When the skin has fully re-epithelialized, usually between 10 and 14 days, an ultraviolet A blocking sunscreen (Skin Tech, Byron Medical, Tucson, AZ) should be introduced, as well as oil free, non irritating mois-turizers and cleansers (Skin Tech). A depigmenting gel, such as Pigment Gel Forte (Physicians Choice, Tucson, AZ), should be introduced to prevent pigmentation for skin types I to IV, starting alternate nights. Patients with skin types 5 require hydroquinone 2.5% to 5.0% with retinoic acid (0.05% to 0.1%) beginning alternate nights. Bleaching creams are continued for 6 to 8 weeks and then tapered off slowly. To overcome the erythema, Skin Tech anti-red tinted sunscreen should be used in all patients.

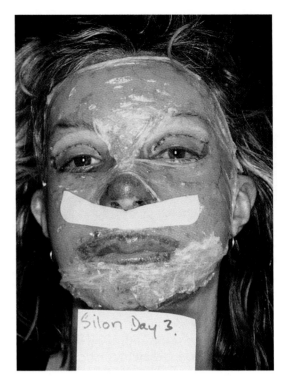

FIGURE 24.11
Appearance 3 days postoperatively with semi-occlusive silicon dressing applied.

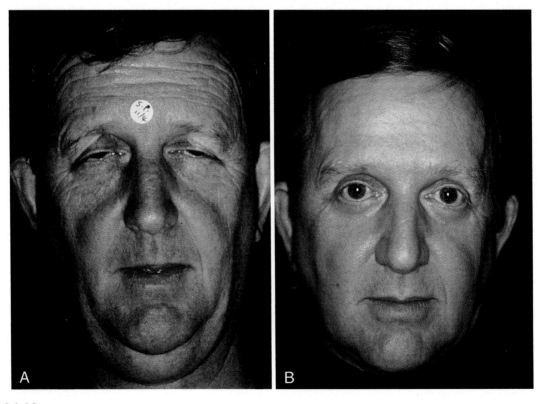

FIGURE 24.12
52-year-old man who underwent transblepharoplasty corrugator resection, endoscopic forehead lift, neck liposuction and full face CO_2 laser resurfacing. A, Preoperative appearance. B, Appearance 6 months postoperatively. (Reprinted with permission from Coleman WP III, et al. Cosmetic Surgery of the Skin. St. Louis: Mosby, 1997.)

RESULTS (FIGURES 24.12–24.15)

Naturally, with all new techniques there is a steep learning curve. Endoscopic forehead lifting and transblepharoplasty corrugator resection combined with CO_2 laser resurfacing was recently performed in a series of 127 patients. In most cases, the results were good to excellent. Poor results occurred early in the series with recurrence of brow ptosis due to inadequate release of the periosteum at the orbital rim. In most cases, decrease in frowning postoperatively was significant with some recurrence over a period of 12 months. Despite this, the ability to frown was still markedly reduced ($\geq$50% at 12 months).

The balance between brow lifting and upper eyelid skin resection was satisfactory in all patients. By

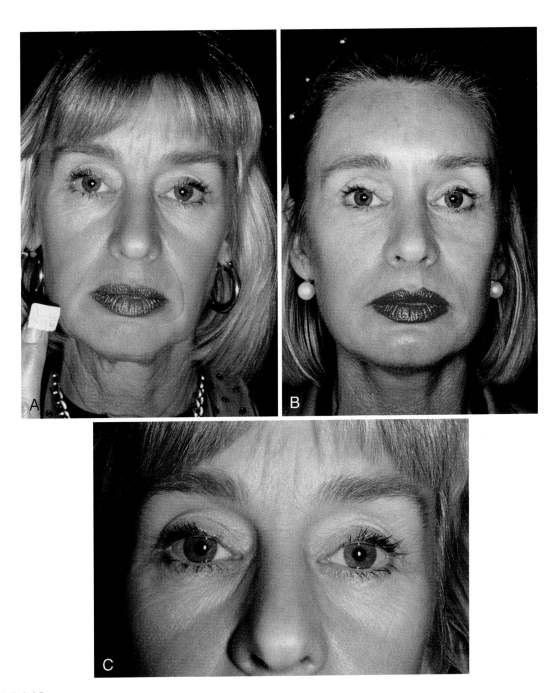

FIGURE 24.13

55-year-old woman who underwent transblepharoplasty corrugator resection, endoscopic forehead lift, lower face and neck lift (superficial muscular aponeurotic system) and CO_2 laser resurfacing of forehead, periocular region and perioral region. A, Appearance of the full face preoperatively. B, Appearance 6 months postoperatively. C, Close up of glabella region preoperatively. (Reprinted with permission from Coleman WP III, et al. Cosmetic Surgery of the Skin. St. Louis: Mosby, 1997.)   *(continued)*

FIGURE 24.13 *(continued)*
D, Close up of glabella 6 months postoperatively.
E, Close up glabella region preoperatively. F, Close up
of patient attempting to frown. (Reprinted with permission from Coleman WP III, et al. Cosmetic Surgery
of the Skin. St. Louis: Mosby, 1997.)

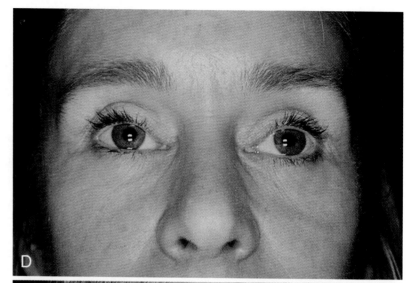

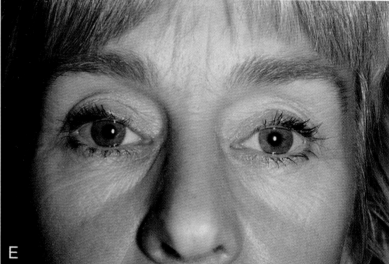

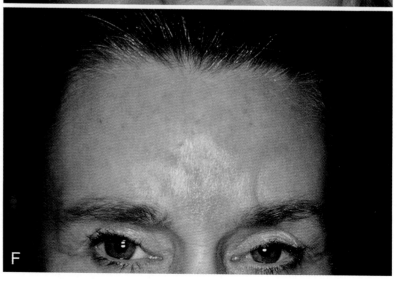

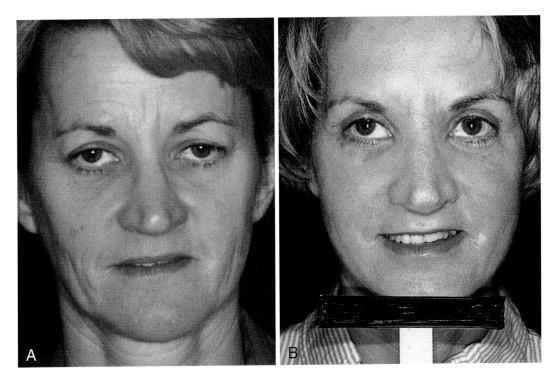

FIGURE 24.14
48-year-old woman with deep glabella creases, heavy eyelids and high forehead who underwent CO₂ laser blepharoplasty, transblepharo-plasty corrugator resection, lateral brow release and full face CO₂ laser resurfacing. A, Preoperative appearance. B, Appearance 11 days postoperatively.

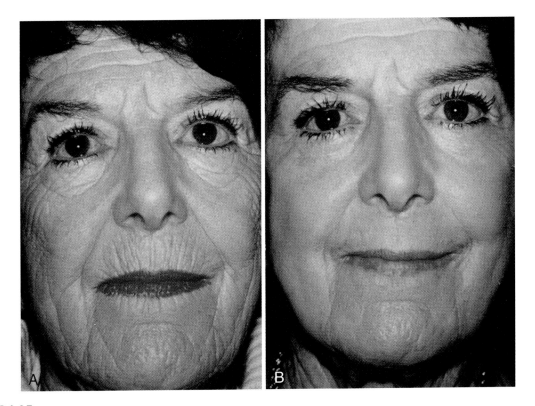

FIGURE 24.15
72-year-old woman who underwent aggressive full face resurfacing without forehead lift or corrugator resection. Note improvement in wrinkles of mouth and cheek, but poor response in forehead and glabella area. A, Preoperative view. B, 6 months postoperative view. (Reprinted with permission from Coleman WP III, et al. Cosmetic Surgery of the Skin. St. Louis: Mosby, 1997.)

combining endoscopic forehead lifting with laser resurfacing, wrinkle lines of the forehead were improved in all patients, including deep glabella lines. Laser resurfacing also produced tightening of forehead skin.

COMPLICATIONS (TABLE 24.9)

Complications of combined endoscopic forehead lifting with laser resurfacing that can occur include:

1. Injury to the supraorbital nerve.
   Because this nerve supplies sensation to most of the forehead, injury to the nerve will lead to significant numbness of the forehead and scalp (to vertex). Partial injury may produce hyperesthesia and itching. This nerve is readily visualized either by direct vision (transblepharoplasty approach) or via the endoscope (scalp incisions). Its accompanying vessels are large. With experience, it should be uncommon to injure this nerve.

TABLE 24.9

COMPLICATIONS OF COMBINED ENDOSCOPIC FOREHEAD LIFT AND CO_2 LASER RESURFACING

1. Injury to the supraorbital nerve
2. Injury to the supratrochlear nerve
3. Injury to the frontal branch facial nerve
4. Inadequate brow lift
5. Recurrence of brow ptosis
6. Recurrence of frowning
7. Asymmetry
8. Infection
9. Bleeding
10. Skin necrosis

2. Injury to the supratrochlear nerve.
   The supratrochlear nerve provides sensation to a small area on the medial aspect of the forehead. The nerve is divided into several branches (coursing within the corrugator muscle), and injury to one or two branches is unlikely to produce significant numbness. However, painful paraesthesia may occur following injury to any of the nerve branches.
3. Injury to the temporal branch of the facial nerve (Figure 24.16).
   This is the most dreaded and serious complication of the endoscopic forehead lift. This branch is located superficially in the superficial temporalis fascia in the temple region. It is therefore imperative to remain below this structure at all times (in the plane between the deep and superficial temporalis fascia) when operating. Using the endoscope to dissect the temporal pocket will ensure that the correct plane is maintained. Also, transition across the temporal crest should be from the temporal to the medial pocket to avoid injuring the nerve.
4. Inadequate brow lift.
   It is impossible to maintain brow elevation unless a complete periosteal release is performed at the orbital rim.
5. Recurrence of brow ptosis.
   Inadequate periosteal release at the orbital rim may lead to recurrence of brow ptosis. Similarly, inadequate fixation or insufficient undermining will not allow maintenance of brow elevation.
6. Recurrence of frowning.
   Since frowning is caused by depressor supercilii portion of the orbicularis oculi and the corrugator muscles, inadequate destruction of these muscles will lead to minimal change in frowning or rapid recurrence. It is easier to obtain a more thorough destruction of frown muscles via the blepharoplasty

FIGURE 24.16.

Danger area illustrated. The frontal (temporal) branch of the facial nerve is superficial as it courses through the temporal pocket. It is in danger of being injured. The green line (end ruler) points to the course of this nerve.

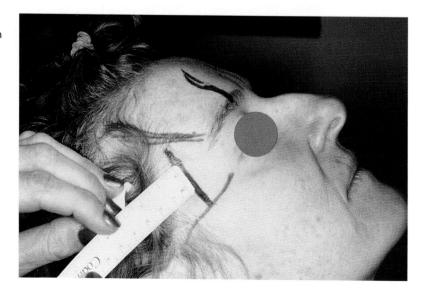

route under direct vision. If muscle ablation is performed via scalp incisions, the use of a fiberoptic CO_2 laser will provide more complete muscle destruction.

7. Asymmetry.
Asymmetry of eyebrows can be avoided by carefully measuring the amount of desired eyebrow elevation on each side. It is often possible to improve pre-existing asymmetry.

8. Infection.
Due to the excellent blood supply in this region, infection is very rare. However, all patients should be given prophylactic antibiotics.

9. Bleeding.
As the region is highly vascular, bleeding may occur leading to hematoma. Careful attention to hemostasis should avoid this problem.

10. Skin necrosis.
As this procedure combines extensive tissue undermining with skin resurfacing, a more careful approach to skin resurfacing is indicated to avoid skin necrosis. However, due to the combination of excellent blood supply to the forehead, maintenance of a subperiosteal plane, and thick skin in this region, skin necrosis is rare. In the author's series, no patient developed skin necrosis.

CONCLUSION

The endoscopic minimal incision brow lift combined with laser resurfacing and blepharoplasty addresses all the components of upper facial aging. The combined approach provides the best opportunity to rejuvenate the upper face. However, experience and technical skill are necessary to produce good results with few complications.

REFERENCES

1. McKinney P, Mossie RD, Zukowski ML. Criteria forehead lift. Aesth Plast Surg 1991;15:141.
2. Connell BF, Lambros VS, Neurohr GH. The forehead lift: techniques to avoid complications and produce optimum results. Aesth Plast Surg 1989;13:217.
3. Raminez OM. Endoscopic techniques in facial rejuvenation. An overview. Part 1. Aesth Plast Surg 1994;18:141-147.
4. Liang M, Narayannan N. Endoscopic ablation of the frontalis and corrugator muscles: a clinical study. Plast Surg Forum 1992;15:54.
5. Matarasso A. Endoscopically assisted forehead-brow rhytidoplasty. Aesth Plastic Surg 1995;19:141-147.
6. Isse NG. Endoscopic facial rejuvenation: endoforehead, the functional lift: case reports, Aesth Plast Surg 1994;18:21.
7. Matarasso A, Matarasso S. Endoscopic surgical correction of glabella creases. J Derm Surg 1995;21:695-700.
8. Hamas R. Endoscopic resection of corrugator muscles for glabella creases. 26th Annual meeting of American Society of Aesthetic Plastic Surgery, Boston, MA. April 21, 1993.
9. Weinstein C. Endoscopic forehead lift. In: Coleman WP III, et al., ed. Cosmetic surgery of the skin. 2nd ed. St Louis: Mosby, 1997:421-427.
10. Raminez OM. Endoscopic facial rejuvenation. Perspect Plast Surg 1995;9:22.
11. Raminez OM. Endoscopic forehead and facelift: step by step, operative technique. Plast Surg 1995;2:129.
12. Raminez OM. Endoscopic subperiosteal browlift and facelift. Clin Plast Surg 1995;22:639.
13. Abramo AC. Anatomy of the forehead muscles: the basis for the videoendoscopic approach in forehead rhytidoplasty. Plast Reconstr Surg 1995;95:1170.
14. Raminez OM, Daniel RK. Endoscopic plastic surgery. New York: Springer-Verlag, 1995.
15. Krize DM. Transpalpebral approach to the corrugator supercilii and procerus muscles. Plast Reconstr Surg 1995;95: 52-60.
16. Ellbogen R. Transcoronal eyebrow lift with concomitant upper blepharoplasty. Plast Reconstr Surg 1983;71:490.
17. Friedland MD, Jacobsen WM, Terkonda S. Safety and efficiency of combined upper blepharoplasties and open coronal browlift: a consecutive series of 600 patients. Aesth Plastic Surg 1996;20:453-462.
18. Gardner ES, Reinisch L, Sticklin GP: In vitro changes in non-facial human skin following CO_2 laser resurfacing: a comparison study. Laser Surg Med 1996;19:379-387.
19. Weinstein C. Carbon dioxide laser resurfacing. In: Coleman WP III, et al., ed. Cosmetic surgery of the skin, 2nd ed. St Louis: Mosby, 1997:152-177.

CHAPTER 25

Resurfacing Complications and Their Management

■ Mitchel P. Goldman
Richard E. Fitzpatrick
Stacy R. Smith

With impressive cosmetic results, pulsed carbon dioxide (CO_2) laser resurfacing of photoaged facial skin has become increasingly popular with physicians and patients. Improved technique and proper instrumentation have made significant complications rare and manageable. Most noninfectious complications, including hypopigmentation, persistent erythema, and scarring are related more to improper technique or instrumentation than to inherent risks of the procedure. On the other hand, infection complicating the procedure during the healing phase may be preventable. This chapter will detail the authors' current protocol for postoperative care of the laser resurfacing patient. It is based on our 5-year experience with more than 2,000 patients treated with the Coherent UltraPulse CO_2 laser (Coherent Laser Corp., Palo Alto, CA). We recognize that, even with this experience, postoperative treatment of the laser resurfacing patient is under evolution as new dressings are developed and techniques are modified to speed epithelialization, maximize rejuvenation, and minimize adverse sequelae.

INFECTION

Infection, along with scarring, ranks among the most feared complications in facial laser resurfacing. Our experience with infection was recently reviewed (1). Much of what follows is summarized from this work.

Infection, unfortunately, is a somewhat common problem in laser resurfacing. In a retrospective review of 395 laser resurfacing procedures performed over a 16-month period, seventeen cases of postoperative infection were documented, an incidence of 4.3%. This compares favorably with the 4.7% (5/106) infection rate found in a multicenter study (2). The frequency and type of organism are listed in Table 25.1. Pseudomonas *sp*. was the most commonly identified pathogen (7/17) followed by S. aureus (6/17). Infections by multiple organisms are the rule rather than the exception, usually gram positive with gram negative, but various combinations are seen including bacteria with Candida *sp*. A single case of Herpes simplex virus (HSV) reactivation was found which occurred despite the use of perioperative acyclovir. The types of microorganisms identified in this study are very similar to those reported for burn injury (3-5). This finding is not a surprise because the resulting wound in laser resurfacing is equivalent to a second-degree burn. However, owing to a laser pulsewidth shorter than that of the thermal relaxation time of the skin, the residual thermal damage zone is relatively small compared with that of a conventional second-degree burn.

Signs and symptoms of infection may begin as early as 48 hours after the procedure or as late as the tenth postoperative day. Eighty percent of infections become symptomatic within 7 days. When infection does occur, pain is by far the most common complaint, being reported by about 50% of patients. A sensation of burning and itching is the second most frequent symptom, reported by approximately one-third of patients. Physical examination

TABLE 25.1

ISOLATES FROM FACIAL RESURFACING INFECTIONS

Rank	Organism	Number of Isolates	Percent
1	Pseudomonas	7	41.2
2	S. aureus	6	35.3
3	S. epidermidis	6	35.3
4	Candida	4	23.5
5	Enterobacter	2	11.8
6	E. coli	1	5.9
7	Proteus	1	5.9
8	Corynebacterium	1	5.9
9	Serratia	1	5.9
10	HSV	1	5.9
	Total Cases	17	100

shows excessive erythema in almost two-thirds of the patients followed by evidence of yellow crust or exudate, pus, erosion, and papules or plaques. Satellite lesions may be seen, indicating candidal infection (Fig. 25.1). Patients may have localized patches of edema, epithelial erosion and mucoid exudate (Fig. 25.2). In rare cases, infection can also be seen with only a complaint of burning and itching and no unusual physical findings. Complaints of pain by the patient should always be taken seriously and infection considered as a cause.

An infection should be suspected and actively looked for in the following situations:

1. When a patient complains of persistent or increasing pain (especially when the new onset of pain is different from the mild sunburn-like stinging experienced by most patients)

FIGURE 25.1

Candidiasis may present as a typical, beefy red patch with satellite lesions as shown here or sometimes as only a subtle, patchy erythema.

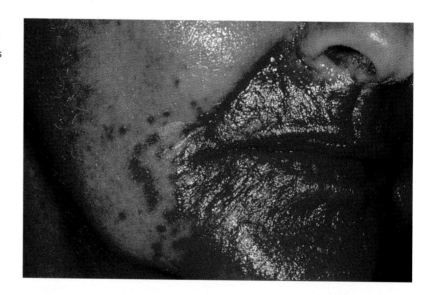

FIGURE 25.2

Patchy erosions with superficial crusts and exudate are commonly seen as signs of infection.

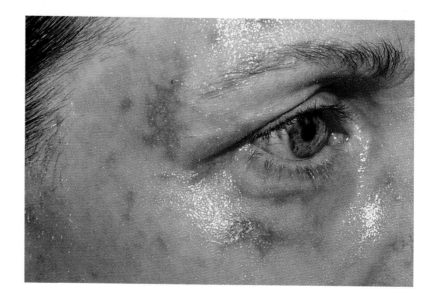

2. If burning or itching is reported beyond the first three days
3. If abnormal erythema, yellow exudate/crust, papules, pustules, or erosion is found
4. If a "reversal of healing" is seen, i.e., the patient reports previously re-epithelialized areas have become eroded. The patient's symptoms are important since physical findings may be as subtle as only patchy erythema or may be obvious and diagnostic in some cases (Fig. 25.3).

If symptoms or signs of infection are experienced, the following diagnostic measures should be undertaken:

1. Review history of previous yeast, bacterial, or herpetic infections, especially any requiring hospitalization
2. Direct smear from the suspected areas for gram stain, Tzanck smear (or immunofluorescence examination for HSV), KOH examination
3. Culture for bacteria, yeast, and herpes virus should be taken from multiple sites

Treatment should begin directly after the cultures are taken without waiting for the laboratory results. Of primary importance is the removal of all occlusive topical treatments, especially petrolatum and any occlusive dressing. If the KOH examination reveals pseudohyphae and/or spores, oral anticandidal treatment should be instituted. We prefer administering a single 400 mg dose of fluconazole. Since half of all candidal infections are mixed with bacterial agents and the majority of bacterial infections are with multiple agents, institution (or change) of a broad spectrum antibacterial agent at the same time is advised. Once the culture result is obtained, treatment should be adjusted accordingly and continued until complete healing of the wound. Patients with diffuse dermal scarring secondary to previous chemical peels or dermabrasion should be treated at least until 2 weeks after all signs and symptoms of infection subside to ensure complete eradication of the infective agents from scar tissue. If there is no improvement or worsening despite good compliance after 3 to 4 days of treatment, all investigations should be repeated and antimicrobials adjusted as appropriate.

The pattern of antimicrobial sensitivities seen suggests that most infections are community-acquired. We have encountered one isolate of Pseudomonas that exhibited the multiple-drug resistance characteristics of a hospital-acquired infection. This patient had symptoms starting on the second postoperative day, the earliest of any in our experience. A single case of methicillin-resistant *Staphylococcus aureus* has also been found.

Early treatment of bacterial infections with appropriate antimicrobials almost always results in an uneventful infection. Herpetic infection or reactivation can be more problematic. Once reactivation occurs, the potential for significant, difficult to treat scarring is great (Fig. 25.4). Prevention with perioperative antiviral medication should be the rule. In patients with a history of frequent (more than once per year) perioral lesion outbreaks, antiviral medications should be started 3 days before the resurfacing procedure. Known factors leading to reactivation of herpetic infections such as local trauma or excessive ultraviolet irradiation are felt to mediate reactivation via prostaglandin synthesis (6). Laser resurfacing leads to significant tissue injury and variations in the local prostaglandin milieu. Thus, resurfacing itself may be a potent factor in herpetic reactivation.

Potential herpetic infection should be rapidly addressed and treated. Initiation or altering of current antiviral regimens should not wait for culture or immunofluorescence results. Valacyclovir or famcyclovir should be used, especially if the patient is already taking acyclovir. Both have better absorption than acyclovir. The

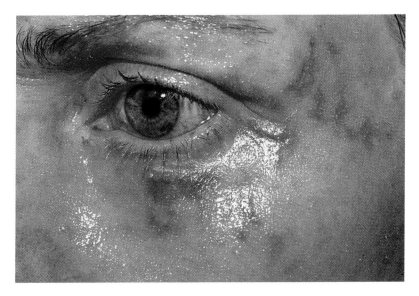

FIGURE 25.3
Excessive patchy erythema is the most common physical sign of infection and is accompanied by pain and/or itching.

FIGURE 25.4
Disseminated herpes simplex may result in atrophic scarring. Pretreatment of all patients with valacyclovir or famcyclovir is warranted to prevent this complication.

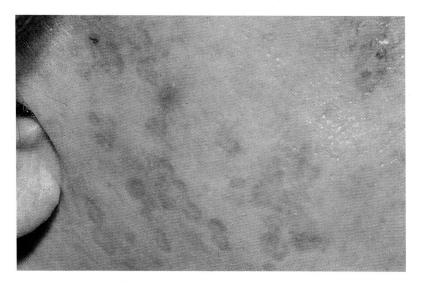

TABLE 25.2

GUIDELINES FOR PREOPERATIVE CARE FOR THE LASER RESURFACING PATIENT

1. Hair, face and hand washing with chlorhexidine (e.g., Hibiclens) for 3 days before the operation.
2. Intranasal mupirocin twice daily, beginning 3 days before and continuing for 7 days after operation.
3. 1% to 2% acetic acid solution, or gentamicin otic, instilled into both external ear canals twice daily, starting 3 days before and continuing for 7 days after operation.
4. Oral fluconazole 400 mg on the day of the procedure for women with history of candidal vaginal infection.
5. Prophylaxis for herpes simplex in all cases starting 1 day preoperatively and continuing for 7 days, using either valacyclovir 250 mg orally 3 times daily for famiciclovir 250 mg orally 2 times daily. Patients with a history of frequent cold sores should begin an antiviral medication 3 days before the procedure and continue for a total of 10 days.
6. Immediate pre-operative cleansing of the face with Septisol followed by thorough rinsing with normal saline.
7. Broad-spectrum, systemic antibiotics such as ciprofloxacin 500 mg twice daily for 7 days starting the morning of surgery.

TABLE 25.3

POSTOPERATIVE GUIDELINES FOR THE LASER RESURFACING PATIENT

1. Frequent (at least every 4 to 6 hours) soaking of the treated area with dilute vinegar solution and previously cleaned and dried towels or disposable gauze. Do not reuse damp towels or wash cloths as they become a source of bacterial contamination.
2. Frequent hand washing with Hibiclens for 7 days postoperatively.
3. Continue oral antibacterial and antiviral agents as prescribed preoperatively.

intracellular half-life of penciclovir, the active metabolite of famciclovir, is twenty times greater than acyclovir (7). Although genuine acyclovir resistance is rare, and resistance to it usually confers resistance to the other acyclic nucleoside analogues, famciclovir should be tried as rare acyclovir-resistant strains will be sensitive to famciclovir. If true resistance is suspected, foscarnet may be required and the experience of an infectious disease consultant should be sought. Ibuprofen or indomethacin may or may not be helpful to limit the extent of herpetic lesions.

Theoretically, patients may acquire wound infections from either areas surrounding or remote to the wound.

Surrounding areas include the scalp, eyes, ears, nose, mouth, and neck. Remote areas that may harbor infective agents range from remote sites on the body (e.g., hands, feet, perineum) to the patient's immediate environment (e.g., spouse, children, friends, pets, soil, water, plants, etc.). However, almost all infective agents from remote areas are transmitted to the wound surface by the patient's hands. Avoidance of gardening activity and physical contact with soil or fresh flowers for two weeks before and after the procedure may help reduce the risk of Pseudomonas colonization as plants are common sources of Pseudomonas. Hand-washing with an antimicrobial soap multiple times daily, starting 3 days preoperatively and continuing until the surface is re-epithelialized (about 7 days) is also recommended. Our most recent pre- and postoperative guidelines are listed in Tables 25.2 and 25.3.

Pre- and postoperative regimens vary among practitioners and contribute greatly to the risk of infection, but other factors may also contribute to the overall risk of infection. These include the total area treated, the use of occlusive dressings and host factors.

The infection rate increases as the size of the treated area increases (3). In our experience, the rate of infection for full face resurfacing has been 8.1% (15/185) while that for partial resurfacing is less than 1% (2/210). The fact that all infections are found between postoperative days 2 and 10 and that the rate of infection increases with the size of the treated areas, confirms the vital barrier function of the intact skin surface. It is remarkable that no infection has been noted when only a single cosmetic unit was resurfaced, even in the perioral area where the chance of contamination by oral flora is high. It is possible that there is a threshold size of treatment area that significantly affects the local and/or systemic immune response of the host. The benefit of obtaining a more uniform cosmetic appearance over the whole face versus the risk of an infection might therefore be considered by both physician and patient until a better way to prevent infections can be devised.

The use of an occlusive dressing immediately following the procedure provides most patients with significant comfort and enhanced healing. However, the occluded, moist environment also provides a medium for growth of both pathogenic and nonpathogenic organisms. To reduce the risk of infection in this setting, several strategies may be considered. First, the duration of occlusion may be reduced to the minimum. Although it has been shown that the crucial period for applying an occlusive dressing in general is the first few days, the optimal duration for occluding the wound resulting from laser resurfacing may not be the same (8). This optimal time for using an occlusive dressing in these patients should be determined in a systematic manner in the future. Second, the occlusive dressing needs to be removed after a few days and then a new dressing reapplied daily after thorough cleansing of the wound surface to reduce bacterial colonization. Third, the ideal type of occlusive dressing is yet to be determined and alternative dressings should be considered (9-11). Furthermore, incorporation of antimicrobials into the occlusive dressing may help reduce the risk of infection (12, 13). However, once an infection is suspected, all occlusive dressings and topical ointments (e.g., Vaseline, Chesebrough-Ponds, Inc., Greenwich, CT) should be removed and withheld.

A defect in the local and systemic immune response also predisposes the patient to infection that can be refractory to treatment. One of our patients who had multiple facial scars from previous chemical peels, developed *P. cellulitis* that was resistant to multiple antibiotics including ciprofloxacin. Investigation after hospitalization for treatment revealed an anergic state that might have been responsible for this refractory infection. A retrospective review of the patient's medical history also revealed a previous hospitalization for *P. pneumonia* years earlier. Extreme caution should therefore be exercised before performing laser resurfacing in the presence of diffuse scarring and/or a defect in host immunity.

The postoperative period is often filled with anxiety for the facial resurfacing patient. If infection occurs, it can dishearten both the patient and the physician. All should remain optimistic. The overwhelming majority of causative organisms are bacterial or Candida *sp.*, and if they are recognized and treated early, they have few sequelae. The time to complete epithelialization and full clearing of erythema may be delayed but the overall result and improvement in photoaging remains equal to that seen in uninfected patients. Even after infection, scarring is rare.

POSTOPERATIVE SWELLING

This adverse sequela is not a true complication, but can be disturbing to patients. It is considered a normal consequence of cutaneous injury and represents the release of histamine and various other factors from dermal and perivascular mast cells. The degree of swelling is related both to the patients' predisposition to swell and to the degree of thermal injury. Rarely, patients may swell significantly intraoperatively. If significant swelling occurs, 125 mg Solumedrol (The Upjohn Co., Kalamazoo, MI) is given intravenously and the patient is placed on a short course of prednisone (60 mg/day for 5 days).

Edema is usually maximal between 48 and 72 hours postoperative and rapidly resolves because of weeping through the denuded skin surface. It usually resolves completely in 7 to 10 days. We advise patients to use a bag of frozen peas on the face (especially in the periorbital areas) for the first day or two to decrease the extent of edema. We have found that the prophylactic use of corticosteroids does not markedly decrease edema.

ERYTHEMA

Erythema is a universal sequela of laser resurfacing and not a complication per se. It represents angiogenesis in response to re-epithelialization and occurs to some degree in all patients. In our experience, it appears to relate to the depth of dermal wounding and occurs to a greater extent and for a longer time in patients with deeper resurfacing procedures. The degree of erythema may correlate positively with the overall degree of improvement in wrinkling. Patients who undergo one or two passes with the UPCO$_2$ laser or who are treated with the Erbium:YAG laser (which vaporizes approximately 10 to 20 μm of tissue with each pass versus 80 to 100 μm per pass with the UPCO$_2$) have less erythema, which lasts for a shorter period of time.

We have found that periorbital erythema is more common at 90 day follow-up than is perioral erythema (14). This may be due to the thicker skin in the perioral area since this area is usually treated with 3 to 4 laser passes versus 1 to 2 passes used in the periorbital region. About 31% of patients will have persistent periorbital erythema at 90 days while 12% of patients will have persistent perioral erythema over a similar time period (14). Patients with Fitzpatrick type I or II skin demonstrate greater erythema, which is felt to be secondary to less epidermal melanin and makes the skin more transparent to the underlying vasculature.

The best treatment for erythema may be no treatment at all and advise the patient to wear a green-tinted cover-up makeup. If treatment is strongly requested, topical nonfluorinated corticosteroids can be used sparingly. Topical antioxidants such as Cellex-C (Cellex-C Cosmaceuticals Inc., Toronto, Canada) can also be recommended.

Rarely, persistent erythema may indicate infection, especially if associated with pruritus as 64% of our patients with infection had this physical finding. However, erythema as a sign of infection has never occurred without coexistent swelling, pustule, erosion or exudate.

HYPERPIGMENTATION

Hyperpigmentation is usually related to the Fitzpatrick skin type and occurs in 20% to 30% of patients with type III skin, and in nearly 100% of patients with type IV skin (14). We have found that almost all episodes of hyperpigmentation resolve in 2 to 4 months and usually respond faster to treatment. Pretreatment with hydroxyquinone preparations, tretinoin, Cellex-C, strict sun avoidance and use of sunscreens will minimize its occurrence. Patients of Asian ancestry are particularly prone to hyperpigmentation. In general, Asian patients do well after laser resurfacing, with pigmentation resolving in 4 to 6 months.

Once hyperpigmentation has occurred, treating it is more of an art than a science. In addition to strict sun avoidance and the use of full spectrum sunscreens with titanium dioxide, various melanocytic cytotoxic agents are helpful. Hydroquinone is directly cytotoxic to melanocytes and is the mainstay of treatment. Tretinoin promotes melanosome transfer and keratinocyte elimination. Azeleic acid, kojic acid and glucosamine inhibit tyrosinase and DNA synthesis. Topical vitamins C and E function as free radical scavengers.

ACNE/MILIA

Acne and milia formation can also occur after laser resurfacing. Acne usually occurs in patients with a history of cystic acne or very oily skin. It is usually exacerbated by using petrolatum-based ointments after treatment, which further occludes follicular ostia. Our impression is that a greater degree of both milia and acne occurs with excessive thermal damage. Perhaps thermal injury leads to a shock effect on sebaceous glands causing their disruption and dedifferentiation of adnexal structures that produced an aberrant reformation of the canal. (A. Shalita, personal communication, 1997).

Despite the cause of acne/milia, treatment is usually successful. First one should minimize the use of petrolatum-based ointments and substitute light creams or lotions such as Cetaphil (Galderma Laboratories, Ft. Worth, TX). Tetracycline or minocycline are also helpful because of their anti-polymorphonucleocyte mobility function. Re-instituting tretinoin and the use of topical benzoyl peroxide soaps may also speed resolution. Finally, gentle comedo/milia extraction can be instituted once weekly.

ITCHING

Although a common complaint, itching, by itself, is rarely a difficult problem. It can be a sign of infection but is then usually accompanied by pain or other physical findings. It often occurs about the fourth postoperative day and may represent an irritant or allergic contact dermatitis to the applied topical agents. True contact allergy to petrolatum has been demonstrated in nonlaser resurfacing patients, but all of our patients with pruritus have used petrolatum-based products later without difficulty (15). Once infection has been ruled out, either by physical examination or culture, the petrolatum should be replaced with a water or glycerin-based emollient such as Cetaphil lotion. In addition, twice daily use of a low potency topical corticosteroid such as aclometasone dipropionate cream will hasten the resolution of symptoms.

HYPOPIGMENTATION

Post-laser hypopigmentation has been estimated to occur in 0.8% of patients surveyed in 1997 by C. William Hanke (personal communication). This is in contrast to an 8% incidence with phenol, 4% to 5% incidence with dermabrasion, and 1% with 35% trichloroacetic acid (TCA)/Jessner's chemical peeling. However, this survey did not include length of follow up. Hypopigmentation is often not apparent for 6 to 12 months. It may be related to the depth of resurfacing since it is usually seen when laser impacts are excessively overlapped by 40% or more or when free-hand resurfacing techniques are used (without computerized pattern generators). Our experience is that this complication is permanent and does not resolve even with the use of psoralen/ultraviolet A light treatment. The only improvement noted in our patients occurred when the patient was retreated with light laser resurfacing without the use of melanotoxic agents in the pre- or postoperative periods.

PETECHIAE

Although it is of almost no long term significance, the appearance of small petechiae often generates much concern by the patient. They appear just as re-epithelialization is complete, conflicting with the patient's desire to return to the public view. Small subepithelial hemorrhages due to the immature basement membrane and undeveloped rete ridges are the cause. They may continue for several weeks after the procedure but clear quickly without treatment.

SCARRING

Erythematous and hypertrophic scars usually occur secondary to excessive depth of tissue injury. This injury is usually the result of excess tissue heating and residual thermal damage well beyond the depth of tissue vaporized by the laser. Incorrect "off" times, high scanner densities (greater than 40%) and failure to keep the handpiece moving during resurfacing are some of the causes that lead to inadvertent overlap or "stacking" of pulses with the resultant accumulation of heat and residual thermal damage.

Scarring may also be seen with higher frequency in patients with prior superficial radiation treatment and with patients who develop a postoperative infection. Obviously, careful preoperative history to rule out predisposing factors and immediate treatment of postoperative infections is mandatory.

The earliest evidence for the development of a scar is usually erythema and pruritus. At this point, the affected area should be cultured to rule out infection and topical high potency corticosteroids should be applied 2 to 3 times daily. If the affected area begins to thicken, intralesional injection of 10 mg/ml triamcinalone with 5-fluorouracil (50 mg/ml) in a 1:9 dilution should begin every 2 to 3 days. Topical silicone dressings should also be applied. If further progression of scarring occurs, we advise using a 585 nm flash-lamp pumped pulse dye laser every 4 weeks. With these techniques, permanent scarring has been avoided.

ECTROPION

Contraction of scarred tissue leads to exposure of the conjunctiva. This avoidable complication usually occurs in patients who have undergone a lower lid blepharoplasty without stabilizing the lateral canthal tendon. Ectropion may also occur if laser resurfacing is performed aggressively in this region. To minimize ectropion, we recommend that the patient's skin elastic recoil be tested (the so called "snap test"). This can easily be accomplished by asking the patient to look straight ahead and pulling down on the infraorbital skin. When released, the lower lid margin should recoil to a normal position in less than 3 seconds. Recoil greater than 3 seconds should be an indication for lateral canthal repair. In addition, laser density should not exceed 20% to 30%

in this region to limit nonspecific thermal damage of dermal tissues.

In summary, most complications and adverse sequelae in laser resurfacing can be minimized through careful technique and close patient observation in follow-up. Patient complaints should be taken seriously and treatment of postoperative infections must occur promptly. When properly performed, laser resurfacing can be a gratifying form of skin rejuvenation.

REFERENCES

1. Sriprachya-anunt S, Fitzpatrick RE, Goldman MP, Smith SR. Infections complicating pulsed CO_2 laser resurfacing for photoaged facial skin. Dermatol Surg 1997;23:527-536.
2. Fitzpatrick RE, Geronemus RG, Grevelink JM, Kilmer SL, McDaniel DH. The incidence of adverse healing reactions occurring with UltraPulse CO_2 resurfacing during a multicenter study [abstract]. Lasers Surg Med 1996;(Suppl 8):34.
3. Yurt RW. In: Mandell GL, Bennett JE, Dolin R, eds. Mandell, Douglas and Bennett's Principles and Practice of Infectious Diseases. New York: Churchill Livingstone, 1995:2761-2765.
4. Phillips LG, Heggers JP, Robson MC, et al. The effect of endogenous skin bacteria on burn wound infection. Ann Plast Surg 1989;23:35-38.
5. Husain MT, Karim QN, Tajuri S. Analysis of infection in a burn ward. Burns 1989;15:299-302.
6. Kurane I, Tsuchiya Y, Sekizawa T, et al. Inhibition by indomethacin of in vitro reactivation of latent herpes simplex virus type I in murine trigeminal ganglia. J Gen Virol 1984;65:1665-1674.
7. Pue MA, Benet LZ. Pharmacokinetics of famciclovir in man. Antiviral Chem Chemother 1993;4(Suppl 1):47-55.
8. Eaglstein WH, Davis SC, Mehle AL, Mertz PM. Optimal use of an occlusive dressing to enhance healing. Effect of delayed application and early removal on wound healing. Arch Dermatol 1988;124:392-395.
9. Torsova V, Chmelarova E, Dolecek R, Adamkova M, Tymonova J. Evaluation of the effects of a new Water-Jel system on specific bacterial and yeast strains in laboratory conditions. Burns 1995;21:47-49.
10. Gerding RL, Emerman CL, Effron D, et al. Outpatient management of partial thickness burns: biobrane versus 1% silver sulfadiazine. Ann Emerg Med 1990;16:347-352.
11. Salasche SJ, Winton GB. Clinical evaluation of a non-adhering wound dressing. J Dermatol Surg Oncol 1986; 12:1220-1222.
12. Sawada Y, Ara M, Yotsuyanagi T, Sone K. Treatment of dermal depth burn wounds with an antimicrobial agent-releasing silicone gel sheet. Burns 1990;16:347-352.
13. Haberal M, Oner Z, Bayraktar U, Bilgin N. The use of silver nitrate-incorporated amniotic membrane as a temporary dressing. Burns 1987;13:159-163.
14. Fitzpatrick RE, Goldman MP, Satur NM, Tope WD. Pulsed carbon dioxide laser resurfacing of photoaged facial skin. Arch Dermatol 1996;132:395-402.
15. Dooms-Goossens A, DeGreef H. Contact allergy to petrolatum. Contact Derm 1983;9:175-185.

CHAPTER 26

The Use of Postoperative Cosmetics

■ Zoe Diana Draelos

The postoperative period is a critical time for the patient during which physical healing must occur with a minimum of emotional trauma. Skin resurfacing procedures uniformly produce a suboptimal appearance that may last hours, as is the case following low strength glycolic acid peel, to weeks, as is the case following trichloroacetic acid (TCA) peel, to months, as is the case following dermabrasion or laser resurfacing. This can be a difficult period for the patient who must answer questions from family and peers regarding which procedure was performed and why. It can be a time of uncertainty when the patient wonders if the skin is healing properly and if the results will meet expectations. The postoperative period also can be uncomfortable until the injured skin heals. The skilled physician must not only demonstrate expertise in the resurfacing procedure, but should also provide skin care and cosmetic recommendations to allow optimum healing with minimal discomfort while addressing the patient's social needs.

The importance of selecting appropriate skin care products and cosmetics in the postoperative period cannot be underestimated. Skin healing occurs best in a carefully monitored environment that can be created or destroyed by substances which are applied to the face. Cosmetics and skin care products must account for the increased percutaneous absorption, heightened skin sensitivity, and postinflammatory pigmentation alterations that may follow resurfacing procedures. Skin care products must prevent infection and encourage reestablishment of the stratum corneum barrier. Cosmetics, on the other hand, must create a socially acceptable appearance while not hindering the healing process. This chapter provides information for the surgeon to formulate a medically sound postoperative skin care protocol for patients undergoing skin rejuvenation procedures.

CUTANEOUS ALTERATIONS FOLLOWING RESURFACING

Resurfacing procedures of all types result in varying degrees of damage to the stratum corneum barrier. Barrier damage can take the form of a mild exfoliation, seen following exposure to 25% to 50% glycolic acid. With glycolic acid peels a few layers of the stratum corneum are removed, but the resulting thinner barrier is largely intact. This thinner barrier may temporarily cause some heightened skin sensitivity, but percutaneous absorption is minimally affected. Skin exposure to 70% glycolic acid or Jessner's solution produces more corneocyte removal, especially in patients pretreated with topical tretinoin. Both skin sensitivity and percutaneous absorption are heightened, but repair occurs rapidly within days. TCA in combination with Jessner's solution, laser resurfacing, and dermabrasion cause complete disruption of the epidermal barrier and cause dermal alterations. Skin sensitivity and percutaneous absorption are dramatically altered for weeks. All trauma to the skin can theoretically produce pigmentation alterations. However, pigment changes are more likely to occur with procedures that cause more epidermal and dermal damage.

Percutaneous Absorption

Alterations in percutaneous absorption immediately following resurfacing procedures allow the dermal vasculature to contact higher concentrations of topical products. This alteration means greater exposure to immune responsive cells and increased systemic absorption of topically applied substances. During the healing phase following resurfacing, care should be taken to avoid substances that are common sources of allergic contact dermatitis. Patients with a low grade sensitivity to a given fragrance or preservative may present with a dramatic reaction if the substance is applied during the postoperative period. Systemic absorption of topical high potency corticosteroids or topical antibiotics is also possible during the healing phase. In general, topical medications should be discontinued until re-epithelialization has occurred.

Heightened Skin Sensitivity

Heightened skin sensitivity occurs to a greater or lesser degree following all resurfacing procedures. As expected, the more unprotected the dermal nerve endings become, the more skin sensitivity is experienced by the patient. It should also be recognized that individual perceptions influence skin sensitivity greatly. In general, topical substances that are cutaneous irritants, such as glycolic acid, lactic acid, and salicylic acid, should be avoided until the skin has recovered. Products containing volatile vehicles, such as isopropyl alcohol or propylene glycol, may cause stinging upon application. Also, cutaneous sensory stimulants, such as menthol or camphor, should not be used. The main criteria for selection of postoperative skin care products and cosmetics should be appropriateness for sensitive skin.

Postinflammatory Pigmentation Alterations

Postinflammatory pigmentation alterations are a common problem following resurfacing procedures of all types. Even peels that induce minor exfoliation can cause hypo- or hyperpigmentation in susceptible skin types. Unfortunately, no method is available that prevents all inflammation associated with resurfacing, but it is possible to select skin care products and cosmetics that minimize postoperative inflammation while providing sun protection.

SKIN CARE FOLLOWING RESURFACING

Skin care following resurfacing has one goal: to hasten reestablishment of the epidermal barrier. This means creating an environment optimal for cellular repair and production of intercellular lipids. There are three intercellular lipids implicated in epidermal barrier function: sphingolipids, free sterols, and free fatty acids (1). In addition, it is thought that the lamellar bodies, containing sphingolipids, free sterols and phospholipids, play a key role in barrier function and are essential to trap water and prevent excessive water loss (2, 3). Perturbations within the epidermal barrier result in rapid lamellar body secretion and a cascade of cytokine changes associated with adhesion molecule expression and growth factor production (4). Interestingly enough, transepidermal water loss is necessary to initiate lipid synthesis and subsequent barrier repair (5, 6).

SKIN CLEANSING

Cleansing in the postoperative period is important to prevent infection, eliminate surgical debris, and remove environmental dirt. Water alone is actually an excellent cleanser, removing 24.2% of surface lipids, while soap and water cleansing removes 35.6% of surface lipids (7). In the immediate postoperative period following deep peeling, laser resurfacing, or dermabrasion, lukewarm water alone may be used, at least for 48 hours. However, some surgeons may wish to add soap to the cleansing routine later.

Modern soap is a blend of tallow and nut oil, or the fatty acids derived from these products, in a ratio of 4:1. Increasing this ratio results in "superfatted" soaps designed to leave an oily film behind on the skin while providing mild cleansing. Bar soaps can be divided into three basic types:

1. True soaps composed of long chain fatty acid alkali salts with a pH between 9 and 10 (Ivory, Procter and Gamble).
2. Combars (combination bars) composed of alkaline soaps to which surface active agents have been added also to achieve a pH between 9 and 10 (Dial, Dial Corp.)
3. Syndet (synthetic detergent) bars composed of synthetic detergents and fillers that contain less than 10% soap and have an adjusted pH between 5.5 and 7.0 (8) (Dove, Unilever, Oil of Olay, Procter and Gamble).

The most appropriate soap in the postoperative period is a superfatted syndet bar because it cleans and produces less dryness than other formulations while causing less surface pH alkalization. The normal pH of the skin is acidic, between 4.5 and 6.5. Applying an alkali soap raises the pH of the skin, allowing it to feel dry and uncomfortable. Healthy skin regains its acidic pH within 30 minutes (9, 10). This is not the case with the damaged skin present following laser resurfacing.

Skin irritation occurs if an alkaline pH is maintained for more than 4 hours. Irritation can occur as a result of frequent cleansing or failure to completely remove cleanser residue from the skin. It is interesting to note that the skin pH rises 1.1 points following washing with water alone, 1.2 points after washing with an alkaline soap, and 0.9 points after washing with a syndet bar (11). Maintaining the natural acidic pH of the skin is important as it inhibits some bacterial and fungal growth (12). The combination of sebaceous and eccrine secretions are also thought to chemically inhibit infection (13).

The mechanical act of washing and rinsing the skin removes contaminants and skin debris, but some surgeons prefer use of a product containing a topical antibacterial. These products are known as deodorant cleansers, and contain triclocarban or triclosan in addition to the surfactants. Triclocarban eradicates gram positive organisms while triclosan eliminates both gram positive and gram negative bacteria. The topical value of these chemicals depends on their concentration and skin contact time. Unfortunately, both topical antibacterial cleansers are skin irritants.

Another product that is of value in the postoperative period is a lipid-free cleanser, named for the absence of fats in the formulation. Lipid-free cleansers are applied to dry or moistened skin, rubbed to produce a lather, and water-rinsed or wiped away without water. Lipid-free cleansers may contain water, glycerin, cetyl alcohol, stearyl alcohol, sodium laurel sulfate and occasionally propylene glycol and leave behind a thin moisturizing film. The cleansers can also be used effectively to remove facial cosmetics and environmental dirt in postoperative patients once initial healing has occurred. Lipid-free cleansers have been shown to cause less cutaneous irritation in photoaged skin (14).

SKIN MOISTURIZATION

Skin moisturization is important in the postoperative period since the barrier to transepidermal water loss has been damaged or possibly removed. Thus, an artificial barrier must be established until re-epithelialization occurs. Skin moisturization requires four steps: initiation of barrier repair, alteration of the surface cutaneous moisture partition coefficient, onset of dermal-epidermal moisture diffusion, and synthesis of intercellular lipids (15). It is generally thought that a gel containing 20% to 35% water allows the stratum corneum to exhibit normal softness and pliability (16).

All moisturizers attempt to mimic the effects of the naturally occurring skin lipids. Lipids present in the stratum corneum include cholesterol sulfate, free sterols, free fatty acids, triglycerides, sterol wax/esters, squalene, and n-alkanes (17). Moisturizers that are appropriate for use in the immediate postoperative period should contain both occlusive and humectant agents (18). Occlusive ingredients function to put an oily film over the healing skin through which water loss is decreased. Common occlusive substances include petrolatum, mineral oil, paraffin, silicone oils, vegetable oils, waxes, fatty alcohols, and lanolin (19).

A commonly used occlusive moisturizer is petroleum jelly alone or as part of a topical antibiotic preparation (Polysporin). Pure petroleum jelly is the most occlusive of the substances previously listed, but still allows sufficient transepidermal water loss for re-epithelialization to occur (20, 21). It is well suited as a postoperative moisturizer since it permeates throughout the interstices of the stratum corneum, allowing barrier function to be reestablished while protecting exposed dermal nerve endings (22). Additionally, petroleum jelly does not contribute to wound infections since it is anhydrous and cannot sustain bacterial growth.

Another concept in rehydrating post surgical skin is the use of humectants. Humectants, by definition, attract water that is drawn from the deeper epidermal and der-

mal tissues to rehydrate the stratum corneum. Water applied to the skin by itself cannot be used as a moisturizer since, in the absence of a humectant, it is rapidly lost to the atmosphere, resulting in more pronounced skin dryness (23). Substances that function as humectants are glycerin, honey, sodium lactate, urea, propylene glycol, sorbitol, pyrrolidone carboxylic acid, gelatin, hyaluronic acid, vitamins, and some proteins (24, 25). Humectants may also allow the flaking, healing skin to feel smoother by inducing swelling (26).

A good postoperative moisturizer should contain both occlusive and humectant ingredients. Humectants alone, such as glycerin, will actually draw moisture from the skin and increase transepidermal water loss under low humidity conditions (27). A well-formulated moisturizer should be worn at all times during the healing phase of skin resurfacing to speed re-epithelialization, decrease skin sensitivity, and prevent scarring.

CAMOUFLAGING AND COSMETIC APPLICATION FOLLOWING RESURFACING

Cosmetic application creates an acceptable appearance while allowing healing to continue. Skin resurfacing procedures produce facial erythema of varying severity and duration. However, it is not advisable for the patient to apply a foundation until re-epithelialization is well underway. Premature cosmetic application may increase facial milia.

Table 26.1 provides general recommendations for the selection of postoperative colored cosmetics. Certainly, the surgeon will need to customize the list to particular

TABLE 26.1

POSTOPERATIVE COSMETIC RECOMMENDATIONS

1. When possible, powder cosmetics should be selected over cream or lotion formulations.
2. All cosmetics should be easily removed by water, no waterproof cosmetics should be selected.
3. Old cosmetics should be discarded and fresh products purchased.
4. Eyeliner and mascara should be black in color.
5. Pencil forms of eyeliner and eyebrow cosmetics should be selected.
6. Eye shadows should be selected from the light earth tones, colors such as tan, peach, light pink, etc. Deep colors, such as blues, purples, and greens, should be avoided.
7. Select cosmetics with physical sunscreen agents, such as micronized titanium dioxide. Avoid chemical sunscreen agents (oxybenzone, methoxycinnamate) until re-epithelialization is complete.
8. Purchase cosmetic products with no more than ten ingredients, if possible.
9. Avoid nail polishes.
10. Select cream or liquid facial foundations based on silicone derivatives (cyclomethicone, dimethicone).

patient needs depending on the resurfacing procedure. The rationale for development of these recommendations is the need to minimize irritation, allergic reactions, and infection in the post surgical patient.

FACIAL FOUNDATIONS

Facial foundation is a pigmented liquid, cream, powder, or paste that is applied to add facial color, blend facial colors, or camouflage unwanted facial color. Selecting a moisturizing liquid or cream foundation can aid in decreasing transepidermal water loss and smoothing down skin scale.

The patient who has undergone a glycolic acid or Jessner's peel may be able to wear facial foundation to blend slight pink tones following the procedure and may appear to have rosier cheeks than normal. However, patients that have undergone deeper TCA peels, dermabrasion, or laser resurfacing will need a higher coverage cosmetic.

Liquid or cream makeups for appropriate camouflaging are similar to those marketed for general use. However, increased amounts of titanium dioxide provide superior coverage. These products also usually contain a higher oil concentration to allow improved wear. The higher oil concentration also prevents the color of the foundation from changing as it mixes with sebum. Products from this category that are appropriate for postoperative patients are listed in Table 26.2 (28). Generally, patients cannot wear this type of foundation until serous drainage has stopped and the amount of peeling skin is decreased. I advise medium depth TCA peel patients to not wear facial foundation for 4 days after a procedure. Dermabrasion and laser resurfacing patients may need to wait 7 to 10 days before applying facial foundation depending on the depth of the resurfacing.

Some dermabrasion and laser resurfacing patients may have complete re-epithelialization in 2 weeks, but also have erythema that can persist for weeks to months. Higher coverage can be obtained with pancake facial foundations, which are packaged in a flat, round container. The pancake foundation is removed from the compact by stroking with a dry sponge for less coverage or a wet sponge for higher coverage. Pancake foundation is composed of talc, kaolin, zinc oxide, precipitated chalk, titanium dioxide and iron oxide (29). This foundation dries quickly and possesses a matte, or dull, finish. Unfortunately, the pancake foundation is easily removed with body warmth and perspiration, but is easy to retouch, if necessary. These products are popular in the television industry to camouflage facial defects.

Cheek color, in the form of powdered blush, can be applied over the facial foundation to better blend facial erythema. It is not cosmetically necessary to completely cover the underlying erythema, in some patients as rosy cheeks are still considered a sign of health.

TABLE 26.2

POSTOPERATIVE FACIAL FOUNDATIONS

Name/Company	Type	Cost[a]	Color Selection	Availability
Continuous Coverage (Clinique)	Cream	+ + +	Fair to medium	Cosmetic counter
Pan-Cake Makeup (Max Factor)	Cream/powder	+	Fair to medium	Mass merchandise
Powdercreme Makeup (Revlon)	Cream/powder	+ +	Fair to medium	Mass merchandise
Dual Finish Creme/ Powder Makeup (Lancome)	Cream/powder	+ + + + +	Fair to dark	Cosmetic counter
Maximum Cover (Estee Lauder)	Cream	+ + + +	Fair to medium	Cosmetic counter
Creme Powder Makeup (Almay)	Cream/powder	+	Fair to medium	Mass merchandise
Ultimate Coverage Makeup (Ultima II)	Cream	+ + +	Fair to medium	Cosmetic counter

[a]Cost: +, $4–5; + +, $5–10; + + +, $10–20; + + + +, $20–30; + + + + +, $30–40.

(Reprinted with permission from Draelos ZD. Cosmetics in dermatology. 2nd ed. Edinburgh: Churchill Livingstone, 1995:78.)

TABLE 26.3

CAMOUFLAGING FACIAL FOUNDATIONS

Trade name	Manufacturer/distributor	Trade Name	Manufacturer/distributor
Astarté	Astarté Cosmetics, Inc. 460 West 34th Street New York NY 10001 USA	Hide and Sleek	RH Cosmetics 80 39th Street Brooklyn NY 11232 USA
Cinema Secrets	Cinema Secrets Inc. 4400 Riverside Drive Burbank CA 91505 USA	Keren Happuch	Keren Happuch, Ltd. PO Box 809 Oconomowoc WI 53066 USA
Columbia Cosmetics	Columbia Cosmetics Manufacturing, Inc. 1661 Timothy Drive San Leandro CA 94577 USA	Keromask Cover Cream	Innoxa Ltd. 202 Terminus Road Eastbourne, Sussex BN21 3DF England
Corrective Concepts	Pattee Products European Crossroads—Bordeaux Building 2829 West Northwest Highway Dallas TX 75220 USA	Laboratoire Dr. Renaud	Renaud Skin Care 1040 Rockland Road Montreal PQ H2V 3A1 Canada
Coverette	Ben Nye Company, Inc. 5935 Bowcroft Street Los Angeles CA 90016 USA	Lady Burd/private label	Lady Burd Exclusive Private Label Cosmetics 73 Powerhouse Road Roslyn Heights NY 11577 USA
Covermark	Lydia O'Leary 1 Anderson Avenue Moonachie NJ 07074 USA	Marvin Westmore Cosmetics	Westmore Academy of Cosmetic Arts 15445 Ventura Boulevard, #8 Sherman Oaks CA 91403 USA
Cover Tone	Fashion Fair Cosmetics 820 South Michigan Avenue Chicago IL 60605 USA	Natural Cover	LS Cosmetics PO Box 32203 Baltimore MD 21208 USA
Cream Makiage	Il-Makiage PO Box 1064 Long Island City NY 11101 USA	Naturalessa	Naturalessa 5-02 Banta Place Fair Lawn NJ 07410 USA
Danielle Cosmetics	Danielle Cosmetics Division Teka Fine Line Brushes, Inc. 3307 Avenue N Brooklyn NY 11234 USA	Patricia Milton Rhetorique	C'est La Vie 3401 Dufferin Street Suite 306 Toronto ON M6A 2T9 Canada
Dermablend	Dermablend Corrective Cosmetics PO Box 3008 Lakewood NJ 08701 USA	Pevonia	Cosmopro, Inc. 320 Fentress Boulevard Daytona Beach FL 32114 USA
Dermaceal	Joe Blasco Cosmetics 1708 Hillhurst Avenue Hollywood CA 90027 USA	Veil	Atelier Esthetique 386 Park Avenue South Suite 209 New York NY 10016 USA
Dermacolor	Kryolan Corporation 132 Ninth Street San Francisco CA 94103 USA	Your Name Cosmetics	Your Name div. of Mana Products 32-02 Queens Boulevard Long Island City NY 11101 USA
Grafton Products	Grafton Products Corporation 25 Butler Street Norwalk CT 06850 USA		

Reprinted with permission from Draelos ZD. Camouflage cosmetics and techniques. Cosmet Toilet 1994;109:75–84.

FIGURE 26.1
Red and green are complementary on the color wheel yielding brown when combined.

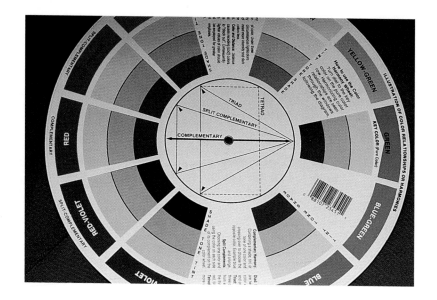

CAMOUFLAGE FACIAL FOUNDATIONS

Occasionally, there is a need for true camouflage facial foundations in deep laser resurfacing and dermabrasion patients, especially dermabrasion patients with severe acne scarring. There are many companies in the United States and Europe who manufacture cosmetics specifically designed for camouflaging purposes. Table 26.3 is a list of some of the more popular products presently available (30).

These camouflage facial foundations require special application and removal instructions. The cosmetic is generally a thick, waxy, cream that is scooped from a jar. Prior to application, soften the product by warming it in the hand. It may be necessary to mix several foundation colors to achieve a match for the patient's skin tone. Generally, no more than three shades should be blended to preserve the quality of the final color. The cosmetic should then be dabbed over the entire face into the hairline, around the ears, and below the chin. A transparent powder should then be pressed into the foundation to yield a matte finish, increase product wear, and impart waterproof characteristics. A properly applied camouflage foundation should wear 8 hours with minimal touch up. Remaining color cosmetics, such as blush, eye shadow, and mascara, can then be applied to reestablish facial landmarks.

UNDERCOVER COSMETICS

Special liquid or cream makeups are available for application under traditional facial foundations. These products are available in green, orange, purple, white, and brown colors. Their use is based on the principle of complementary colors on an artist's color wheel (Fig. 26.1). The combination of two complementary colors yields brown. For example, the erythema following laser resurfacing can be

TABLE 26.4

COMPLEMENTARY COLORED UNDERCOVER COSMETICS

Undercover Cosmetic Color	Skin Lesion Color	Postoperative Dermatologic Abnormality
Green	Red	Erythema
Orange	Blue	Acute bruise
Purple	Yellow	Resolving bruise
White	Brown	Post-inflammatory hyperpigmentation
Brown	White	Post-inflammatory hypopigmentation

more readily camouflaged by applying a green undercover cosmetics (Table 26.4). Bluish-purple postoperative bruising can be improved by applying a peach colored undercover product before foundation application. The yellowish discoloration of a healing hematoma can be camouflaged with a purple undercover cosmetic.

SUMMARY

Proper selection of cosmetics and skin care products in the postoperative period is important to patient satisfaction and optimal healing. A patient who can quickly resume normal activities following resurfacing will more likely feel that the procedure has been successful. This positive attitude helps contribute to a better convalescent period. Furthermore, careful selection of cleansers, moisturizers, and cosmetics can actually aid in the re-epithelialization process by creating an environment appropriate for healing. The surgeon's skill is an important part of the final resurfacing result, but postoperative care is equally important in ensuring the best possible outcome.

REFERENCES

1. Elias PM. Lipids and the epidermal permeability barrier. Arch Dermatol Res 1981;270:95-117.
2. Holleran WM, Man MQ, Wen NG, Gopinathan KM, Elias PM, Feingold KR. Sphingolipids are required for mammalian epidermal barrier function. J Clin Invest 1991;88:1338-1345.
3. Downing DT. Lipids: their role in epidermal structure and function. Cosmet Toilet 1991;106:63-69.
4. Nickoloff BJ, Naidu Y. Perturbation of epidermal barrier function correlates with initiation of cytokine cascade in human skin. J Am Acad Dermatol 1994;30:535-546.
5. Jass HE, Elias PM. The living stratum corneum: implications for cosmetic formulation. Cosmet Toilet 1991;106:47-53.
6. Holleran W, Feingold K, Man MQ, Gao W, Lee J, Elias PM. Regulation of epidermal sphingolipid synthesis by permeability barrier function. J Lipid Res 1991;32:1151-1158.
7. Morganti P. Natural soap and syndet bars. Cosmet Toilet 1995;110:89-97.
8. Wortzman MS, Scott RA, Wong PS, Lowe MJ, et al. Soap and detergent bar rinsability. J Soc Cosmet Chem 1986;37:89-97.
9. Prottey C, Ferguson T. Factors which determine the skin irritation potential of soap and detergents. J Soc Cosmet Chem 1975;26:29.
10. Wickett RR, Trobaugh CM. Personal care products. Cosmet Toilet 1990;105:41-46.
11. Morganti P. Natural soap and syndet bars. Cosmet Toilet 1995;110:89-97.
12. Peck SM, Rosenfeld H, Leifer W, Bierman W. Role of sweat as a fungicide. Arch Dermatol 1979;39:126-146.
13. Wheatley VR. The nature, origin and possible functions of the cutaneous lipids. Pro Sci Sec TGA 1963;39:25.
14. Mills OH, Berger RS, Baker MD. A controlled comparison of skin cleansers in photoaged skin. J Geriatric Dermatol 1993;1:173-179.
15. Jackson EM. Moisturizers: what's in them? How do they work? Am J Contact Dermatitis 1992;3:162-168.
16. Reiger MM. Skin, water and moisturization. Cosmet Toilet 1989;104:41-51.
17. Brod J. Characterization and physiological role of epidermal lipids. Int J Dermatol 1991;30:84-90.
18. Baker CG. Moisturization: new methods to support time proven ingredients. Cosmet Toilet 1987;102:99-102.
19. De Groot AC, Weyland JW, Nater JP, eds. Unwanted effects of cosmetics and drugs used in dermatology, 3rd ed. Amsterdam: Elsevier, 1994:498-500.
20. Friberg SE, Ma Z. Stratum corneum lipids, petrolatum and white oils. Cosmet Toilet 1993;107:55-59.
21. Grubauer G, Feingold KR, Elias PM. Relationship of epidermal lipogenesis to cutaneous barrier function. J Lip Res 1987;28:746-752.
22. Ghadially R, Halkier-Sorensen L, Elias PM. Effects of petrolatum on stratum corneum structure and function. J Am Acad Dermatol 1992;26:387-396.
23. Rieger MM, Deem DE. Skin moisturizers II The effects of cosmetic ingredients on human stratum corneum. J Soc Cosmet Chem 1974;25:253-262.
24. De Groot AC, Weyland JW, Nater JP, eds. Unwanted effects of cosmetics and drugs used in dermatology, 3rd ed. Amsterdam: Elsevier, 1994:498-500.
25. Spencer TS. Dry skin and skin moisturizers. Clin Dermatol 1988;6:24-28.
26. Robbins CR, Fernee KM. Some observations on the swelling of human epidermal membrane. J Soc Cosmet Chem 1983;37:21-34.
27. Idson B. Dry skin: moisturizing and emolliency. Cosmet Toilet 1992;107:69-78.
28. Draelos ZD. Cosmetics in dermatology. 2nd ed. Edinburgh: Churchill Livingstone, 1995:78.
29. Wilkinson JB, Moore RJ. Harry's cosmeticology, 7th ed. New York: Chemical Publishing, 1982:304-307.
30. Draelos ZD. Camouflage cosmetics and techniques. Cosmet Toilet 1994;109:75-84.

APPENDIX A

Commentary on Wound Healing

■ David J. Margolis

The purpose of this section is to review the chapters on wound healing and to try to create a conceptual framework of wound healing as it relates to skin resurfacing procedures. The chapters on wound healing in this monograph include *Skin Response to Chemical Peeling* (Chapter 5), *Skin Response to Abrasive Resurfacing* (Chapter 9), and *Skin Response to Laser Resurfacing* (Chapter 13). To make clear any potential conflicts of interest, the author of this summary is not a cosmetic surgeon, but a clinical epidemiologist interested in the treatment of chronic wounds.

A REVIEW OF ACUTE WOUND HEALING

Wound healing is a tightly regulated process. It involves interactions of keratinocytes, fibroblasts, endothelial cells, neutrophils, lymphocytes, macrophages, and platelets. These interactions are mediated by cytokines, growth factors, selectins, matrix proteins, integrins, proteases, and inhibitors. And, in fact, there are probably other cells and mediators involved that have not been identified. I feel confident in stating that, while a lot has been learned about these interactions, even more still needs to be learned. Wonderful summaries and books on the pathophysiology of wound healing are available (1-5).

In brief, acute wound healing can be divided into three overlapping phases (3, 4). These phases are the inflammatory phase, the tissue regeneration phase, and the remodeling phase. The inflammatory phase is the starting point and commences immediately after tissue injury. Tissue injury causes plasma leakage. Plasma contains fibrinogen which is cleaved by thrombin to form fibrin. Fibrin cross-links and serves as a provisional matrix. Within the matrix, platelets are trapped and

then degranulate. The degranulation of platelets causes the attraction and activation of polymorphonuclear leukocytes, lymphocytes, macrophages, and fibroblasts. These cells are required to clean the wound and begin to repair the wound environment.

The changes to the wound environment caused by the inflammatory cells result in alterations to the integrins of the keratinocytes. Simply, integrins serve as points of interaction and attachment between cells or cells and matrix proteins. Initially there is a loss of the hemidesmosome binding of the keratinocyte to laminin via integrins $\alpha6\beta4$ (6). Migration of keratinocytes occur because of the formation of integrins $\alpha5\beta1$, $\alpha v\beta6$, $\alpha v\beta5$, and $\alpha2\beta1$ (1). These integrins, in association with actinomycin filaments in the keratinocyte, allow the keratinocytes at the edge of the wound to migrate into the wound. With the aid of the actinomycin filament, the keratinocyte grasps and crawls over the provisional matrix at the integrin points of attachment. Furthermore, this passage of keratinocytes through the provisional matrix, a fibrin swamp, is aided by the production of proteolytic enzymes (e.g., plasminogen) (1, 4). The proteolytic enzymes help to clear a path for the keratinocyte. These proteolytic enzymes are activated by tissue plasminogen activator (tPA) and uroplasminogen activator (uPA) in the migrating keratinocyte (e.g., plasminogen is activated to plasmin). These processes are also regulated by growth factors which include keratinocyte growth factor (KGF), transforming growth factor alpha (TGF-α) and epidermal growth factor (EGF). Once the wound is covered with keratinocytes, the keratinocytes stop migrating and differentiate, often returning the epidermis to its prewounded structure and function.

Granulation tissue forms beneath the migrating keratinocytes. Granulation tissue is a composite of fibroblasts and endothelial cells. Like keratinocytes, fibroblasts also change phenotype. While the senescent fibroblast phenotype binds to collagen type-1 fibers, the new phenotype expresses integrins capable of crawling over the fibrin matrix. The phenotype includes the presence of integrins $\alpha 3$ and $\alpha 5$ in the cell wall and the creation of an actinomycin cytoskeleton (6). These two cellular constructs are required for migration of the fibroblasts and fibroblast aided wound contraction, which is a helpful and efficient method of decreasing the size of the wound. Cytokines involved in the migration and maturation of fibroblasts include fibroblast growth factor (FGF), platelet derived growth factor (PDGF), and TGF-beta (TGF-β). It initially takes the fibroblast a few days to be activated, but once activated they are quicker to respond to further wounding. Angiogenesis, the formation of new blood vessels, is dependent on endothelial cell migration and maturation. These processes are controlled by cytokines, such as FGFs and vascular endothelial growth factor (VEGF).

The final phase of wound repair is the remodeling phase. It continues for several weeks after the wound clinically appears to be healed. This phase overlaps with the tissue regeneration phase and is controlled by interactions between cells, such as fibroblasts, cytokines, such as FGF and TGF-β, and components of the extracellular matrix (1, 4). The matrix during this phase evolves from mainly being composed of fibronectin to hyaluronic acid to proteoglycans and finally, to collagen. The evolution of the extracellular matrix increases the strength of the dermis. For example, at the end of this phase, wounds are about 60% to 70% as strong as nascent tissue, but are only 20% as strong as nascent tissue when they first appeared clinically to be healed (7). Wound contraction also occurs during this phase by actin containing myofibroblasts.

A REVIEW OF THE PERTINENT CHAPTERS

The chapter by Dr. C.B. Harmon (Chapter 9), discusses the surgical planing of the skin. Surgical planing creates a superficial wound that heals by secondary intention. If the abrasion does not extend too deeply into the reticular dermis, healing appears to be free of scar. In addition, if the planing does not extend deep enough to fully destroy a cutaneous appendage, that appendage will also regrow. The author nicely translates the clinical exam as it relates to the phases of wound healing (summarized above). Most notably, he differentiates between dermabrasive resurfacing and scar revision with dermabrasion. For the latter technique, he claims that if the secondary intention healing of dermabrasive scar revision is superimposed on the remodeling phase of the "primary intention" healing wound (e.g., 6 to 8 weeks after wound closure), then there may be complete elim-

ination of the visual evidence of the scar. He notes that the mechanism for this effect is unknown, but histologically there may be improved collagen bundle formation and collagen topography.

The chapter by Dr. H.J. Brody (Chapter 5), discusses the use of chemical agents to produce partial thickness wounds that heal by secondary intention. Again, if these wounds are to heal scar free by secondary intention they should not extend below the cutaneous appendages. Depth of the peel is dependent on skin pretreatment, the concentration of the agent used (e.g., trichloroacetic acid), and the total time the agent is active and in contact with the skin. Since the wounds are shallow, keratinocytes can migrate from the wound edge and from the cutaneous appendages. Dr. Brody advocates the use of topical agents to promote and accelerate wound healing. The compounds that he feels augment acute wound healing include polymyxin sulfate and zinc bacitracin, petrolatum, aloe vera, and tretinoin applied prior to wounding. He recommends against the long term use of topical corticosteroids.

The chapter by Drs. Cox and Cockerell (chapter 13), discusses the response of the skin to laser resurfacing. These authors differentiate between intrinsic and extrinsic aging. Intrinsic aging of the skin (aging due to the passage of time), causes minor changes in the skin by histopathologic criteria. These include slight epidermal thinning and, in the dermis, loss of elastin and ground substance. In contrast, extrinsic aging of the skin (aging due to photodamage) causes more dramatic change in the skin. In extrinsically aged skin, the epidermis and dermal-epidermal junction are flattened, there are fewer cutaneous appendages, and the dermis has less collagen, fibroblasts, and elastin than in non-photodamaged skin. Furthermore, Drs. Cox and Cockerell nicely describe the depth of destruction caused by CO_2 laser and chemical peels and note that dermal scarring as measured by histologic criteria (e.g., direction of collagen bundles) is more likely to occur with the deeper dermal wounds that are associated with increased laser energy.

AN APPLICATION

So what have we learned about wound repair and why do these procedures result in successful cosmetic outcomes? How can we apply what is known about the pathophysiology of acute wound healing to the cosmetic procedures discussed in this book? A curious reader should make several observations. First, the majority of the studies on the pathophysiology of acute wound healing were conducted on mice, rats, and pigs with full thickness excisional wounds. Do these animals and does the depth of the experimental wound mimic the human condition that occurs after a "skin resurfacing?" Second, since the cutaneous environment for these procedures is usually actinically damaged older skin, is wound healing affected by age? Finally, should the emphasis of a cosmetic surgeon be on the healing process or preventing scarring?

In general, adult human dermal wounds repair and do not regenerate. However, some fetal wounds do not appear to scar and, therefore, may regenerate (8). Whether a fetal wound scars depends on the gestational age of the fetus, the location and depth of the wound, and the species of experimental animal. The phenomenon of regeneration is felt to be due to the wound environment (e.g., amniotic fluid), the cellular regulation of the extracellular matrix/collagen (e.g., high concentration of hyaluronic acid, earlier production of collagen in the fetus than the adult), more active fetal fibroblasts, and the relative lack of an inflammatory response in the fetus.

It has been generally believed that the elderly have impaired wound healing. However, recent reviews on the effect of age on wound healing have shown that this fact is not well substantiated in humans (2). Furthermore, plastic and cosmetic surgeons often report that scars are more cosmetically acceptable in older adults than younger adults. What is known about wound healing in the elderly is that there is a diminished inflammatory response, a delay in the start of the proliferative phase of healing, decreased responsiveness of fibroblasts to cytokine growth factors, and a delay in angiogenesis (2). However, the dermal organization of the scar is superior in the older adult as compared to the younger adult (2, 9). This may be in part due to decreased inflammatory response and a decrease in fibroblast responsiveness to TGF β1 and β2 (9, 10). It may be possible that epidermal destruction and papillary dermal destruction common to these skin resurfacing procedures is sufficient to activate dermal repair and remodeling in the elderly, but not sufficient to induce a brisk inflammatory response. Therefore, wound healing in these individuals might mimic the fetal wound healing process resulting in an improved, minimally scarred, epidermis and dermis.

Although the pathophysiologic mechanism responsible for the cosmetic improvement noted from skin resurfacing wounds has not been well described, the cosmetic outcome has been quantified and studied. As an example, a recent study by Bernstein et al may begin to answer this pathophysiologic quandary (11). Six elderly women with actinically damaged skin were randomized to receive either vehicle or 20% citric acid (CA) lotion on each forearm. After 3 months of application, 4 mm punch biopsy specimens were obtained within the treatment site (i.e., CA or vehicle). Immunohistochemical staining quantified by image analysis revealed an increase in glycosaminoglycans in the CA treated forearm. The epidermis was also thicker in the CA treated forearm. A conclusion from the study could be that agents which cause minor epidermal change can re-

sult in dermal and epidermal structural improvement, perhaps by the mechanism outlined above. This type of response has also been noted for retinoids and alpha hydroxy acids (12, 13).

In summary, chemical peels, dermabrasion and laser resurfacing of the skin result in superficial wounds of the dermis. The cutaneous environment for these procedures is usually the actinically damaged skin in the older adult and the wounds are usually superficial to partial thickness wounds. The epidermis is replenished from the border of the wound and any appendages that survived the wound inducing injury. The dermis, may also improve after these procedures. Why the dermis improves after skin resurfacing has not been well explained. However, it has been well established that regeneration of the dermis after wounding is possible in the fetus. This seems to occur because the fetus is in a sterile environment and probably has fibroblasts that do not require cytokine stimulation to work efficiently (8, 10). In contrast, the adult lives in a dirty environment and has fibroblasts that need excessive stimulation in order to repair the wound, perhaps, before the wound becomes infected. The augmentation of dermal fibroblast function is partially controlled by TGF β1 and β2. The older individual has very poorly responsive fibroblasts and is unable to make large quantity of TGF β1 and β2, so these wounds may heal slowly but the fibroblasts is able to repair the dermis without extensive stimulation by TGF β1 and β2 (8, 9, 14-16).

CONCLUSION

In conclusion, the acute wound healing process has not been extensively studied for the superficial wounds described in this monograph. The procedures causing these wounds tend to be performed in older individuals or in sites of recent injury (e.g., scar revision). The favorable effects seen in these patients post wounding are likely related to the age of the patient, depth of injury, keratinocyte and fibroblast phenotype, wound matrix and local wound cytokines.

REFERENCES

1. Martin P. Wound healing—aiming for perfect skin regeneration. Science 1997;276:75-81.
2. Ashcroft GS, Horan MA, Ferguson MW. The effects of ageing on cutaneous wound healing in mammals. J Anat 1995;187:1-26.
3. Clark RAF. Cutaneous tissue repair: basic biologic considerations. J Am Acad Dermatol 1985;13:701-725.
4. Clark RAF. Wound Repair: Overview and General Considerations. In: Clark RAF, ed. The molecular and cellular biology of wound repair. New York: Plenum, 1996:3-50.
5. Mast BA. The Skin. In: Cohen IK, Diegelmann RF, Lindblad WJ, eds. Wound healing. Biochemical and clinical aspects. Philadelphia: WB Saunders, 1992:344-355.

6. Clark RA, Ashcroft GS, Spencer MJ, Larjava H, Ferguson MW. Re-epithelialization of normal human excisional wounds is associated with a switch from alpha v beta 5 to alpha v beta 6 integrins. Br J Dermatol 1996;135:46-51.

7. Levenson SM, Geever EF, Crowley LV, Oates JF, Berard CW, Rosen H. The healing of rat skin wounds. Ann Surg 1965;161:293-308.

8. Ferguson MW, Whitby DJ, Shah M, Armstrong J, Siebert JW, Longaker MT. Scar formation: the spectral nature of fetal and adult wound repair. Plast Reconstr Surg 1996;97:854-860.

9. Ashcroft GS, Horan MA, Ferguson MW. Aging is associated with reduced deposition of specific extracellular matrix components, an upregulation of angiogenesis, and an altered inflammatory response in a murine incisional wound healing model. J Invest Dermatol 1997;108:430-437.

10. Longaker MT, Whitby DJ, Ferguson MW, Lorenz HP, Harrison MR, Adzick NS. Adult skin wounds in the fetal environment heal with scar formation. Ann Surg 1994;219:65-72.

11. Bernstein EF, Underhill CB, Lakkakorpi J, et al. Citric acid increases viable epidermal thickness and glycosaminoglycan content of sun-damaged skin. Dermatol Surg 1997;23:689-694.

12. Griffiths CEM, Russman AN, Majmudar G, Singer RS, Hamilton TA, Voorhees JJ. Restoration of collagen formation in photodamaged human skin by tretinoin. N Engl J Med 1993;329:530-535.

13. Lavker RM, Kaidbey K, Leyden JJ. Effects of topical ammonium lactate on cutaneous atrophy from a potent topical corticosteroid. J Am Acad Dermatol 1992;26:535-544.

14. Shah M, Foreman DM, Ferguson MW. Neutralizing antibody to TGF-beta 1,2 reduces cutaneous scarring in adult rodents. J Cell Sci 1994;107:1137-1157.

15. Khaw PT. Antiproliferative agents and the prevention of scarring after surgery: friend or foe? Br J Ophthalmol 1995;79:627.

16. Khaw PT, Occleston NL, Schultz G, Grierson I, Sherwood MB, Larkin G. Activation and suppression of fibroblast function. Eye 1994;8:188-195.

APPENDIX B

Survey of Chapter Authors

The survey included the following questions:

1. Indicate the percent of your total resurfacing practice for each modality: laser, dermabrasion, and superficial, medium, and deep peels (See Appendix B, Table 1)
2. Which resurfacing laser do you use? Why?
   Summary of responses:
   A. The Coherent UltraPulse laser (Coherent Laser Corp., Palo Alto, CA) was the most commonly used laser (9 of 15 respondents). The most often reasons cited for this choice were:
      - Best tissue response with collagen tightening
      - Best safety profile, availability (through rental companies)
      - Ease of use with a computer pattern generator scanner
   B. The SilkTouch/FeatherTouch laser (Sharplan Laser Inc., Allendale, NJ) was the second most common choice (4 of 15 respondents). The reasons for this choice were:
      - An instrument with great efficiency and clean removal of the epidermis
      - Good for deep wrinkles and acne scarring
      - Lower cost with same results
3. Physicians were asked to estimate the rate of complication in their own practice for laser, peels, and dermabrasion. (See Appendix B, Table 2)
4. In addition, physicians were asked through a series of questions about the laser complications they had seen from other physicians.
   Summary of responses: (14 respondents)
   A. Four physicians had seen more than 25 complications as referrals,
      Four physicians had seen 10 to 25 complications as referrals,

Six physicians had seen less than 10 complications as referrals.
The distribution of complications was much different than that of their own practices.
   B. From most to least common, the complications included:
      Scar, hypopigmentation, persistent erythema, infection, allergic reaction, and corneal abrasion
   C. The most common reason for the referral complication was felt to be "too aggressive" technique. Second most common reason was "poor physician understanding of pre- and postoperative care." Also cited were "poor quality laser" and "no obvious error."
   D. The most common specialty to send a complication was plastic and reconstructive surgeons with ophthalmologists running second.
5. Finally, the physicians were asked a group of questions about postoperative laser care.
   Summary of responses:
   A. Twice as many experts used occlusion.
      - The most common occlusive dressing used was Silon (Biomed Science Inc., Bethlehem, PA.)
      - Most common time period that the occlusive dressing was left on was 2 to 3 days.
   B. The most common ointment used in after care was Vaseline (Chesebrough-Ponds, Inc., Greenwich, CT)
   C. Step-down care recommended with the use of ointment for 10 days and then a cream formulation.
   D. Most recommended make up application at 10 to 14 days after the procedure.
   E. Pre- and Postoperative topicals used.
      - Retin-A (Ortho Pharmaceutical, Rariton, NJ) was the most common topical used and was started 4 weeks before laser treatment and resumed 4 weeks after.

- Alpha hydroxy acid lotion was the second most common topical used and was started 4 to 6 weeks before treatment and resumed 4 weeks after.

- Cellex-C (Cellex-C Cosmaceuticals, Toronto, Canada) was used by about ⅓ of respondents. It was started 2 weeks before treatment and resumed 2 weeks after.

TABLE 1

PERCENT RESURFACING PRACTICE

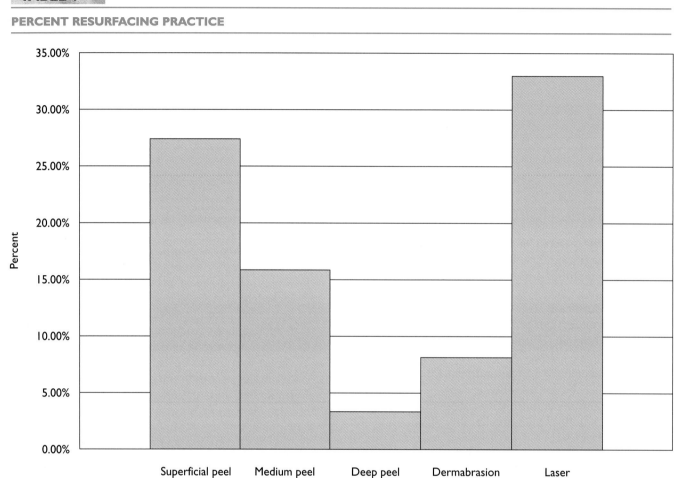

This graph illustrates an important trend. A few years ago superficial peels would have been the most common type of resurfacing done. Laser resurfacing now tops the list. One precaution in evaluating this data: the surveyed population consisted of resurfacing experts who might get a higher percentage of deep resurfacing than other practitioners.

TABLE 2

COMPLICATION FACTORS

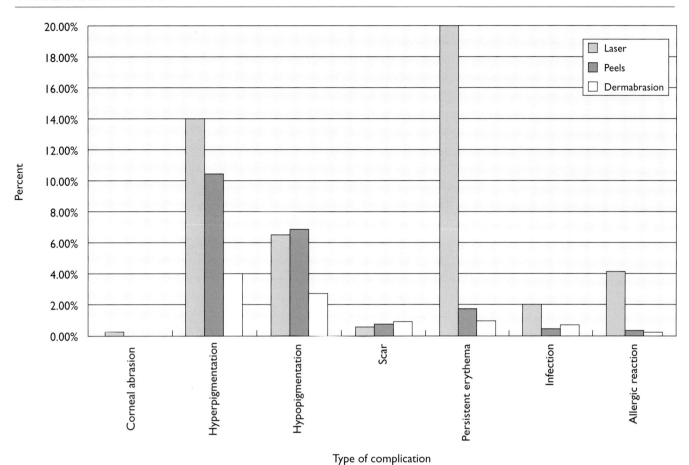

Survey respondents estimated the rate of these complications for laser, peels, and dermabrasion in their practice.

INDEX

Page numbers in *italics* denote figures; those followed by t denote tables

benefits of, 196
  types of, 196
complications from, 271-272, 299
moist, after phenol-based peel, 81
Drug(s), phototoxic and antiseizure, as factor in cause of melasma, 73
Drug interactions, anticipating and avoiding, 8
Dry eye, 254, 256, 272
Dry ice peels. *See* Carbon dioxide (CO_2) ice peels
Dye lasers, electromagnetic spectrum, *156*, 156t
Dynamic *vs.* static skin changes, 217-218, 258
Dyschromia, 11, 82
  chemical peel for, 65
  indications and peel depth for best response, 72, 73t

E

E. coli, 296t
Ectropion formation
  after blepharoplasty, 267-268, *268*, 272
  after laser resurfacing, 172, 173t, 174t, 175, *175*, 271, *272*
  treatment, 301
Eczema, as contraindication to laser surgery, 173, 173t
Edema
  after dermabrasion, minimizing, 107
  after dermasanding, 135
  from CO_2 laser, 268, *269*
  periorbital, following chemical peel, 80
  postoperative, minimizing, 40, 61, 299
Egyptians, skin resurfacing by, 3, 4, 18, 71
Elastin, rate of loss per year of adult life, 144
Elastin degeneration, 40
Elastosis, solar, 11
Elderly, impaired wound healing in, 313
Electrocautery
  for small eyelid lesions, 246
  zones of thermal damage with, 162
Electromagnetic spectrum, 155, *156*, 156t
Electron microscopy, 144
Elta, 190
EMLA, 104, 112, 264
Endoscopic equipment, 284
Enophthalmos, after blepharoplasty, 272
Enterobacter, 296t
Epidermal growth factor (EGF), 311
Epidermal maturation, 40
Epidermal pigment, response to treatment, 65
Epidermolysis, 45
Epinephrine, 77, 104
  for dermabrasion, 112
  during dermasanding, 128, 130
Epithelial cell migration rate, hydration of the wound bed and, 37
Erbium:YAG laser, 187, 197
  benefits of, 197
  for benign eyelid lesions, 267
  effects of, research on, 167-168
  electromagnetic spectrum, *156*, 156t
  for eye resurfacing, 248
  immediate tissue effects, 165, *166*, 197
  neck resurfacing with, 186
  risk of infection to operative team, 197
  thermal diffusion time, 159
  tissue interaction with, 162, 163t
  See also Laser resurfacing; Laser systems, comparison of

Erythema
  after dermasanding, 123
  from CO_2 laser, 268, *269*
  prolonged
    after dermabrasion, 108
    after laser treatment, 174, 174t167
    after phenol-based peel, 84
  resolution of, laser *vs.* phenol-based peel, 82
  treatment, 299-300
Estrogen-progesterone therapy
  as factor in cause of melasma, 73
  and pigmentary changes after chemical peel, 83
Eucerin cream
  after dermabrasion, 107
  after laser resurfacing, 191
  effect on epidermal migration, 76t
  effect on re-epithelialization, 39, 39t
Excimer lasers, 200
  electromagnetic spectrum, *156*, 156t
Exfoliation, as adjunctive agent in chemical peeling, 58t
Exposure time, laser resurfacing, 157-158
Extinction length, 157, 158
Eye, chemical irritation to, during chemical peel, 80
Eye irrigation solution, 80
Eye protection, during laser surgery, 177, *178*, *259*, 259-260, *260*
Eye shields, 260, *261*, *267*, 284
Eyelid crease, marking before brow lift, 284
Eyelids. *See* Blepharoplasty; Periorbital areas

F

Face (upper), aging, major components of
  gravity, 277
  muscle activity, 277-278
  sun damage (photoaging), 278
Face (upper), aging of, major components of, 278t
Facelifts, 11, 12
  on previously peeled skin, 76, 84
  recent, as contraindication to chemexfoliation, 74, 74t
  scarring after, 84
Facial architecture, restoring, 12
Facial foundations, 306, 306t, 307t, 308
Facial nerve
  injury to, 292
  marking before brow lift, 284
Facility, 24
Famcyclovir, 109, 238, 297-298, 298t
Fat, orbital, 264-265, *265*
Fear of the procedure, dealing with, 30
Feathering, laser resurfacing technique for, 186
FeatherTouch laser, 163t, 247, *247*, 268, 287
  immediate tissue effects, 165t
Fetal dermal regeneration, 313
Fibrel, for soft tissue augmentation, 222, 233
Fibrillogenesis, rewounding during, 94
Fibrin, role of in granular tissue formation, 91
Fibrin-fibronectin matrix, 89
Fibroblast growth factor (FGF), 312
Fibroblasts, 38
  accumulation and proliferation, 37, 92
  effects of LELs on, 198, 199t
  role of, 144, 312
Fibronectin, 37, 38
  role of in granular tissue formation, 91

Fibroplasia
  after dermabrasion, 90
  after medium depth peel, 69
Fitzpatrick's classification of sun-reactive skin types, 46, 49t, 72t
  best skin types for laser resurfacing, 173, 173t
  types suitable for phenol-based peels, 72
Flash-lamp pumped pulse dye laser, 301
Flexan dressing, 190
  imprints of, 272
Fluconazole, oral, 298t
Fluence, 157
Fluor Ethyl, 104
Fluorescent marker, to assess uniformity of chemical peeling, 51
5-Fluorouracil, 8t
  effect of, 208
  vs. Jessner's solution plus 35% TCA, 63
Forehead creases, 277-278
Forehead rejuvenation
  CO_2 laser resurfacing, rationale for, 280, 280t
  endoscopic minimal incision brow lift
    combined with CO_2 laser blepharoplasty, 280, 280t
    combined with CO_2 laser resurfacing
    anesthesia, 284
    closure of eyelid incision, 287
    CO_2 laser resurfacing, 287
    and CO_2 laser resurfacing of other regions, 287
    complications, *292*, 292-293, 292t
    equipment, 284
    fixation of the forehead, 287
    indications for, 281, 281t
    marking the patient, *283*, 283-284
    and neck liposuction and submentoplasty, 287
    postoperative care, 287-288, *288*
    preoperative assessment, *281*, 281-282, 281t, *282*
    preoperative patient counseling, 282-283
    preparing scalp incisions, 284
    procedure, 284, *284-286*, 286
    rationale for, 280, 280t
    results, 289, *289-291*, 292
    scalp incisions, 286-287
  ideal approach to, 279, 279t
  lines, soft tissue augmentation for, *221*, 233
  traditional methods
    open forehead lifting, 278-279, 278t
    traditional blepharoplasty, 279
Frank epidermolysis, due to glycolic acid, 10
Free acid concentrations of commercial products, 52, 53t
Freezing agents, prior to dermabrasion, 97, 104
Freon skin degreaser, 51
Frequency, pulse delivery, 182
Frosting after chemical peel
  after phenol-based peel, 81
  end point of Jessner's solution, *61*
  time for maximal reaction, 60
Frown lines. *See* Glabellar frown lines
Frown muscles, 277
Frowning, recurrence of, after treatment, 292-293
Full face photoaging skin, with perioral and periocular rhytides, combination treatments for, *211*, 211-212, *213*

U

UltraPulse 5000 CO$_2$ laser, 162, 163, 163t, 238, 246, 267, 287
  clinical response to, 151-152
  cutaneous effects, comparative histology of, 146-149, *147, 150*
  feathering techniques with, 186
  immediate tissue effect, 165t
  multi-center trials, results of, 167
  perioral technique with, 185-186
  thermal effects of, 150-151
  zones of ablation and thermal damage, compared, 189
Ultraviolet light, pigmentary response to, 72t
Unna, Paul, 54
Unna's paste, modified, 54, 54t
Uroplasminogen activator (uPA), 311
U.S. Food and Drug Administration (FDA), 218

V

Valacyclovir
  for herpes simplex virus, 83, 297, 298t
  prophylactic treatment with, 109
Valium, before dermasanding, 129
Vapor transport rate, biosynthetic dressings, 190
Vascular endothelial growth factor (VEGF), 312
Vaseline, after laser resurfacing, 190, 315
Verrucae, as contraindication to laser surgery, 173, 173t
Vicodin, for postoperative pain, 135
Vigilon dressing, 190
Visual refractive errors, correcting with excimer lasers, 200

Vitamin A. *See* Tretinoin
Vitamin A & E ointment, 191
Vitamin C, topical
  postoperative use of, 81, 192, 300
  preoperative skin care with, 81
Vitamin E, topical
  adverse reactions to, 191
  for hyperpigmentation, 300
  increased bleeding and, 103
Vitiligo, 11
  as contraindication to laser surgery, 173, 173t
  and permanent loss of pigment, 31
Vitronectin, role of in granular tissue formation, 91

W

Wallscreen, dermasanding by, 123
Warts, electrocautery for, 246
Water, as diluent in phenol solution, 75, 75t
Whitfield's ointment, 20
Wlpe, defined, 51
Wire brushes, dermabrasion, 104, *105*
Wound healing, 311-313
  after laser resurfacing, 189
    closed treatment, 189-190
    maintenance of skin, 191-193
    open treatment, 190-191
  fetal wound scars, 313
  hydration and, 76, 76t
  improving management of, 195-196
  response to LEL light, 199
  stages of
    angiogenesis, 38
    coagulation and inflammation, 37, 311
    collagen removing, 38

    granulation tissue formation, 38, 311-312
    medium depth peel, 69
    re-epithelialization, 37-38, *38*, 312
      medications that affect, 39-40, 39t
  topical agents that promote, 312
Wrinkles. *See* Rhytides

X

Xanthelasmas, 267
Xenon-chloride lasers, 200
Xerosis, 18
X-rays, cutaneous injury from, 144
Xylocaine
  for dermabrasion, 112
  during dermasanding, 128, 130, *131*
  for postoperative pain, 189

Z

Zinc bacitracin, 312
Zinc oxide, 54, 54t
Zithromax, 176
Zones of thermal damage, induced by CO$_2$ lasers, 150
Zones of thermal tissue alteration, 159
Zyderm I; Zyderm II; Zyplast, 218, *219,* 220, 232
  complications of, 218, 220
  contraindications to, 218
  for lip augmentation, 233
  technique, *220,* 220-222, *221*
  for treatment of horizontal forehead lines, *221,* 233
  vs. Fibrel, 222